LIBRARY
LEWIS-CLARK STATE COLLEGE
LEWISTON, IDAHO

D0215015

WITHDRAWN

MIGRATION, ILLNESS AND HEALTH CARE

JENNY ALTSCHULER

WITH A CHAPTER BY RACHEL HOPKINS

macmillan education palgrave

© Jenny Altschuler 2016
Chapter 7 © Rachel Hopkins 2016

All rights reserved. No reproduction, copy or transmission of this
publication may be made without written permission.

No portion of this publication may be reproduced, copied or transmitted
save with written permission or in accordance with the provisions of the
Copyright, Designs and Patents Act 1988, or under the terms of any licence
permitting limited copying issued by the Copyright Licensing Agency,
Saffron House, 6–10 Kirby Street, London EC1N 8TS.

Any person who does any unauthorized act in relation to this publication
may be liable to criminal prosecution and civil claims for damages.

The authors have asserted their rights to be identified as the authors of this work
in accordance with the Copyright, Designs and Patents Act 1988.

First published 2016 by
PALGRAVE

Palgrave in the UK is an imprint of Macmillan Publishers Limited,
registered in England, company number 785998, of 4 Crinan Street,
London, N1 9XW.

Palgrave Macmillan in the US is a division of St Martin's Press LLC,
175 Fifth Avenue, New York, NY 10010.

Palgrave is a global imprint of the above companies and is represented
throughout the world.

Palgrave® and Macmillan® are registered trademarks in the United States,
the United Kingdom, Europe and other countries.

ISBN 978–1–137–37850–7 paperback

This book is printed on paper suitable for recycling and made from fully
managed and sustained forest sources. Logging, pulping and manufacturing
processes are expected to conform to the environmental regulations of the
country of origin.

A catalogue record for this book is available from the British Library.

A catalog record for this book is available from the Library of Congress.

Printed and bound by CPI Group (UK) Ltd, Croydon, CR0 4YY

To the refugees who are risking all in the hope of a better future for themselves and their families

CONTENTS

ACKNOWLEDGEMENTS

Jenny Altschuler

This book draws on conversations about illness and migration with many people. I am indebted to the clients with whom I have worked for trusting me with their stories of what it means to be ill and caring for a loved one in the context of having moved from one country to another. I am also indebted to the people who agreed to participate in research focused on the impact of migration from South Africa to the UK during the apartheid era.

I would also like to thank Rachel Hopkins and Karen Sennett with whom I worked at the Killick Street Health Centre, Brian Rock and Julian Stern for the opportunity of working with the Hackney Primary Care Psychotherapy Consultation Service, colleagues at the Tavistock Clinic, particularly Barbara Dale and John Byng-Hall, Wendy Hollway and Ann Phoenix who supervised my research on migration, as well as the many other colleagues, supervisees and friends who shared their personal and professional insights and helped me grapple with aspects of experience that are not only important to me but to them, including: Nazee Akbari, David Amias, Jocelyn Avigad, Kate Daniel, Gwynneth Down, Celia Falicov, Harriet Galgut, Naomi Hartree, Helene Joffe, Ellie Kavner, Evelyn Katz, Deborah Khoder, Britt Krause, Rachel Lasserman, Gail Lawrence, Sue Lonsdale, Merle Mahon, Mary Macleod, Rabia Malik, Elaine Mayon-White, Tim Nedas, Carmel Sher, Gail Schrire, Adam Steingold, Dave Saunders, Gary Stiefl, Dianne Taylor, Charlie Tilly, Dennis Walder and Ester Usiskin-Cohen.

I am also indebted to colleagues working abroad for the opportunity of engaging with their personal and professional experiences of migration, illness and political conflict. This includes colleagues working in post-conflict Kosovo, as part of the sub-Saharan paediatric HIV/AIDS network (PATA), in the Middle East and the Trust board and team of the One to One Children's Fund, including David Altschuler, Georgia Burford, Lawrence Gould, Kevin Gundle, Michael Harding, Lauren Jacobson, Russell Mishcon, Emily Tunnycliffe and Nathalie Renaud who facilitated this work. I would also like to thank Zarlasht Halaimzai, Talya Feldman and Ariana and Jeff Faris who helped David and I set up the Refugee

Trauma Initiative, a project for refugees and volunteers in Idomeni, Northern Greece. My thanks as well to Palgrave – to Stephen Frosh who edited my first two books (*Working with Families Facing Chronic Illness* and *Counselling and Psychotherapy at Times of Illness and Death*), to Catherine Gray who suggested that I write this book and to Peter Hooper and Louise Summerling for their support in taking this book forward.

Special thanks to my parents, Jack and Sarah, whose personal and family stories inspired my interest in understanding how migration has influenced who we were and have become as a family, to my sister Eileen, brothers Brian and Stanley and your partners Keith and Lori: your own thoughts about living apart from one another, particularly at times of illness and death, have challenged me to think more deeply about the impact of migration and belonging for siblings. Likewise, I would like to thank Sylvia, Raymond, Sue, Bernard and Majella for sharing the parallels with your own migration.

Last, but far from least, are my thanks to David and our children Gabriel and Marla, who together with Francesca and Anna have shared so much of this journey and whose interest, challenging questions, IT support and reminders of life outside have kept me going when writing has felt endless.

Rachel Hopkins

I would like to thank, firstly, Jenny Altschuler for inviting me to contribute a chapter in this book. I greatly valued the support of my family, particularly my husband, Duncan Minty, and my mother, Juliet Hopkins. There are also many whose wisdom has helped me, notably Barbara Dale who supervised my original MA thesis, John Launer who introduced me to the ideas of narrative and systemic theory and Britt Krause whose work I greatly admire, as well as all at the Tavistock Clinic. My greatest debt, however, is owed to my patients who have shared their stories with me and from whom I have learned the most, and am still learning.

1

INTRODUCTION

> Attending to the situation of the migrant at times of illness and death is to open ourselves to the coming together of two of the most radical thresholds of bodily estrangement and vulnerability: the movement across territories and from life to death. (Gunaratnam, 2013, p. 2)

The phenomenon of international migration is not new: migrations have occurred throughout human history, beginning with the movements of the first human groups from origins in East Africa to their current location in the world. However, the forces of globalization, economics, political conflict and growth of the Internet and social networks offering news of life elsewhere mean more people are on the move now than at any other time in history. In 2013, the International Organization for Migration estimated there were 232 million international migrants[1] worldwide, with nearly 50% living in the more developed countries of the world (IOM, 2013). This is predicted to rise to 405 million by 2050.

This pattern is reflected in Britain as well: in 2014 approximately 12.5% of the population was born abroad, compared with 8% in 2001. The net long-term migration to the UK was estimated to be 260,000 for the year ending June 2014, with immigration of people from the EU countries increasing by 45,000, and non-EU by 30,000. Until recently, most migrants were assumed to be adult men. However, as reflected in the UN International Migration Report, 48% of all migrants in 2013 were women and 15% were under the age of 20.

For much of the twentieth century, the numbers migrating to and from the UK were roughly in balance, and from the 1960s to the early 1990s the number of emigrants was often greater than the number of immigrants. Over the last two decades, both immigration and emigration have increased to historically high levels, with immigration exceeding emigration by more than 100,000 every year since 1998. More than 13 million of the UK population (20.3%) were either foreign national (7.8%) or foreign-born (12.5%) on 1 January 2014. In 2014, 13% of people migrating to the UK were British nationals, 32% were nationals of other EU countries and

45% were nationals of non-EU countries. This means just under half of migrants entering the UK in 2014 were subject to immigration control. The UK's migrant population is concentrated in London. Around 37% of people living in the UK who were born abroad live in the capital city (Hawkins, 2015).

Experiences of migration vary considerably, influenced for example, by whether the decision was chosen or forced, the country one leaves and reception in the country to which one moves (Falicov, 2013; Fortier, 2002). Similarly, experiences of illness vary, influenced by such factors as the particular nature of the condition in question, the treatment available, access to practical and emotional support, and prior experiences of loss (Rolland, 1994; Altschuler, 2011). Nonetheless, even if one is able to transcend the disruption these experiences present to oneself and relationships with others, both forms of experience will be accompanied by some sense of loss and disarray, questions about bodies and embodiment, identity, memory, the remaking of memory, risk and resilience.

The speed of contemporary migrations, the numbers involved and the fact that they relate to areas with distinct disease profiles pose complex challenges to migrants, their non-migrant kin,[2] and the health care systems of their countries of origin/migration[3] and destination/settlement.[4] Despite the importance of migrant labour to many sectors, including health and social services where migrants are needed to fill highly skilled as well as the low-skilled positions (such as domestic care for sick and elderly people), the policies and regulations of the UK and most EU countries are becoming less rather than more accommodating of migrants.

Studies of the so-called 'health migrant effect' suggest that those who leave tend to be the healthier, stronger and more resilient members of their society and are relatively healthy compared with the non-migrant population of the country to which they move (McDonald and Kennedy, 2004; Razum, Zeeb and Rohrmann, 2000). This is not the case for others, particularly refugees and asylum seekers. In many situations, poverty and language barriers mean it is difficult to find employment: as a result people accept more hazardous work and are therefore more vulnerable to injury and other occupational health hazards (Gushulak, Pace and Weekers, 2010; Jayaweera, 2014; Rechel et al., 2013).

Likewise, depending on the countries one moves to and from, migrants may be more vulnerable to certain communicable and non-communicable conditions. Migrants' health is more likely to be compromised when the condition is stigmatized. For example, the UK has seen an increase in migrant-associated infectious disease, including HIV where the majority of people with heterosexually acquired HIV infection are from sub-Saharan

Africa. While most health care services are well equipped to treat HIV/ AIDS from a medical perspective, fear, stigma and institutional barriers (including lack of cultural understanding and language barriers) mean African migrants tend to access HIV services at a later stage of disease than non-Africans, impacting on the quality of care they need and are able to receive (Burns et al., 2007).

Even where migrants are entitled to free health care, inadequate information regarding their rights to services presents barriers to accessing care and treatment, impacting on the possibilities of healing and survival (Hargreaves et al., 2008; Norredam, Mygind and Krasnick, 2006; Priebe et al., 2011). Sadly, it is often the more vulnerable migrants who are unable to access health care and do not understand their entitlements in the host country and in transit (Kirmayer et al., 2011).

The health risks for undocumented migrants are particularly high as they experience greatest problems in accessing health services and in many countries are expected to cover the full costs of medical treatment. Moreover, concerns about the possibility of being sent home mean that those who can afford this, use private services, where they are unlikely to be asked for any official form of identification, but this can mean being seen by unregistered health care workers (Dixon-Woods, Cavers and Agarwal, 2006; Woodward, Howard and Wolffers, 2013).

However, other than in screening of migrants to prevent the spread of communicable disease more prevalent elsewhere, concerns about the costs to the health care system and 'brain drain' of medical staff that resource-starved countries face, limited attention has been paid to the health implications of migration. The reluctance of many countries to sign the UN Convention on the Rights of Migrants (ratified in 2003) is indicative of a more widespread unwillingness to take account of the ethical as well as public health dimensions of migration (Jayaweera, 2014).

Indeed, in the midst of polarized debates about the risks and benefits of global capitalism and migration, there seems to be little space for thinking about ill, disabled and dying migrants and their families, about the pain, feelings of estrangement and loss that accrue over a lifetime, and the effects this can have on subsequent generations (Gunaratnam, 2013). Likewise, little thought is given to the challenges health care professionals face when language and cultural barriers mean it is difficult to communicate. Although this is starting to change, with the exception of health care professionals working in certain inner city settings, few have been trained to address the consequences of migration for experiences of illness, including the challenges of working with people who are extremely isolated and are struggling to adapt to a different social and geographic environment where constructions of illness, healing and health care are very different to what they were 'back home'. Similarly, few feel equipped to address the particular challenges of refugees[5] and asylum seekers,[6] including the effects trauma can have on interactions with health care professionals and others in positions of authority (Hargreaves and Friedland, 2013; Kelly, Morrell and Sriskandarajah, 2005).

There has been a corresponding lack of thought about the positions of health care professionals who are themselves migrants: the challenges one faces in maintaining one's sense of professional competence when qualifications are not recognized, the hurdles one needs to cross to qualify for registration, of having to adjust to a health care system where the paradigms of treatment, styles of communicating and approach to patient–doctor relationships are different to those of the country in which one trained and worked, and the complex feelings aroused by caring for others when one is unable to 'be there' to offer practical and emotional support for one's own parents, siblings and children when they are ill, distressed or dying.

Growing concerns about the human rights and health care of migrants have led to the signing of a number of legally binding international treaties and resolutions, including the World Health Organization (WHO) 'Resolution on the Health of Migrants' (WHO, 2008) endorsing the commitment to develop and implement more effective methods for monitoring the health and health care of migrants, establishing practices, legal systems and policies sensitive to the positions of migrants, and reducing the level of discrimination which migrants from black and minority ethnic groups face. However, while most governments see health as an essential human right, there is still a considerable gap between stated resolutions like this and reality on the ground (Jayaweera, 2014; Rechel et al., 2013).

One explanation may lie in the fact that policies related to migration tend to be developed in 'silos' with different, often competing, goals, and pay little attention to health (Zimmerman, Kiss and Hossain, 2011). Other explanations are that the pace of worldwide migration might have outstripped capacity to respond. Similarly the myth that most migrations are successful and desire to avoid facing the loss and fragmentation that so often accompany experiences of migration may have led to underplaying the more complex emotional and health challenges migrants and their families face.

However, it is also possible that this gap reflects a reluctance to engage with the position of those deemed to be outsiders. For example, one of the consequences of migrations from Africa, the Caribbean and the Mediterranean is that the incidence of certain forms of inherited conditions such as sickle-cell anaemia and thalassaemia in Britain has increased (Modell et al., 2007). Lack of experience in dealing with these conditions means that in some situations diagnostic, treatment and counselling services fall short of what is wanted and needed. Since these conditions are more prevalent amongst people from black and ethnic minority groups, studies indicating that people with sickle-cell anaemia do not always receive sufficient pain relief suggest that some of this shortfall relates to racism (Elander, Beach and Haywood, 2011; Nelson et al., 2013).

With these issues in mind, this book aims to extend understanding of what it means to be located and dislocated through migration and the ways in which these experiences inform and are informed by experiences of illness, offering recommendations for clinical practice. Particular attention is paid to migrations to and from the UK; however, the book draws on a wider body of academic and clinical studies and raises issues that apply to other forms of migration. Although it is intended to be for health care professionals and academics and researchers interested in the interface between migration, illness and health care, the concerns and questions discussed within this book are likely to be of interest to policy makers as well.

This opening chapter outlines the aims, anticipated readership and structure of the book, and the academic, professional and personal experience upon which the ideas, questions and recommendations presented here are based. Chapter 2 reviews what is currently known about migrancy and health. Chapter 3 discusses developments in theorizing and researching experiences of culture, language barriers and discrimination, and the implications for health care. Chapters 4 and 5 focus on illness and migration respectively, outlining the common threads and key concerns arising from the academic literature and clinical experiences.

The next three chapters draw these more generic discussions together by focusing on the intersection between migration and illness. Chapter 6 looks at the multiple ways in which experiences of migration, experiences of cultural diversity, language barriers and discrimination can inform responses to childhood and adult illness and death, and the reverse, with examples drawn from inpatient, palliative care, outpatient clinical work and supervision. In Chapter 7, Rachel Hopkins draws on her experience as a GP in discussing the challenges and more positive opportunities of working in a primary health care clinic where a high percentage of the population are first- or second-generation immigrants. Chapter 8 addresses an aspect of health care that has received little academic or clinical attention: the migration of health care professionals, including implications for the health care services of the countries they leave and move to, as well as the professional and more personal dilemmas they and their colleagues face. Statistics produced by the Health and Social Care Information Centre indicate that in 2015, 14% of clinical staff working for the NHS and in community health services were foreign nationals and/or trained abroad, in other EEA[7] countries or so-called Third World countries, increasing to

26% for doctors and 39% for doctors on the specialist register (Health and Social Care Information Centre, 2016). As such, this chapter is likely to resonate with your experience as health care professionals, or the experience of your colleagues. The concluding chapter draws these themes together in presenting recommendations for the future.

Informed by systemic theory, the book draws on the assumption that although many aspects of migration and illness are deeply personal, personal experiences affect and are affected by interactions with the people with whom we are most intimately connected, the discourses dominating the wider socio-economic and political context, as well as the practical realities of everyday life. It is also informed by the narrative-based idea that in order to make sense of experiences, we develop 'stories' about these experiences. However, as one story is unable to portray the full complexity of events, particular constructions of reality are privileged over others: consequently other stories or constructions of experience are possible, including less pathologizing constructions of reality (White and Epston, 1990). Emphasis is placed on separating the person from the problem: people are assumed to have skills, abilities, values, commitments, beliefs and competencies that can assist them in changing their relationship with the problems that influence their lives.

The ideas raised here draw on developments in theorizing and researching migration, illness, experiences of culture, racialization and other forms of discrimination. Although attention is paid to common threads of experience, emphasis is placed on the heterogeneity of experience, including the differences between migrations that are chosen or forced, differences related to the medical condition in question, to particular family dynamics, personal resources and genetics, as well as the broader contexts of people's lives, including class, racialization, gender and sexual orientation.

In addition, the book draws on clinical and personal experience. One of the first times I realized what a profound effect migration can have on experiences of illness and health care was when, as a newly appointed family therapist working for a hospital-based psychosocial liaison team, I was asked to see Rani, a 14-year-old girl who had been sent from Pakistan to the UK for treatment shortly after the diagnosis of end-stage renal failure. The decision to seek treatment in the UK arose from her family's concerns about the quality of care she could access in Pakistan. However, it was also informed by the fact that her father had been working in the UK for a number of years, and was living with cousins who could offer her and her father support over the course of her treatment. Although Rani's mother applied to join her daughter, her application was refused until much later.

The medical team that referred Rani felt she was extremely withdrawn and thought she and her father were finding it particularly difficult coming to terms with how ill Rani was. Consequently much of our initial work focused on the illness. It was only after meeting her and her father several times that I was able to see that in the immediacy of a medical crisis, I and the rest of the renal team had overlooked the fact that Rani was not only having to come to terms with the diagnosis of renal failure, the need for dialysis and risks to her future health, she was having to do so in a context that was foreign to her, where she was unable to speak the language or turn to the person who had been her primary source of support until then: her mother. We had also overlooked the challenges her father was facing in assuming primary responsibility for aspects of parenting that had previously been part of his wife's domain. I cannot speak for my colleagues, but looking back I suspect that this initial 'blindness' related to my position as a relatively recent migrant, to my desire to fit in and avoid drawing attention to my own position as an outsider by focusing on the personal and family disruptions that arise from experiences of migration.

The ideas raised in this book also draw on my subsequent work with immigrant parents facing life-limiting illness in an outpatient mental health clinic, in primary health care settings where a high proportion of the patients are first- and second-generation migrants and refugees and a drop-in service for destitute asylum seekers, many of whom are experiencing symptoms of post-traumatic stress disorder. They also draw on my supervision of medical and non-medical health care professionals working in a range of inpatient and outpatient services, and the experience of setting up and mentoring staff working with families affected by political conflict in Kosovo and in refugees camps in Northern Greece.

Over the course of this work, many professionals have expressed discomfort about situations where cultural and language barriers led to misunderstandings and difficulties in providing the collaborative care they see as best practice. Others have spoken about the value of being able to learn about other constructions of health, experiences of family, and responses to loss and trauma, and the need to 'dig deeper' in order to develop some sense of shared understanding. A number of professionals born outside the UK and/or from black and minority ethnic groups have used supervision to reflect on their own experiences of moving from one cultural and health care setting to another, discrimination and the struggle to engage with the suffering of those who treat them with disdain.

However, the book draws on more personal experience as well, on my father's stories of his family leaving Lithuania to escape oppression and settling in Ireland for ten years before moving to South Africa after his aunt was injured in an anti-Semitic pogrom,[8, 9] my mother's stories about boarding a ship to leave Lithuania at the age of 6, of trying to hide that her 3-year-old sister had chicken pox to avoid their being prevented from sailing and how she had played relatively carefree on deck unaware of her own mother's premonition that she would never see her parents again: they were killed when the Nazis invaded their village.

It also draws on my experience of being cared for by a woman who, in common with many black South African women during apartheid, moved from her village to a larger city to care for my siblings and me in order to support her family financially, leaving her own children in the care of her mother. Although she saw her children on her 'days off', and they came to visit from time to time, I suspect we had no conception of how painful it was looking after someone else's children, particularly children privileged as white, while unable to care for one's own children. The book is also informed by my own experience of migrating, on memories of the mixed feelings of anticipation, relief, sadness and guilt of leaving apartheid-based South Africa, of the confusion, isolation and excitement of establishing a new life in Britain, bringing up children in a country that was different to that of my own childhood without the support or constraints of extended family, making friends, rebuilding a sense of professional identity and working in a markedly different system of health care. However, it also draws on the discomfort of knowing that other than during periods of heightened crisis I was unable to offer my parents and siblings the hands-on support they needed at times of illness and death. Like many of the people with whom I work, I have wondered about the impact of migration on my children's lives: when asked, my son has said that he felt a sense of belonging to South Africa as well as the UK, and my daughter that when she was younger, being with family from South Africa felt like being with people who were 'of my blood but not of my life'. Since they have both worked abroad and married partners with connections elsewhere, stories of migration are likely to inform the experiences of the next generation as well.

Before moving on, it is important to note that, because this book focuses on the links between migration, illness and health care the terms migrant, immigrant, non-migrant, refugee and asylum seeker are used. However, I hope it is apparent from what is written that Rachel and I recognize that migration is only one aspect of experience: our beliefs, hopes, decisions and actions are informed by many other areas of life, including our positions as family members, friends, professionals and members of the various communities with which we are connected. It is also important to emphasize that although the book draws on actual clinical cases and research interviews, details have been changed to ensure anonymity.

2

LINKS BETWEEN MIGRANCY AND HEALTH

The diverse nature of migrant experiences means that attempts to understand the links between migrancy and health have yielded contradictory findings. A wide body of research and clinical studies suggests that, overall, the outcomes for physical and mental health are worse for non-UK born individuals residing in the UK compared to the rest of the UK population. However, others suggest that changes in the health and health behaviours of migrants are not as marked or linear as generally assumed, and cannot be understood without considering other factors, including socio-economic circumstances and the immigration regulations of the countries to which migrants move (Gushulak, Pace and Weekers, 2010; Thomas and Gideon, 2013).

Some of these contradictions relate to difficulties in monitoring and recording migrant health, differences in definitions of 'the migrant' and using concepts like ethnicity as a proxy for migrant status. Consequently, this chapter begins by discussing the complexities of monitoring migrant health and entitlements to health care, before discussing key trends emerging from studying physical and mental health.

Monitoring migrant health

One of the complications in understanding the links between migrancy and health is that there is no universally accepted definition of 'migrant' that takes account of the full complexity of people whose lives are located and dislocated through migration. According to UNESCO, the term migrant refers to 'any person who lives temporarily or permanently in a country where he or she was not born, and has acquired some significant social ties to this country'.[10] Likewise, the International Organization for Migration (IOM) defines the migrant as someone who has resided in a foreign country for more than one year irrespective of the cause, voluntary or involuntary, and means, regular or irregular, of migrating (IOM, Glossary on Migration, International Migration Law Series No. 25, 2011). Although 'migrant' is often understood to cover cases where the decision to migrate is taken freely for reasons of 'personal convenience', without the intervention of an external compelling factor, it is generally used to refer to any kind of movement of people, whatever its length, composition and causes, including the migration of refugees, displaced persons, economic migrants and persons moving for other purposes, including family reunification.

However, the UNESCO, IOM and most other definitions fail to mention how long one needs to live in the country before the term is not applicable. Nor do they take account of 'oscillating', 'circular' and temporary migrations, namely that many people (including students, businesspeople, seasonal farm workers and other economic migrants) move back and forth; of 'medical migrations'[11] where people seek medical treatment in another country; and internal migration (for example, people who move from rural to urban areas), which is estimated to involve four times as many people as international migrations (Crooks et al., 2010; Ormond, 2013). Consequently, their positions are not reflected in research or debates about migrant health and health care (Carballo and Mboup, 2005; Zimmerman, Kiss and Hossain, 2011). In addition, these definitions do not take account of children who were born in the UK, are UK nationals whose parents are foreign-born or foreign nationals, despite the fact that they tend to be regarded as part of the migrant population.

There is also little agreement on which term should be used to denote this positioning: although dictionary definitions distinguish between 'immigrants', people who are settling or intend to settle in their new country, and 'migrants', who are temporarily resident, the terms 'immigrant', 'migrant', 'foreigner', 'foreign by birth' and 'of foreign citizenship' tend to be used interchangeably in academia as well as public debate.

Another complication relates to record keeping: other than with respect to infectious diseases more prevalent elsewhere, such as tuberculosis (TB), hepatitis and HIV/AIDs, health care systems of the UK and most other EU countries do not identify people according to migration status and medical files rarely contain this information (Juhász, Makara and Taller, 2010).

Increasingly, researchers are required to produce evidence on the patterns and causes of ethnic inequalities in diverse arenas of health, social and economic wellbeing. This might help to ensure that all sectors of the population have equal access to services. However ethnicity cannot be used as a proxy for migrancy as many people who identify themselves as belonging to minority ethnic groups were born in Britain, and many migrants would not be defined (or define themselves) as belonging to a minority ethnic group. Moreover, researching inequalities between ethnic groups presents other ethical and methodological challenges: ethnic identities and categories are not static but complex and fluid.

Furthermore, the political sensitivities associated with data collection, including fears about personal data being forwarded to immigration authorities and used to invoke racism, mean that placing greater emphasis on monitoring migrant status could reduce migrants' readiness to seek medical care. Consequently, it is important to ensure that the focus and approach of research fits with the views of the target groups. It is also important to pay attention to sampling, data generation and analysis in describing and explaining differences between ethnic groups, to avoid the possibility of misleading and harmful interpretations. Whilst identifying problems more common amongst minority groups may mean it is more possible to recognize and address gaps in service, it has the potential to portray minorities as weaker. Similarly, whilst analysing differences has the potential to bring discrimination into increased visibility (for example, by illustrating the way in which Western norms pathologize people with a different cultural background), the very act of analysing differences can result in perpetuating the categories and stereotypes one is seeking to dispel.

Another complication is that most studies of the links between migrancy and health compare the rates of illness and morbidity and/or mortality of migrants with those of the native-born population. However, particularly in studies of physical health, the oversampling required for statistically relevant data means that findings arising from large-scale studies have often been skewed. Initial attempts to trace the links between migrancy and mental health were hampered by other methodological problems, including the lack of standardized diagnostic criteria and comparisons with the general host population rather than with people seen by a mental health care professional. Although this is less true of recent research, much of what is known is based on small and often skewed samples, which increases the likelihood of contradictory findings (Kirkbride and Jones, 2011; McKay, Macintyre and Ellerway, 2003; Rechel et al., 2013; Ruiz, Maggi and Yusim, 2011). In addition, much of the existing evidence focuses on ethnic group rather than migration variables such as country of birth, length of residence in the UK or immigration status (Jayaweera, 2014).

Entitlement to health care

As migrants and health care providers are often unsure about entitlements to health care, it is important to clarify that currently, regardless of immigrant status, in accordance with the National Health Service Act of 2006, the Human Rights Act of 1998, the Equality Act of 2010, the National Health Service (Charges to Overseas Visitors) Regulations, the Immigration Act of 2014 and Regulations on the Immigration Health Charge of 2015 (National Health System, 2015) anyone has access to:

- Registration with a general practitioner (GP), at discretion of the GP

- Accident and Emergency care

- Genito-urinary medicine and family planning clinics

- Mental health admission under the 1983 Mental Health Act

- Antenatal care[12]

- Hospital care for urgent conditions.[13]

In addition, according to the Department of Health (2015) migrants are entitled to full National Health Service (NHS) health care during asylum claims and until they receive a final refusal. Where asylum has been refused but a fresh claim is being made, or the Home Office is unable to return a person to their country they are entitled to receive Home Office accommodation, support and full NHS care. Where asylum has been refused and the person no longer receives Home Office housing or support, GPs are required to register the patient but secondary care is more difficult to access. Depending on the situation and the conditions of their visa, students may have full entitlement to NHS treatment.

The registration and treatment of undocumented migrants and people with a visitor's visa are at the GP's discretion. Refugees are often registered on a temporary basis because they are seen as highly mobile and unlikely to be in the area for long. However, the likelihood of mobility is highly inflated. Moreover, this practice prevents access to past records, if they exist, and removes any financial incentives to undertaking immunization and cervical smear tests. Some primary care trusts advise GPs to avoid registering people who are not deemed to be 'ordinary residents'. Despite this, the General Medical Council, Royal College of General Practitioners and British Medical Association (BMA Ethics, 2012) recommend doctors treat patients according to need and consider registering all vulnerable people living in their catchment area.

At this point in time, there are some differences in entitlements across Britain. In England, Wales and Northern Ireland, migrants are entitled to emergency treatment in a walk-in centre free of charge, but are charged if referred on to an outpatient clinic or admitted to hospital. Treatment for certain communicable conditions such as TB, cholera, gastroenteritis, malaria, meningitis and pandemic influenza is free throughout the UK. Treatment for HIV/AIDS is also free in England, Scotland and Northern

Ireland. However, in Wales, although there is no charge for testing for the HIV virus and counselling following a test, one may have to pay for subsequent treatment and medication. In England and Northern Ireland, refused asylum seekers who are not receiving United Kingdom Border Agency financial support are denied free secondary health care, including pregnant women, families with young children, people with terminal illness and survivors of sexual violence. Although some might be able to pay for secondary services, this is beyond the reach of most people.

Most of the evidence on barriers to health care draws on local and small-scale qualitative studies. Nonetheless, these studies have identified important areas of concern. For example, several have found that many migrants are unfamiliar with how the health care systems operate (particularly new migrants), and that they suffer from a lack of access to reliable transport and poor services in the areas of deprivation where many recent migrants live; cultural insensitivity amongst some front line health care providers; insufficient support with translation; and confusion about entitlement to services – among service providers as well as migrants whose immigration status is unclear (Johnson, 2006; Phillimore et al., 2010; Scheppers et al., 2006). Some of these barriers (including limited access to accurate information, language and transport) affect the lives of longer established migrants as well.

Particular attention has been paid to the barriers faced by irregular migrants and those with uncertain immigration status. This includes people who overstay their visas, refused asylum seekers, those who have been trafficked and spousal migrants escaping domestic violence. As outlined earlier, according to current government rules, these categories of people are not entitled to certain services, for instance free hospital care other than for emergency care or HIV treatment, in most areas of the UK. Moreover, according to the UK Immigration Act of 2014 which redefined the terms of 'ordinary residence', all new 'temporary' entrants (including workers on the points-based system and their dependants, family members joining British citizens or permanent residents, and international students) will need to pay an additional charge as part of their entry visa fee to access NHS services (Grove-White, 2014; Phillimore et al., 2010). It is predicted that there will be additional restrictions in the rights of undocumented migrants and of UK-born children of undocumented parents to some services currently granted on humanitarian and public health protection grounds, for example free access to Accident and Emergency services (Jayaweera, 2014).

Statutory as well as non-statutory agencies have expressed particular concern about the risks associated with lack of, or confusion around, entitlements to health care among vulnerable groups, including pregnant women and children, and the ramifications of denying women access to maternity and infant health services (Oliver, 2013). For example, although NHS maternity treatment is classed as immediately necessary and should not be based on a patient's ability to pay, the cost can run into several thousand pounds. Whilst some hospitals are less vigilant about pursuing payment, the users of these services are still liable for charges and pursued for unpaid bills they cannot afford.

As a result, many migrants and asylum seekers avoid seeking antenatal care until the later stages of their pregnancy for fear of the high costs and being arrested or thrown out of the UK, give false names and 'disappear' after their first antenatal appointment, relying on informal and more precarious forms of care. The delay in seeking care can result in suffering problems in childbirth that could have been averted earlier – for example, through scans alerting pregnant women and professionals to areas of concern. This may account for the fact that studies of maternity care and pregnancy outcomes identified asylum seekers and refused asylums seekers as especially vulnerable (Bollini et al., 2009; Gideon, 2013). An additional complication is that, in common with other NHS staff, midwives are expected to act as 'border officials' to determine who is eligible for free NHS care at a time when their primary attention should be focused on the mothers-to-be (Shortall et al., 2015).

Furthermore, dispersal policies make very little allowance for the health care and social needs of pregnant women, specify no time limit for dispersal during pregnancy and see women as eligible to be moved elsewhere within two weeks of giving birth. This should have changed with the introduction of new guidelines in 2012. However a study commissioned by Maternity Action and the Refugee Council found that most of the women who were dispersed or relocated during pregnancy had reported feeling unwell during pregnancy; two-thirds had their first contact with a midwife later than the NICE guidelines; over half described suffering from mental health conditions such as depression, anxiety, flashbacks and very high levels of stress; and two had attempted suicide during pregnancy (Feldman, 2013).

Likewise, midwives reported a high prevalence of serious underlying health conditions including diabetes, HIV, other sexually transmitted diseases and female genital mutilation (FGM), as well as particular problems of pregnancy, including severe headaches, elevated blood pressure and repeated urinary tract infections. They also reported a disturbingly high incidence of mental health problems among the dispersed and pre-dispersed women they had looked after, many of whom had spent considerable time in initial accommodation where they were subjected to unhygienic and unsafe conditions before being moved on. In addition, the antenatal care most of these women received had been interrupted as a result of dispersal mainly due to difficulties in registering with GPs. This can have serious consequences for women with conditions like diabetes and hepatitis where regular monitoring and treatment needs to be sustained during pregnancy (Bragg, 2013).

Fewer studies focus on migrants' uptake of treatment. However, the studies that have been conducted emphasize the importance of taking account of other aspects of experience, such as ethnicity, socio-demographic factors and, as discussed in greater detail in Chapter 4, diversities in cultural constructs of health and illness: this includes understanding how the belief in fatalism affects the uptake of immunizations and screening. Socio-economic factors are also important to bear in mind as poor nutrition and lack of access to welfare benefits, good quality housing and transport to care facilities in the more deprived areas affect the wider determinants of health (Jayaweera and Quigley, 2010; Marlow, Wadle and Waller, 2015; Webb et al., 2004).

However, debates about access and barriers to health care touch on moral, political and financial questions about the boundaries of responsibility: while most governments see health as an essential human right, there is still considerable debate about the extent to which non-citizens should share the same rights and entitlements to health care as citizens (Haour-Knipe, 2013).

Migration and physical health

Genetic, behavioural and environmental factors mean there are many differences in the prevalence and frequency of disease between certain populations. Migration to areas where rates of prevalence and frequency are markedly different allows for the transfer or elaboration of these differences and redistribution of the disability burden, with considerable implications for the treatment and prevention of disease and for health services, training and the professionals entrusted with providing health care (Crisp and Chen, 2014; Hargreaves and Friedland, 2013). As a result, health care professionals can find themselves dealing with adverse health outcomes that originate outside of their jurisdiction and health care planning, and with people whose health is far worse than the locally born population. This is particularly complicated where there are differences in health care beliefs, practices, and presentations of illness, and where literacy levels are lower than the host population, as is true of some people from developing countries that move to Britain.

One of the main findings arising from studies of the link between migration and physical health is that migrants tend to seek medical care for the same health concerns as the rest of the UK population. However, although this is not the case with all conditions, overall the health outcomes for non-UK born individuals residing in the UK are worse when compared to the UK population. The economic hardship, unemployment and poor housing many face on arriving affect the likelihood of developing communicable and non-communicable diseases (Rechel et al., 2013; Zimmerman, Kiss and Hossain, 2011). In some cases migration increases the risks of developing conditions that are prevalent amongst the rest of the population: for example, in a study of referrals to two genito-urinary clinics in the UK, 10 per cent of new referrals involved recent migrants from Eastern and Central Europe (Burns et al., 2009). Some migrant groups are at greater risk of developing hereditary conditions, for example sickle-cell anaemia, and contagious conditions more prevalent elsewhere than is usual in the UK, such as TB, Hepatitis and HIV/AIDS (Abubakar, Stagg, Cohen, et al., 2012; Health Protection Services, 2011). Lifestyle, cultural traditions related to food and circumstances subsequent to migration mean that some migrants have a higher risk of developing non-communicable diseases, including diabetes and coronary conditions (Dreyer et al., 2009; Ujcic-Voortman et al., 2012).

In other cases migrants and their children are vulnerable to the health consequences of practices that are valued and regarded as obligatory 'back home' but are unacceptable and/or illegal in the UK. For example, according to an NHS Choices briefing, over 20,000 girls under the age of 15 in the UK are estimated to be at risk of female genital mutilation (FGM), and the health of 66,000 women has been compromised by FGM.[14] FGM involves the partial or total removal of external female genitalia for non-medical reasons which can cause severe and long-lasting damage to physical and emotional health, increasing the likelihood of birth complications and consequently the health of their children (MacFarlane and Dorkenoo, 2014). Although FGM has been a criminal offence in the UK since 1985, more recent legislation (The Serious Crime Act 2015) has been introduced to strengthen the protection of girls and women against whom such an offence has been committed, increasing the penalty for committing such an act or supporting someone inflicting this on themselves. This appears to have increased awareness of UK legislation against and penalties for FGM: a study of attitudes to FGM amongst communities where this practice is common found that between 2010 and 2013 opposition had increased, particularly among younger women, although some women, particularly those who are older, continue to support this practice. Young men brought up in the UK tend to oppose or report being unaware of FGM, while older men's attitudes range across the spectrum. Although there has been a significant decline of FGM on religious grounds, it continues to be associated with cultural identity (Bindel, 2014; Brown, 2013).

'Healthy migrant effect' and paradox of assimilation

One of the other issues arising from analysing the link between migration and health relates to what has been called the 'healthy migrant effect' (and in the US the 'Hispanic paradox'), that, regardless of whether the move is temporary or permanent, migrants tend to be healthier than the population they originate from, and the population of the country to which they move, including people of similar ethnic backgrounds (McDonald and Kennedy, 2004; Razum, Zeeb and Rohrmann, 2000; Rechel et al., 2013).

For example, in one of the earlier studies of migrant health, Bennett (1993) found significant differences between immigrants and people born in Australia, with immigrants exhibiting lower rates of chronic vascular disease than the host population. Similar findings arose from studies of Latin American, Chinese and South Asian migrants to Canada (Nair et al., 1990) and Turkish nationals migrating to Germany (Razum et al., 1998). Likewise, a large number of studies of migrations to the UK, European countries and the USA found migrants had lower overall mortality rates than the respective local population, despite the fact that in each of these contexts, migrants tend to be characterized by low socio-economic status and working in unhealthy jobs, factors more usually associated with unfavourable health behaviour, opportunities and outcomes (Deboosere and Gadeyne, 2005; Singh and Hiatt, 2006).

This pattern has been attributed to the protective effects of genetics, conditions in migrants' country of origin, and self-selection, namely that people who are chronically ill and disabled are less likely to be able to migrate. It is also possible that research figures are skewed by the fact that, where this is financially viable and there is access to better support, some people who become seriously ill after moving return to their country of origin for treatment and/or to die (Ormond, 2013). Nonetheless, experiences of and responses to illness are far from uniform, and vary depending on such factors as the particular nature of the condition in question. For example, in a study of migrants living in the Netherlands, migrants from Turkey, Morocco, Surinam, Netherlands Antilles and Aruba were found to be 50% less likely to develop most forms of cancer than the host population, but the chances of developing stomach and liver cancers were greater (Stirbu et al., 2006).

However, over time, the migrants' health advantage tends to diminish in what Rumbaut (1997) calls the 'paradox of assimilation', as reflected in the correlation between length of stay and incidence of low-birth weight in infants, risky behaviour in adolescents, cancer, anxiety, depression and general morality. Rates of morbidity and mortality tend to converge or become worse than the host population in relation to the incidence of conditions such as cardiovascular diseases, lung and prostate cancer, chronic obstructive pulmonary diseases, cirrhosis, pneumonia and influenza (Fennelly, 2005; Singh and Miller, 2004). In some cases, the incidence of disease and mortality is higher for second-generation in contrast with first-generation migrants, for example in relation to several forms of cancer (Deboosere and Gadeyne, 2005; Singh and Hiatt, 2006; Singh and Siahpush, 2002).

The change from health advantage to disadvantage has been attributed to acculturation, including the loss and in some cases discarding of resources that enhance health (such as familiar social networks, cultural practices, employment in the same field), stresses of settlement wearing down one's resilience and a tendency to adopt the poor health behaviours and lifestyles of the host culture (Noh and Kaspar, 2003). For example, a large-scale review of migrations to six European countries found obesity (which increases one's risk of developing diabetes) to be higher amongst migrant children than the host population (Labree et al., 2011). Whilst other factors are likely to be implicated as well, in a cross-sectional comparison of 3- to 12-year-old children from sub-Saharan Africa living in Australia the risks of becoming obese were less amongst children who maintained traditional lifestyles than those who were more assimilated (Renzaho, Swinburn and Burns, 2008).

Nonetheless, it is misleading to cluster different migrant groups together. For example, although an earlier study found that overall migrants from the Indian sub-continent had a higher rate of mortality from coronary heart disease than the white majority population and other minority groups in the UK (Balarajan and Soni Raleigh, 1993), subsequent research found a considerable difference between South Asian migrants: rates of mortality were highest for people from Bangladesh, followed by people from Pakistan and thirdly from India (Balarajan, 1996; Bhopal and Usher, 2002). Similarly, Agyemang et al. (2009) found the incidence of coronary heart disease to be lower amongst migrants from African countries than those from European countries. In addition, although the incidence of cancer amongst many minority ethnic groups is lower than that of the majority white population, the mortality rates are higher, attesting to the importance of understanding barriers to health care (Ben-Shlomo, 2008; Moller et al., 2008).

It is important to avoid framing the experience of particular people as indicative of the complexity of the situations of everyone who fits under this umbrella, whether this involves viewing all women as particularly vulnerable or assuming that more privileged women from less developed countries can speak for all women from that country (Yuval-Davis, 1997). Indeed, although migrant women are often presented as heavy users of health and social care services, relying on social housing and additional welfare benefits (Hargreaves and Friedland, 2013), an increased percentage of migrant women are the primary breadwinners for their family, many of them working in the health services and education and looking after the children of the population of the country to which they move (Anderson, 2001; Ehrenreich and Hochschild, 2003; Lutz, 2008). Furthermore, many women who have the right to claim health and social care services find it difficult to access these services.

Racism and other forms of discrimination

As will be discussed in greater detail in Chapter 4, although geneticists have long argued that the boundaries used to mark 'race' do not reflect clear biological differences, 'race' tends to be treated as if it is inherited and with discernable biological and physical markers; instead, 'race' is constructed through the discourses that dominate the socio-political and cultural contexts and the material realities of daily living. Consequently, this book uses racialization – the term given to the process of ascribing racial identities to a relationship, social practice or group that does not identify itself as such – or, as above, uses inverted commas in referring to 'race'. This is particularly important in considering the links between migrancy, health and access to care across different racialized and ethnic groups, as it is often difficult to separate experiences of migration from the consequences of racism and other forms of discrimination (Salway et al., 2011).

For example, a survey of mothers who gave birth over a two-week period in England in 2009 revealed that in comparison with white UK-born women, black and minority ethnic (BME) women born outside the UK started antenatal care later, received poorer information provision and were less likely to be treated with respect by staff (Redshaw and Heikkila, 2011). Similarly, the UK Confidential Enquiry into Maternal Deaths (2006–2008) found that the mortality rate of black African mothers, a high percentage of whom were recent migrants including refugees and asylum seekers, was almost four times that of white women. Risk factors for maternal mortality included lack of antenatal care, late booking for first appointments (particularly among mothers of African-Caribbean and Pakistani ethnicity), little or no fluency in English and inadequate access to interpreters (Lewis, 2011).

Likewise, the Millennium Cohort Study (2001–2002) found that 7.1% of mothers born abroad who gave birth in the UK received no antenatal care, compared to 2.4% of UK-born mothers, and that particularly high proportions of Pakistani and Bangladeshi migrant mothers received no antenatal care. However, the strongest predictors of no antenatal care were not country of birth, ethnic group, or, in the case of migrants, length of residence in the UK, but socio-demographic factors including younger age, lower educational level and occupational class, and living in an area where at least 30% of the population were from BME categories (Jayaweera and Quigley, 2010).

Elsewhere, experiences of discrimination and inequities take a different form. For example, Irish immigrants are one of the largest immigrant groups in the UK and have the highest mortality ratio of all first-generation immigrants, with raised levels of mortality persisting into the second generation, regardless of which part of Ireland their parents originated from or whether one or both parents were Irish (Harding, Rosato and Teyhan, 2009; Marmot et al., 2010; NCAT/FIS, 2012; Raftery, Jones and Rosato, 1990; Tilki et al., 2009; Wild et al., 2006). This pattern has been attributed to the use of alcohol as an accepted method of coping with stress, economics, the relatively unsettled nature of many Irish migrants, and links between deprivation, ethnicity, age, gender (male) and late diagnosis amongst the Irish community in Britain. However, despite increased rates of mortality amongst Irish first- and second-generation migrants, most studies investigating differences in the screening uptake or in help seeking behaviour (for example, in relation to cancer) of minority ethnic groups aggregate the Irish into the host white population (Cuthbertson, Goyder and Poole, 2009), focus on visible minorities (Waller et al., 2009), South Asian communities (Karbani et al., 2011; Szczepura et al., 2008) or pay limited attention to ethnicity (Weller et al., 2007). As a result, preventative and treatment programmes have paid insufficient attention to the health and health care challenges of Irish immigrants and their children (Federation of Irish Studies, 2011).

Crenshaw (1969) coined the term 'intersectionality' in arguing that rather than different aspects of identity (for example, 'race', gender, ethnicity, migration and socio-economic position) having an additive effect on experience, these different factors and aspects of identity are continually and mutually constituting each other. Consequently, in trying to make sense of the links between migration, health and inequalities in access to, and the quality of care across different racialized and ethnic groups we need to consider how gender is raced, 'race' is gendered, and the intersection between migration, illness, racialization, gender and socio-economics.

Socio-economic factors

Many health discrepancies are less evident after controlling for socio-economic status: indeed, in many situations, a poorer socio-economic status may be a reflection of migration experiences. For example, although this is not always the case, migrants are often a minority with lower social status, experience higher rates of unemployment, poverty and homelessness, and are less able to access medical care than members of the host population (Carballo and Mboup, 2005; Davies, Basten and Frattini, 2009). Similarly, although the UK and many other European countries have seen an increase of migrant-associated TB, because many migrants live in cheap, overcrowded places where there is a greater risk of the spread of respiratory conditions the increase is likely to relate to socio-economics and cramped accommodation (Abubakar et al., 2012; Gilbert et al., 2009).

Likewise many migrants, particularly those who are unauthorized, work in low-skilled, poorly paid, high-risk and temporary positions that pose significant risks to health, for example in construction, mining and agriculture: this may explain why the incidence of occupational accidents is two-thirds higher for migrants (Carballo and Mboup, 2005; Elkeles and Seifert, 1996; Hard, Myers and Gerberich, 2002). In addition, migrants are particularly vulnerable to worldwide downturns in the economy, for example as a result of increased restrictions to the admission of new migrant workers, non-renewal of visas, job losses, reduction of working hours in sectors that employ migrants (including unauthorized migrants), and xenophobic beliefs that migrants are taking jobs away from the people to whom they 'rightfully belong': the locally born population (International Organization for Migration, 2011).

Where residency is determined on the basis of employment, people tend to continue to work despite being ill or badly injured, compounding the damage caused by the initial injury (Aronsson and Gustafsson, 2005; McKay, Craw and Chopra, 2006). It is also difficult to prioritize one's own health when one is responsible for sending funds home to pay for the basic essentials of everyday life or one's child's education (Haour-Knipe, 2013). Moreover, the combination of social circumstances, distrust of the medical profession and fear of being exposed to the migration authorities mean there is often a delay in seeking care, impacting on the process of diagnosis, treatment and chances of recovering (Pont et al., 2009; Haour-Knipe, 2013; Papadopoulos et al., 2004). Consequently, there tends to be a dichotomy between the health of documented and irregular/forced migrants, as those who are highly skilled and legally entitled to remain have fewer health problems.

Migration and mental health

As with physical health, it is impossible to understand the impact of migration on mental health without taking account of the variability of migrant experiences and wider aspects of people's lives, including the particular circumstances of the country one leaves, reception in the country to which one moves, family dynamics, socio-economics and exposure to racialization and other forms of discrimination.

The numbers of immigrants who go on to establish a settled and successful family life attest to the enormously positive impact migration can have. In many cases migration offers an opportunity to establish greater emotional wellbeing: this is particularly likely when living in a country dominated by political conflict where one is at risk of, or has undergone, imprisonment, where stigma means one is unable to acknowledge one is gay or has mental health problems and where family dynamics mean there seems to be no other possibility of claiming a greater sense of independence.

Disruptions to relationships with one's country of origin and non-migrant family, changes in social status, the absence of a familiar social network, the feelings of inadequacy associated with experiences of exclusion and being unable to communicate in the main language of the country in which one is living can threaten one's sense of 'ontological security'. Giddens (1991) coined the term 'ontological security' in discussing the stable mental state derived from a sense of continuity in regard to events in life: he argues that stability is reliant on the ability to give meaning to experiences, meanings that are founded on experiencing positive and stable emotions, and avoiding chaos and anxiety.

Living in an area where there are high numbers of migrants from the same society can act as a buffer against stress, providing support and a positive sense of ethnic identity. However, this is less sustainable in a racist, discriminatory society, particularly when migrants are settled in an area where they are perceived as a threat (Tilki, 2006). Moreover, maintaining contact with one's compatriots is not feasible where there is a policy of dispersal. Although disruption to one's sense of ontological security is likely to be difficult for most people, this tends to be particularly difficult when one moves from a collectivist society to one that is more individualistic (Bhugra and Becker, 2005).

Unless there are other opportunities to maintain a positive sense of identity, feelings of disruption can give rise to generalized anxieties, losing trust in one's abilities, affecting one's interest in engaging with others, withdrawal, loneliness, depression, anxiety, hopelessness and resorting to alcohol, drugs and suicidal behaviour (Iliceto et al., 2013). Some people experience mental health problems before migrating. For example, in a study focused on Turkish-speaking immigrant women in London, 13.4% reported having had mental health problems before. However, experiences of depression, nervousness and isolation subsequent to arriving in the UK meant the rates of mental health problems increased to 47.2% post-migration (Hatzidimitriadou and Cahir, 2013).

The inextricable links between physical and mental health mean that, particularly during the initial period of resettlement, it is not unusual for migrants to report with psychosomatic and stress-related symptoms including peptic ulcers, dermatitis, migraines, backache and tightness of the chest, symptoms that can affect the ability to integrate and work (Butler et al., 2015; Kirkcaldy et al., 2005; Sundquist et al., 2000; Ullman et al., 2013). Similarly, difficulties in adjusting to life in a new context can result in relying more heavily on comfort eating (which increases the risks of diabetes) and chemical comforters like alcohol, cigarettes, other drugs, and, in the case of isolated men, resorting to the services of sex workers, all of which carry distinct health risks.

Nonetheless, despite considerable economic hardship, the mental health profile of many migrants is better than the generation born subsequent to migrating. Possible explanations include research artefacts such as selection bias, a protective effect of traditional family networks, racism and an elevated frequency of substance abuse amongst those born subsequent to migration (Cantor-Graae and Selten, 2005; Escobar, Hoyos and Gara, 2000).

Risks of schizophrenia

Considerable attention has been paid to exploring the risks of schizophrenia amongst migrants. In one of the earliest studies, Ødegaard (1932) found a twofold increase in first admission rates for schizophrenia amongst Norwegians who moved to the United States compared with native-born Americans and Norwegians, with a peak between 10 and 12 years post-migration. This has been replicated in subsequent research: several studies indicate that people who moved from the Caribbean, Ireland, Pakistan, India and Poland to the UK were at greater risk of developing schizophrenia and relapsing than the locally born population (Jarvis, 1998; Selten, Cantor-Graae and Khan, 2003). However, it is also important to bear in mind that in most countries immigrants' pathways to psychiatric care involve longer delays in seeking and accessing professional help, a lower probability of medical referral, frequent involvement of the police, emergency services and high proportions of compulsory and secure-unit admissions.

Growing recognition of the heterogeneity of migrant experience resulted in attempts to identify the symptom profiles of particular migrant and ethnic groups, and factors contributing to risk and protection. An extensive review of the literature indicates that globally first- and second-generation migrants are at greater risk of developing schizophrenia where they are from a developing versus developed country and where the majority of the population is black (Cantor-Graae and Selten, 2005). This finding is reflective of studies of the experiences of first- and second-generation migrants in the UK and elsewhere in Europe (Fearon et al., 2006). Amongst certain groups, the risks appear to be less for the first generation but elevated in relation to the next: for example, Bhugra (2000) found the rate of schizophrenia amongst first-generation immigrants from Trinidad to be lower than people born in the UK and the rates of schizophrenia as well as suicide higher amongst the second generation.

It has been argued the increased risk is suggestive of a biological vulnerability (Cochrane and Bal, 1987). However, the rates of schizophrenia in one of the areas from which large numbers of migrants come, the Caribbean countries, are similar to the rates for the indigenous UK population, and lower than rates for immigrants from that region. Similarly, the risks for parents and siblings are about the same in both populations. Furthermore, this pattern is not specific to African-Caribbean immigrants (who are themselves ethnically diverse) but evident among African-born black immigrants, and, to a lesser extent, immigrants from Asian countries. It has also been suggested that because cultural and language barriers mean misunderstandings are more likely, these increased rates reflect an over-diagnosis of schizophrenia. However, this pattern is not evident in all situations where language and cultural differences exist (Hickling, 2005). Moreover, neither of these explanations can account for the increased rate amongst second generations and why the rate is not higher for all migrant groups (McKay, Macintyre and Ellerway, 2003).

As schizophrenia strikes families at all levels of society, personal, genetic and family characteristics are likely to be implicated. Nevertheless, although social disadvantage may not be a sufficient or a necessary cause for developing schizophrenia, it is difficult to refute suggestions that poor housing, overcrowding, lack of defensible space, areas of high levels of crime and illicit drug use play a significant role as well (Cooper, 2005). Similarly, as the incidence of schizophrenia in first- and second-generation black Caribbeans in the UK is substantially higher than that of the white British-born population, racism and other forms of discrimination are likely to inform the aetiology of the condition as well (Pinto, Ashworth and Jones, 2008).

Suicide and suicidal ideation

Many of the challenges discussed in considering the aetiology of schizophrenia are relevant to understanding the factors that could contribute to suicide, including the challenges posed to disruptions of self, family and wider experience of life, financial difficulties and exposure to racism and other forms of discrimination. It is difficult to establish an accurate picture of worldwide trends in suicide because many African, Middle Eastern and Central and South American countries do not report suicide rates to the World Health Organization (WHO).

Research based on the UK, other European countries, the USA and Australia indicate that the risks of suicide and suicide attempts vary across the different receiving countries and tend to mirror trends within migrants' country of origin (Bursztein Lipsicas et al., 2012; Ide et al., 2012; Voracek and Loibl, 2008). In the Netherlands, Pottie et al. (2014) found that suicidal ideation was lower across adolescents of most ethnicities, with the exception of Turkish and South Asian Surinamese female adolescents. However, overall, the risks of suicide appear to be highest amongst immigrants from Northern and Eastern Europe and lowest for those from the Middle East and Southern Europe. These differences have been attributed to a higher consumption of alcohol amongst immigrants from Northern and Eastern Europe, and the importance migrants from the Middle East and Southern Europe tend to place on traditional values, family and religion. For example, religious affiliation offers access to communal events and a sense of being connected with others. Most Southern European and Middle Eastern religions adopt a negative stance towards suicide (Koenig, 2009; Ratkowska and De Leo, 2013).

The length of time spent in the country to which one moves is also important. In line with previous national studies on Asian and Latino Americans' suicide-related outcomes (Borges et al., 2009; Duldulao, Takeuchi and Hong, 2009; Fortuna et al., 2007), in a large-scale study of people from the six biggest Asian American ethnic groups, suicidal ideation was associated with the length of one's life spent in the USA (Wong, Vaughen, Liu and Chang, 2014). However, the links between suicidality and having spent a greater proportion of one's life in the United States was weaker among Chinese, Japanese, Korean and Vietnamese Americans relative to non-Chinese, non-Japanese, non-Korean, and non-Vietnamese Asian Americans respectively. In contrast, the association was stronger among Indian Americans than among non-Indian Americans. It is difficult to discern the reasons for these disparities. However, to some extent, these findings mirror the rates of suicidal ideation in the countries in which people had grown up (Jeon et al., 2010; Lester, 2006).

Gender appears to be an important factor. Globally, the suicide rate for men is higher than for women. One exception is China where the reported rate for women is higher. However, as China only documents suicide fatalities for a small percentage of the nation, and independent studies produce estimates that conflict with official statistics, reported rates of suicide are likely to be inaccurate (Law and Liu, 2008). The other exception is amongst Asian women. Bursztein Lipsicas and Makinen (2010) found that South Asian women who had migrated to the UK were three times more likely to attempt suicide. Likewise, van Bergen et al. (2006) found that Asian women migrants living in the Netherlands were four times more likely to commit suicide than locally born women of a similar age. These findings have been attributed to difficulties in acculturation and marginalization. Many Asian women follow their primary provider (usually their father or husband) and are poorly educated and have little understanding of the language and culture of the host country. As such they tend to remain on the periphery of society: this is not only extremely isolating but limits the possibilities of learning the language and understanding the values of the country in which they live. The more highly educated women face a different challenge: having to balance their father and husband's desire for them to be intelligent, have a career and fulfil traditional female roles with their own personal and professional aspirations (Hicks and Bhugra, 2003).

Another issue to bear in mind is that cultural differences in expressions of distress and the shame some groups associate with acknowledging distress mean that depression, anxiety and other affective disorders tend to be under-reported, under-diagnosed and under-treated: indeed, despite the fact that people who attempt, or succeed in committing, suicide are more likely to be suffering from stress, they are less likely to have been diagnosed as mentally ill, are frequently overlooked by and/or do not present their concerns to their GP (Ineichen, 2008).

As with adults, children and young people's experience of migration range from extremely beneficial, as where the move is voluntary and offers access to better education and social support, to damaging, as when children move clandestinely with parents, other caretakers, on their own and/or are confronted with racism (Chase, 2013; Hernandez, Denton and Macartney, 2007; Mendoza, Javier and Burgos, 2007). Very few studies look at suicidal behaviour in culturally diverse first- and second-generation immigrant youth. Moreover, those have been conducted do not differentiate between ethnic minorities and immigrants. As with adults, overall the risks for migrants are higher than those for the locally born population. However, this varies according to ethnicity and country of settlement. For example, several studies found that Ethiopian youth who migrated to Israel were more likely to commit suicide than other immigrant populations (Shoval et al. 2007; Walsh, Edelstein and Vota, 2012), and children of Moroccan immigrants living in Rotterdam were found to be three times as likely as Dutch children to commit suicide, while those born to immigrants from Turkey were five times as likely (Carballo and Nerukar, 2001). Likewise, Surinamese immigrant children and adolescents, particularly girls in the Netherlands, were found to have a suicide rate three times higher than that of Dutch children (van Bergen et al., 2006).

The increased rates of suicide appears to be linked with length of time in the new country, intergenerational communication, conflicts with parents, both parties' difficulties in negotiating their sense of identity in relation to at least two socio-cultural contexts, racism and other stressors related to migration (Bursztein Lipsicas and Makinen, 2010). Nevertheless, mental disorder remains one of the strongest indicators, particularly affective disorders, substance abuse, behavioural disorders and antisocial behaviours (Beautrias, 2000).

As with other forms of mental problems, very little academic attention has been paid to the suicide risk of non-migrant kin. However, the high rates of suicide in areas of rural Ireland with high rates of migration suggest that there is an increased risk of suicide amongst 'left behind' kin as well (Laouire, 2001). Likewise, Borges, Breslau and Aguila-Gaxiola (2009) found an increase in suicidal ideation and suicide attempts amongst Mexicans following the migration of a close family member, and Gao et al. (2010) found an increase in rates of suicide ideation amongst adolescents who remained in China under the care of other relatives, particularly amongst boys. However, although some studies suggest that 'left behind' children are at increased risk of developing psychological problems, as in studies of the wellbeing of left behind children in China (Cheng and Sun, 2014), Ghana, Nigeria and Angola (Mazuccato et al., 2014), others suggest that this is not necessarily the case (Parrenas, 2005). Likewise, although there is evidence that 'left behind' parents have an increased tendency to become depressed in later life, other studies refute these findings (Abas and Prince, 2015; Abas et al., 2009). These findings attest to the homogeneity of migrant experiences and the importance of understanding the factors that contribute to resilience as well as risk.

Dementia

The numbers of older immigrants in the UK are rising, as reflected in the ageing of immigrants who arrived after the Second World War. Despite this, relatively few studies consider whether migration increases the risk of developing dementia and depression, and those that do tend to be small and lack concurrent controls. This is an unfortunate omission: factors such as socio-economic deprivation and uncertainty surrounding immigrant status and old age mean many migrants are particularly vulnerable. There have been some attempts to look at the links between ethnicity and age-ing: however, ethnicity cannot be used as a proxy for migration. Moreover, these studies fail to differentiate between migration status, ethnicity and racialized categories.

Even if one has never moved country it can be extremely difficult deal-ing with the reality that you or a loved one are becoming increasingly confused, attempting to cover up lapses in memory and undergoing the changes in personality that are indicative of dementia. Depending on the form of dementia, many people retain some of their abilities and feel an emotional connection to others and their environment, even when the condition is fairly advanced. Nonetheless, they and people with whom they are most connected will be faced with multiple and progressive experiences of loss and, in the case of the affected person, with a loss of confidence, self-esteem, independence and autonomy, of social roles and relationships, the ability to continue with hobbies and the skills of daily living such as cooking and driving.

However, this is more complicated when one has moved as the envi-ronment in which one lives is unfamiliar. Social care is critically important in the care of dementia (Henwood and ellis, 2015). Because long-term memory tends to deteriorate more slowly than short-term, talking about the past can help in holding on to who one is and has been. However, unless one is connected with people from one's country of origin, this is not feasible for migrants.

It is difficult to access appropriate care when the individual and their loved one/carer have little understanding of how the health services oper-ate and the resources available to them and their family. It can also be more difficult to recognize dementia as a certain level of confusion could be discounted as a response to the challenges of transitioning from one country and society to another. For medical professionals, dementia is more difficult to diagnose when the person is isolated and no one has any understanding of how they had lived their lives before.

As reflected in discussing the links between migration and other forms of discrimination, it is important to take account of the inter-section with racism and other forms of discrimination. For example, a higher percentage of older as well as younger people from Afro-Caribbean countries develop dementia than the host white population of the UK (Adelman et al., 2011). However, cultural factors appear to have a significant effect on experiences of dementia as well: particular religious beliefs and cultural practices (including practices related to personal care, food and beliefs about social support and family respon-sibility to the elderly) can affect the course of the condition by offering some protection against the more distressing consequences of losing one's memory and, in the case of carers, of witnessing the person one loves being 'chipped' away by dementia (Iliffe and Manthorpe, 2004; Manley and Mayeax, 2004). Language is also important: for example, the likelihood of recognizing symptoms as indicators of dementia is reduced where there is no concept or word to denote dementia, as with many South Asian languages (Azam, 2007).

Reports presented to a recent All-Party Parliamentary Group on Dementia (2013) found evidence of good practice in many areas. However, in some areas health care professionals working with dementia were found to lack cultural sensitivity and were experienced as hostile and racist, limiting people's readiness to seek the care they needed. Other studies indicate that within black and minority ethnic communities, people's understanding and knowledge about Alzheimer's, other forms of dementia and available services is limited. Although certain cultural groups (for example, the Chinese) tend to be more accepting and view dementia as a normal consequence of ageing, the stigma associated with other cultural groups is far higher than is currently the case for the rest of the UK population (Moriarty, Sharif and Robinson, 2011). There is also evidence to suggest that some people do not seek additional support because they feel pressurized by the local community to shoulder responsibility for caring for people with dementia on their own, particularly where the culture places emphasis on the family's responsibility to care for their own (Lievesley, 2010; Rauf, 2011). Since these are modifiable risk factors, preventative work is vital to reduce the burden of dementia amongst these communities.

In many areas voluntary sector organizations provide culturally appropriate support to older people. As many people working for these organizations are from the same cultural groups as the people with whom they are working, they are likely to have insider experience of their own or their parents' migration as well. However, they often lack formal training in providing dementia care. Consequently shared learning between specialist and voluntary services could go a long way towards improving services for people with dementia from black and minority ethnic groups, including immigrants.

Refugees and asylum seekers

People become refugees and asylum seekers because they are forced (directly or indirectly) to leave and seek refuge in another geographic locality as a result of political and/or military actions. In and of itself, becoming a refugee is not a psychological phenomenon: it is a socio-political and legal phenomenon which can have significant implications for psychological and in many cases physical health (Papadopoulos, 2007). Refugees face many of the health challenges discussed above. However, they also face challenges specific to their experiences as a refugee. The dislocation involved in being forced to flee persecution, parting from family, friends and homeland, and moving to what is hoped to be a safer place means their needs may range from the basics of food and shelter to the need for love, a sense of belonging and self-esteem, impacting on physical as well as emotional wellbeing (Papadopoulos, 2007; Papadopoulos et al., 2004).

Refugees are also vulnerable to health risks which arise from the stuttering, informal and in many cases dangerous nature of their journey, including travelling in overcrowded, unsafe vehicles and exposure to extremes of temperature (Kelly, Morrell and Sriskandarajah, 2005). Many find themselves stuck in countries which are not their final destination, where they enter some form of limbo, prevented from continuing, desperate to avoid being sent back and living in difficult, often unsafe circumstances where desperation can give rise to aggression as is currently the case in the camps of Calais and Northern Greece, where the rates of violence towards women and children, and inter-ethnic violence, are high.

The challenges are even greater when leaving has to be kept secret and a third party is paid to assist in the process, where residency is illegal and migrants are at risk of being exposed and abused by employers. Women are particularly vulnerable as they are open to sexual exploitation and may be pressurized to pay in sexual 'favours' (Carballo and Mboup, 2005; Zimmerman et al., 2006).

Factors such as economic deprivation and political conflict mean refugees are unlikely to have received good or any health care in their country of origin, particularly where health care provision is poor or has collapsed. In areas with a high prevalence of infectious diseases, political and social unrest tends to disrupt immunization, treatment programmes and nutritional health, increasing the likelihood of developing anaemia and rickets (Jayaweera, 2014). Political unrest and access to less developed health care can mean chronic diseases like diabetes, hypertension and dental problems have not been diagnosed or treated before (Burnett, 2002; Pottie et al., 2011). In addition, people caught up in armed conflict and/or survivors of torture who have experienced significant injuries, including the loss of a limb, are unlikely to have received appropriate care and are therefore more disabled than might have been the case (Williams and Van der Merwe, 2013).

As discussed in relation to other migrants, many refugees arrive in relatively good physical health. However, difficulty in accessing appropriate and timely health care, confusion about entitlement to health care services, problems in registering and accessing primary and community health care services and obstacles related to language barriers can mean their health deteriorates quite rapidly. For example, research suggests that the uptake of services for sexually transmitted diseases, antenatal care and pregnancy outcomes amongst refugees and asylum seekers is lower than the rest of the population, which may reflect barriers to accessing these services by women (Bragg, 2013; Gaudion, McLeish and Homeyard, 2006; Lewis, 2011). Although there is a lack of prevalence data, the same is true of services for women affected by FGM and domestic violence (Refugee Council, 2015).

There is also evidence that rates of blood pressure problems and strokes amongst refugees are higher than the norm: this finding is understood to be a consequence of traumatic experiences in the past as well as specific difficulties related to their situation in the UK, including language barriers and racism (Connelly, Guy and Rudiger, 2006).

In some cases, family and friends died while trying to escape or during the course of their journey, evoking feelings of 'survivor'[15] guilt that interfere with the possibility of mourning and accepting death. Mourning is particularly difficult when the hazardous nature of one's journey means it was impossible to observe cultural and religious practices one values to mark and honour the deceased and ensure their safe passage into the afterlife (Ben-Ezer, 2006; Englund, 1998). In other cases, the need for secrecy and uncertainty about loved ones' whereabouts means refugees do not know when close family or friends are seriously ill or have died until much later. Even if they hear in time, it may be too risky to contact their family or return to mark their death (Gunaratnam, 2013).

In common with adults, the consequences for refugee children and young people range from extremely beneficial to damaging, as when children move clandestinely with parents, other caretakers or on their own (Chase, 2013), and when parents are too traumatized to engage with their children and children seek affection from strangers with dangerous consequences. Following their arrival, schools can play a significant role in promoting psychosocial adjustment and cognitive growth. They also offer parents the opportunity to engage with other parents which can be so helpful when one is isolated. However, heightened levels of anxiety, hypervigilance and flashbacks related to past traumatic experiences can interfere with the possibility of learning and adapting to a new school environment.

Hardly surprisingly, the rates of psychiatric morbidity and post-traumatic stress disorder (PTSD) of unaccompanied minors are greater than the rates for the rest of the population (Chase, 2013; Hopkins and Hill, 2008). This is likely to relate to the fact that the absence of a parent or another trusted adult means that there is greater risk of being exposed to violence, child trafficking, exploitation, sexual and other forms of abuse, and of being forced into begging, drug dealing or prostitution (Fazel et al., 2011; Huemer, Karnik and Steiner, 2009). Even when the move has been less catastrophic, the stresses of leaving, having to adapt to a new environment, coping with uncertainty alone and living with a foster family who have little understanding of one's culture and what one has been through can mean children and young people experience a pervasive sense of anxiety, powerlessness and frustration, and as such engage in risky behaviour such as skipping school, drug taking and joining up with older disenfranchised youth.

Asylum seekers are a relatively small percentage of migrants in the UK. However, the loss of family and friends, social status, choice and control and the isolation, uncertainty and housing difficulties the majority face mean they are particularly vulnerable. A considerable proportion live on benefits below poverty level. Consequently, many of the problems they experience overlap with those of other deprived or marginalized low-income groups. People who have been through refugee camps will have been exposed to communicable disease, poor nutrition and sanitation, and abuse. Some spend time awaiting a decision about their status in detention camps where it becomes 'acceptable' to resolve conflicts through violence and prioritize the positions of men over those of women and children, triggering feelings related to prior experiences. Undocumented migrants, including those who are trafficked, are particularly vulnerable given their dependency on the trafficker. Moreover, although women trafficked to work in a sex industry are at risk of developing health problems related to their work as well as abuse by those who control them, they tend to avoid reporting this for fear of being deported.

Living with the consequences of violence

40 year-old Akia came to a drop-in centre for asylum seekers at a time when he was reapplying to be accepted as an asylum seeker. Although he had arrived in the UK 10 years before, uncertainty about his right to remain, disturbing flashbacks from the past and a range of physical symptoms (including stomach pain and excessive sweating) meant that his life remained dominated by feelings of anxiety, grief and anger, feelings that related to experiences in his home country, Uganda, and experiences subsequent to arriving in the UK. What Akia found even more painful was that there were times he felt overwhelmed with rage and hit out without realizing so tried to distance himself from his 3- and 5-year-old UK-born children. Although this was aimed at protecting his children from feelings he found difficult to control, they thought their daddy would not play with them because they had done something wrong.

As reflected in Akia's case, studies of the Holocaust, survivors of other forms of genocide and political conflict indicate that being forced to flee under traumatic circumstances does not only affect the individual but can have a profound effect on interactions with the next generation (Braga, Mello and Fiks, 2012; Derluyn and Brockaet, 2008).

Experiences of torture and political violence mean that it is not unusual for people to experience increased levels of physical pain, symptoms of PTSD, depression and a pervasive sense of anxiety (Craig, 2007; Feldman, 2006; Johnson and Thompson, 2008; Nutkiewicz, 2007; Silove et al., 2002). Although counselling can be helpful, amongst certain cultural groups the stigma associated with mental illness means there is a virtual taboo against expressing emotional distress or accessing help; moreover, in many languages (for example, Somali) there is no word for 'counselling'.

Throughout the globe, sexual violence has long been used as a weapon of war. It is widely recognized that refugee women are more likely to have experienced violence than any other population of women (Johnson, 2006); with limited opportunities to seek protection in their own countries and restrictions to international travel, many survivors of sexual violence are forced to risk the possibility of further sexual violence in their quest to seek safety, as reflected in accounts of women who have been raped and forced to 'exchange' sex for safe passage to the UK (Kelly and Spencer, 2006; Refugee Council, 2015).

When survivors of sexual violence do seek help, they are not always able to access female interpreters. Moreover, although the UK criminal courts recognize that the trauma of rape can cause feelings of shame and guilt, on arrival an asylum seeker is immediately obliged to tell a stranger (a representative of the UK Border Agency) of any violence that might substantiate her claim to asylum to avoid being detained.

As might be expected, there is a strong link between exposure to conflict-related violence, sexual violence, and sexual and reproductive health. For example, a recent study of Syrian women who fled to Lebanon found evidence of poor reproductive health, including delayed entry to antenatal care, pregnancy and delivery complications and poor birth outcomes (Masterson et al., 2014). Although 30% of the respondents said they had experienced violence and abuse, over 64% failed to seek medical care subsequent to this experience, suggesting the actual number exposed to violence and abuse was far greater. The majority attributed their experience of violence to the armed forces. However, extensive evidence of an increased prevalence in intimate partner violence in situations of political and military conflict suggests that some of the violence is likely to have taken place at home (Clark et al., 2010; Saile et al., 2013).

Older refugees

Until recently, most mainstream policies and research paid little attention to the distinct challenges of refugee and asylum seeking women (Coombes, Hutton and Lukes, 2006). The first comprehensive overview of refugee women's experience was carried out in 2002 (Dumper, 2002) and strategic guidance for supporting refugee women was developed by the Refugee Council in 2005 (Dumper, 2005), neither of which included a focus on older women. Likewise, very little attention has been paid to the distinct positions of older women refugees. This is unfortunate as an increased percentage of older refugees are women. Moreover, although women from cultures where they are not permitted to go out without a chaperone are at risk of becoming isolated, regardless of their age, the increased rates of physical frailty and reduced mobility experienced in later life means this is more likely when women are older. The mobility of older women is restricted further by the fact that despite some shifts in gendered assumptions, caring for vulnerable family members continues to be seen as women's work.

This is particularly problematic as social isolation tends to have negative consequences for emotional wellbeing, increasing the likelihood of mental health problems like depression, stress, anxiety, and a lack of confidence. Moreover, there is growing evidence of a strong link between social isolation and physical ill health. For example, in a large-scale study of women with breast cancer, those who were socially isolated were five times more likely to die of the disease than people who were more connected with family and friends (Price et al., 2001). People who are socially isolated are more likely to develop changes in their immune system, leading to a condition called chronic inflammation: although short-term inflammation is necessary to heal after a cut or an infection, if this persists, the likelihood of developing cardiovascular disease and cancer increases. Similarly, exposure to psychosocial stressors tends to elicit increases in negative affect and blood pressure (BP). Ruminating about a stressor after the crisis is over is associated with delayed recovery (Cacioppo et al., 2006; Hawkley et al., 2010; Valtorta and Hanratty, 2012). Given that older age is associated with greater BP reactivity to psychosocial stressors, rumination (which is more likely when one is lonely) may be more detrimental to the recovery of older adults than younger adults (Robinette and Charles, 2014). People who are socially isolated are also more prone to wake up during the night, resulting in less restorative sleep and daytime fatigue. Although these issues are relevant to all refugees, as older adults tend to be more socially isolated, they are likely to be particularly vulnerable to these risks. An added problem is that although many non-statutory refugee organizations and bicultural advocates can and do play a part in assisting older refugees in registering with a GP, older refugees tend to find it particularly difficult to access appropriate care (Connelly, Guy and Njike, 2005).

There is evidence to suggest that the experiences and needs of older people who left their country of origin when they were young are very different to that of people who moved when they were older. However the differences are not necessarily that great. Even if one moved some time before, the losses associated with growing older can re-evoke experiences of loss and trauma related to the past (Connolly, Guy and Rudiger, 2006). It is also important to bear in mind that the experiences of particular cultural groups tend to be different, depending on such factors as the way in which that group is viewed in the UK, access to people who are from the same country, and the extent to which political conflict affects the possibility of transnational communication and travel. In some cases, it is difficult to draw a clear boundary between migrants who are and are not refugees: the Tamils' long history of persecution in Sri Lanka means that people who came as migrants some time back may have had similar experiences to more recent refugees.

Resilience

It is commonly assumed that people who are resilient experience few or no negative emotions displaying optimism in all situations. This is not the case: resilience relates to the ability to balance negative emotions with positive ones, to navigate one's way through crises and utilize effective methods of coping. Although individual characteristics are important experiences of resilience are bound up with relationships with others. Indeed, resilience is best understood as a process rather than a trait, and can be developed in virtually anyone (Rutter, 2012). Indeed, despite the enormous difficulties with which refugees are confronted, individual resilience, subjective experience, access to social support and opportunities to experience agency inform responses to potentially traumatizing events (Alayarian, 2015; Pat-Horenczyk et al., 2009). Where people are protected from significant harm, are able to receive appropriate humanitarian assistance and housing and find appropriate employment the transition may be less problematic. For example, in a study of long-settled refugees from the former Yugoslavia living in Germany, Italy and the UK, the prevalence of mental disorder was informed by the level of trauma to which people had been exposed socio-economic status, education and post-migration circumstances played a significant role in alleviating stressors associated with their experience as refugees (Bogic et al., 2012). Similarly, over a third of Somali refugees living in London were identified as experiencing or having experienced a mental disorder, in many cases PTSD. However, there was a lower prevalence of PTSD amongst those who did not use khat[16] and were in employment or education (Bhui et al., 2006).

Likewise, Orton et al. (2012) found many HIV-positive asylum seekers whose residency in the UK was undetermined were enormously resourceful in dealing with the challenges they faced despite living in an unfamiliar environment with far less access to taken-for-granted social support, where feelings of isolation were exacerbated by stigmatizing attitudes to HIV, where they are trapped in the asylum system and reliant on HIV treatment to stay alive: this resourceful behaviour included staying busy and drawing on personal faith and the support of HIV care providers and voluntary organizations. As this study suggests, having survived enormous hardship, many people are extremely resilient and manage with minimal or no additional help: indeed, despite or possibly because of the pain, disorientation, disruption and loss, traumatic experiences can lead to re-evaluating priorities, a change in lifestyle and increased resilience (Alayarian, 2015).

Although many refugee children remain scarred by the experience, this is not always the case: many children, including unaccompanied minors, experience great pride and increased agency from helping to support their families by seeking a better life abroad (Thomas and Gideon, 2013). Children's experiences are informed by the responses of the people with whom they are most connected: memories and the consequences of violent events are embedded in social experiences (Panter-Brick et al., 2015). This may explain why, even though former child soldiers have an increased risk of developing symptoms of post-traumatic stress, depression, aggression and clinically significant behavioural and emotional problems (Duarte, 2008), in a study of returnee child soldiers who had been caught up with war in Uganda, those who had lower exposure to domestic violence, whose families were in a better socio-economic position, who perceived spiritual support and experienced less guilt and desire to seek revenge were more resilient, attesting to the importance of understanding the factors contributing to resilience (Klasen et al., 2010).

Recommendations for practice

In 2004, the WHO, International Organization for Migration (IOM), Standing Committee of the Hospitals of the EU (HOPE) and Migrants Rights International endorsed 'The Amsterdam Declaration', aimed at ensuring hospitals are more responsive to ethnic, cultural, linguistic and other social differences of patients as well as staff. Similar priorities were outlined in the Resolution on Migrant Health by the WHO in 2008 and a subsequent consultation on its implementation (WHO, 2010).

The NHS is well placed to provide migrant-sensitive health services. However, despite many examples of good practice, there is considerable variability in access and the extent to which services meet the needs of the people concerned. Consequently more proactive steps are required:

- **Monitoring migrant health:** The NHS needs to record additional information in routine data collection in order to develop a better understanding of migrant health and health care, including migration status, employment (or some other proxy for socio-economic status), country of birth, duration in the UK and access to health care. Likewise, additional research is needed to establish the particular health needs of different migrant groups.

- **Policy and legal framework:** In order to address the confusion and inconsistency in how policies are applied and enhance collaboration between the various services, there needs to be national focal point for migrant health within the Department of Health or Public Health England which is mirrored at a local level in order to coordinate migrant health responses.

- **Improving migrant-sensitive health care:** Greater emphasis needs to be placed on researching and sharing best practice amongst practitioners as well as the commissioners of health services. There needs to be greater investment in training aimed at increasing health care professionals' awareness of the experiences of migrants, trauma, racism and other forms of discrimination, the use of interpreters, and health disparities and inequalities (including gender-related inequities) to ensure services are culturally sensitive. Trainings are also needed in addressing the particular needs of refugees and asylum seekers, and to ensure all front line health professionals have an accurate understanding of entitlements to health care.

- **Community engagement, clarification of needs and resource allocation:** Greater emphasis needs to be placed on establishing a clearer understanding of the needs of particular migrant and ethnic groups. This is likely to require changes in communication, organizational routines and allocation of resources, including greater engagement with stakeholders (including patients, families and representatives of local community organizations) and advocacy groups knowledgeable about migrant and minority ethnic group issues, particularly where there is distrust of the medical system.[17]

However, it is important to acknowledge that in a country with limited resources for distribution (free health care) and an increasingly ageing population, where views range between xenophobia and a strong identification with and sympathy for migrants, questions about the health care of immigrants touch on complex political as well as human rights concerns.

3

INDIVIDUAL AND FAMILY EXPERIENCES OF ILLNESS AND DEATH

The diagnosis of a life-limiting illness tends to have a profound effect on one's experience of self and relationship with others (Bury, 1982). Finding out one has a life-limiting condition (or that one's child or another loved one is seriously ill, significantly impaired and/or may die) can give rise to a range of powerful emotions including shock, anger, anxiety and fear: fear of the pain and other symptoms associated with the disease, of losing control, becoming increasingly dependent, intolerant, driving one's partner (or another loved one) away, and of dying. Being ill confronts one with changes in experiences of embodiment, with the confusion of becoming someone different even though one is still the same person (Swoboda, 2006). This sense of disruption is not only relevant to situations of actual illness: many 'previvors' report a similar sense of disruption on being told they have a genetic predisposition to developing life-limiting conditions, as for example when blood tests reveal mutations to the BRCA 1 or 2 gene, signifying one has hereditary breast-ovarian cancer syndrome (Hamilton, Moyer and Lobel, 2009).

Some people respond by drawing on beliefs and memories that help to maintain a sense of continuity between the past, present and future. In other cases, illness becomes a 'turning point' (Le Shan, 1989), opening up the possibility of changes that lead to a more comfortable and fulfilling experience of self and relationship with others. However, many find this is not possible: the diagnosis, manifestations of the condition and consequences of the treatment mean it is impossible to hold on to other aspects of identity, giving rise to a sense of estrangement and diminishment of who one is (Gagnon, 2010). Even where one's health improves, the challenges individuals and family face may mean life continues to be consumed by loss and despair, whereby certain aspects of experience such as shame, dependency, anger and resentment crowd out the possibility of everything else with questions of 'Why me?', 'Why now?' and 'Why this condition?' and an awareness of the gap between who one was, is now and still longs to be (Rolland, 1994; Roose and Neimeyer, 2007; Russell, White and White, 2006).

Even where people appear to adjust with relatively little difficulty, illness tends to confront individuals and their families with challenges that are unknown to others, including the challenges of living with ongoing uncertainties; of having to rework personal and family boundaries, roles and responsibilities; negotiating the demands of the illness with other family demands; balancing acceptance with some sense of hope; and holding on to an identity that is not fully consumed by illness. As reflected below, factors influencing the ways in which individuals and families respond include current and prior experiences of loss and trauma, gender, age, positions in the life cycle, socio-economics and the discourses that dominate the society in which one lives.

Loss

Despite the fact that illness can become an opportunity for introducing beneficial changes, all experiences of illness are accompanied by some sense of loss and disarray. Experiences of loss may relate to the physical consequences of the condition; including symptoms of chronic pain, nausea, dizziness, fatigue and numbness. However, it can be just as (or even more) difficult dealing with the emotional consequences; for example, living with ongoing uncertainty and situations where anxiety, exhaustion, pain and regret result in lapses in behaviour and outbursts of emotion that shatter the image one has of oneself, and who one aspires to be. Likewise, it can be extremely difficult dealing with the relational consequences: indeed, the pain of watching a loved one suffer and difficulties in meeting one's own and others' expectations of being together 'in sickness and in health' mean it may be impossible to disentangle experiences of 'self-loss' from 'other-loss' (Weingarten, 2013).

Attachment theory has had a profound effect on current understandings of loss. Drawing on studies of infants separated from parents, Bowlby (1969/1999) proposed that infants need to be close to their main caretaker for reasons other than food and comfort: to feel secure, and that their ability to explore the world depends on the development of a secure base. By drawing attention to the damaging consequences of separation in early life, Bowlby's work led to substantial changes in the care of children in hospital.

Subsequent studies have found that where there is a history of secure attachment we are more able to negotiate the losses encountered later. In contrast, where attachment has been less secure, we tend to be more vulnerable to the potentially destructive consequences of subsequent loss, including illness, disability, death and migration (Holmes, 2001). Moreover, even where there is a history of secure attachment, particular experiences can mean that it is more difficult to deal with subsequent loss, as for example when diagnosed with a condition that led to the death of one's parent or another close relative (Rolland, 1994). Likewise, unresolved grief in response to a miscarriage or stillbirth can affect prenatal attachment in subsequent pregnancies (Forray et al., 2014; O'Leary, 2004).

Byng-Hall (1995) drew on attachment theory in outlining how experiences of family inform the internalized models ('family scripts') we draw on in responding to and making sense of our lives. These experiences can leave us with the desire to give our children the sort of care we were able to receive when young (a 'replicative script'), or the opposite: to protect our children from facing similar experiences (a 'corrective script'). Sadly this is not always possible. Situations of heightened emotion can result in responding in a way that mirrors the internalized model of parenting we have wanted to avoid, giving rise to actions that feel like a betrayal of ourselves as well as our children. This is reflected in situations where parents who have worked hard to ensure that, unlike themselves, their children are not brought up in a hostile environment find themselves acting aggressively or withdrawing when they feel depleted as a result of chemotherapy or pain.

Kubler-Ross (1970) proposed that we go through a series of stages in coming to terms with loss including *denial* (a conscious or unconscious refusal to accept the facts, information and reality of the situation), *anger* (anger at ourselves and/or others), *bargaining* (with whatever spiritual source we believe in), *depression* (a preparatory form of grieving accompanied by sadness, regret, fear and feelings of uncertainty) and *acceptance* (evidenced by greater emotional detachment and objectivity), suggesting that responses which are adaptive at a certain stage may be problematic at another. For example, although denial can be helpful in managing the confusion that often sets in following the diagnosis of a life-limiting condition, if continued, denial can isolate family members at a time when there is so much to gain 'from the intimacy of knowing that one knows what the other knows, even if what one knows is not what one would ever want to know' (Weingarten, 2013, p. 98).

However, responses to loss are far more varied than Kubler-Ross suggests: for example, following the diagnosis of a life-limiting illness, some of us try to deny what is happening, some prepare for the worst, and others oscillate between periods of intense grief and being able to get on with other aspects of life. Coming to terms with loss is more complicated when a partner's frailty means one assumes responsibility for aspects of family life that had previously lain in the domain of the other, leading to an increased sense of agency and self-esteem.

Similarly, coming to terms with loss is more complicated in relation to 'disenfranchised loss', when the loss 'cannot be openly acknowledged, publicly mourned, or socially supported' (Doka, 1999, p. 37), as with the suicide of a loved one or a stigmatized condition that can be transmitted sexually, like HIV/AIDS. It is also more complicated when the status of the condition as a legitimate illness is questioned and one has to fight to be seen as a 'truth teller', as is currently the case with conditions like chronic fatigue syndrome, fibromyalgia and what are regarded as 'medically unexplained symptoms' (MUS), symptoms for which no organic cause can be found (Frank, 1995; Swoboda, 2006). It is also more complicated when the loss is ambiguous; for example, when someone is physically present but emotionally absent, as where someone looks the same but their condition results in significant cognitive deficit:

Marian experienced extensive brain damage as a result of a motor accident. Although she had been in a coma for more than five years, her husband and adolescent children continued to live in limbo. In working with this family, rather than helping them to mourn and achieve some form of closure, it was more important to focus on the losses they were facing, and what needed to change before they felt ready to move on with their lives.

In situations like these, regarding the affected person as a real presence with an identity that extends beyond disease and deficit can help in maintaining some sense of continuity. As with Marian's family, difficulties tend to arise if this means failing to adjust to the person's altered level of functioning (Boss and Carnes, 2012). This is particularly complicated when there are times when the affected person appears to be rational and coherent and others when they act inappropriately:

Anita understood that her husband Sam's behaviour towards her was a consequence of early onset dementia. However, there were times when she became overwhelmed with anger and acted in ways she regretted later including swearing and pushing him fairly aggressively. Her anger was fuelled by the fact that although Sam had several affairs over the course of their married life, she found herself compromising her working life in order to look after him. It was only when she was able to come to terms with the loss of the life she had hoped for, her own motivation in staying with him, and shift from viewing her role from that of a wife to a carer, that it was possible to find a better balance between her new role and prioritizing her own needs (which included recruiting the services of a professional carer).

Mourning is also more complicated when one is told a loved one has died but one cannot be sure, as is the experience of refugees who hear that the family they left behind were killed but there is no proof of this. For example, following the war in Kosovo, many families were faced with coming to terms with the absence and probable death of loved ones:

> Resmira was told her husband was dead by someone who saw him being killed and buried in a mass grave in Serbia. However, because his body was never returned she found it impossible letting go of the hope that he had escaped and would return home one day. Although she found this sustaining, it was confusing for her children who heard from others that their father was dead. Faced with conflicting realities they were forced to make sense of the death of their father without her help.

Confronted with situations of loss and uncertainty we cannot understand, it is not uncommon to blame ourselves, project what we fear or hate onto someone else, or an entirely different situation (Benjamin, 1998; Klein, 1975). In situations of illness, this may involve distancing ourselves from our own bodies, viewing the body as an unreliable but indispensible vehicle rather than integral to our identity: this is reflected in the tendency to talk about the affected body part in a depersonalized way, as in 'the breast', and 'the skin' rather than using the more personal 'my'. Blaming others limits the possibility of understanding the consequences of our actions. In contrast, becoming consumed with self-blame can result in distancing ourselves from the person who embodies feelings of guilt (for example, one's ill child) and/or compensating by failing to provide realistic limit setting. For example, when one parent is terminally ill or has died it is not unusual for the other parent to accept behaviour they would have previously regarded as inappropriate in order to avoid conflict and keep the peace: Another response is to blame the health care system.

> Stella was reluctant to discipline her daughter when she became increasingly aggressive after her father died, which included hitting her mother. The combination of anger, shame, confusion and the desire to avoid alienating her daughter meant that Stella held back on telling anyone or reprimanding her. However, failure to set realistic boundaries resulted in an escalation of hostility, limiting the possibility of her daughter experiencing the emotional containment she needed from her mother.

The tendency to blame (or feel blamed) is more likely when the condition when the condition evokes considerable fear: Castro and Farmer (2005) found that the stigma associated with HIV/AIDs in Haiti reduced, and uptake of testing increased, following the introduction of anti-retroviral medication which meant that HIV/AIDS was not necessarily a death sentence. Blame is also more likely where the condition is poorly understood, hereditary or where deterioration in health could relate to a lifestyle choice, for example with conditions where there is an established link with smoking (as with lung cancer and certain respiratory conditions), alcohol abuse (cirrhosis) and where stress is seen as a major contributor (as with many heart and gastric conditions).

I would not want to dispute the notion that lifestyle and dietary factors can affect one's health. However, placing full responsibility on the affected person ignores the multi-factorial nature of the aetiology of most conditions, impacting on the uptake of preventative services and treatment: research focused on people with heart disease suggests that some delay seeking medical care because they believe they will be criticized for failing to take better care of their health (Richards, Reid and Watt, 2003). When the ill person is a child, parents are more likely to be held accountable; however, although parents do carry considerable responsibility for their children, regarding parents as fully responsible ignores the role of the environment and interactions with other adults and peers (Weingarten, 1994).

Trauma

Some experiences of illness are not only deeply distressing, but traumatic, as for example when one is unable to breathe or loses control of one's bowels in a public setting, and, in the case of parents, when one cannot protect a newborn baby or older children from multiple invasive procedures, including repeated blood tests and life-saving medication with potentially problematic side effects.

A wide body of studies based in the fields of neurobiology, endocrinology, immunology and psychology indicate that faced with a perceived harmful event we tend to react with a general discharge of the sympathetic nervous system which primes us to fight or flee or, if neither is possible, freeze: the capacity to think becomes paralysed in trying to reduce the unmanageable quantities of excitation that pour through the protective shield with which we tend to surround ourselves (Karr-Morse, 2012). This is particularly likely when age, size or other vulnerabilities mean one is unable to move or it would be dangerous to do so. The memory of the trauma appears to be held in a specific memory network and is therefore not integrated into one's long-term memory stores (Joseph, Williams and Yule, 1997). However, it can resurface in the form of an unintended re-experiencing of symptoms and recall of the traumatic event. An added complication is that lack of understanding about the physiological responses (for example, the adrenalin rush and increased heart rate) that accompany flashbacks adds to the terror these situations evoke (Ehlers, Hackman and Michael, 2004).

The magnitude of the event informs the likelihood of developing symptoms of post-traumatic stress disorder (PTSD). Responses are also informed by peri-traumatic factors (including the exact nature of the immediate threat, cognitions, fear and dissociation at the time of the event), appraisal processes, what happens after the event (including the responses of others), whether one has had opportunities to discharge the energy that builds up, social support, personality and the emotions driving the ongoing appraisal of the event (Hunter et al., 2015).

In a recent review of the research and clinical literature, Bienvenue and Neufeld (2011) concluded that PTSD was far more common amongst survivors of critical conditions than is assumed. For example, symptoms of PTSD have been identified amongst people who have been diagnosed and treated for various forms of cancer (Kangas, Henry and Bryant, 2002) and subarachnoid haemorrhage (Powell, Kitchen and Heslin, 2002). Several studies have found a link between PTSD, the development of certain conditions and poorer health outcomes (Doerfler, Paraskos and Piniarski, 2005). Similarly, pre-trauma experiences and premorbid characteristics including a previous life of adversity and/or history of substance abuse (Klutz et al., 1994), previous mental health difficulties (Czarnoka and Slade, 2000), individual characteristics such as a repressive coping style and a tendency for negative affect (Brydon et al., 2009) increase the likelihood of developing PTSD in response to illness. In addition, threats in the present can trigger responses that relate to the past, resulting in intrusive emotions, sensory phenomena, autonomic arousal and physical reactions (Fisher, 2014):

> While having blood tests prior to a hip replacement, Anna started to shake and sweat, became nauseous and left the hospital as soon as she could. When asked if she had experienced these symptoms before, Anna realized they were markedly similar to the symptoms she experienced following breast surgery five years previously when the development of septicaemia resulted in her becoming confused, feeling unable to eat, and bringing up a mixture of food and blood. Consequently, although it was important to help Anna make sense of her experience at a verbal and emotional level, it was also important to work towards re-regulating her physiological response to this memory, which included exploring where these feelings were located in the body (in this case in her chest).

It was previously believed that young children were far more resilient than adults when faced with potentially traumatic events, including persistent stress and fear. However, current research and clinical experience suggests that depending on the particular circumstances (including the responses of parents and other caretakers), children are at greater risk of becoming traumatized (Karr-Morse, 2012; Levine and Kline, 2007). Whilst research in this area is limited, there is also evidence to suggest that adverse experiences in childhood can lead to enduring abnormalities in stress-sensitive biological systems (through protracted experiences of raised levels of cortisol and/or the erosion of telomere), increasing the risk of developing a number of adult health conditions (Danese et al., 2009).

Reflecting on traumatic experiences can help one make sense of these experiences. However, it is often best to wait until the person feels safe enough to do so (Fisher, 2014), and, as indicated above, work towards re-regulating the physiological responses that exposure to potentially traumatic situations evokes, for example through relaxation techniques, eye movement desensitization and somatic experiencing (Levine and Kline, 2007; Shapiro and Laliotis, 2010).

The possibility of the past affecting responses to the present is particularly important to bear in mind when one knows or suspects there has been physical or sexual abuse (Herman, 1997); for example, having to lie still while a drip is inserted can re-evoke feelings related to past experiences of being unable to escape while something is inserted into one's body. Likewise, for people who have been incarcerated or tortured, feeling helpless and seeing one's body become increasingly emaciated can trigger flashbacks of previous experiences of powerlessness and emaciation, giving rise to medically unexplained pain (Nutkiewicz, 2007). An added complication is that where aspects of the illness or treatment trigger memories that have been blocked out, and/or feelings of shame and guilt have meant these experiences were kept secret, it is difficult for one's partner, children and friends to know what is wanted and needed.

Nature of actual condition and treatment

As discussed earlier, experiences of illness are informed by a wide range of factors, including cultural beliefs, practices, the discourses dominating the socio-political context in which one lives, habitual responses to challenging situations and prior trauma. However, they are also informed by the actual condition, including the particular nature of the onset, course, prognosis, level of incapacitation and treatment (Rolland, 1994).

For example, where the onset and course is gradual, as is often the case with multiple sclerosis, Duchenne muscular dystrophy and various forms of dementia, families are usually able to mobilize in an unhurried way. However, because gradual changes are less obvious, responses to the condition may be complicated by feelings of regret, guilt and frustration about the delay in diagnosis, particularly where confusion about changes in behaviour meant relationships had become increasingly fraught.

Where the onset is more acute, as with a stroke, certain aspects of readjustment, problem solving and emotional demands are likely to be similar. However, families need to mobilize more rapidly and whilst the initial crisis is likely to require considerable adjustment, once the condition has stabilized the family is faced with altering their roles to take account of the change in the affected person's functioning.

Where the course is more progressive, the individual and families have to adapt to new changes repeatedly. In contrast, where the condition is episodic or relapsing, periods of good health enable some activities and rituals to be maintained or restored. Because transitions tend to require a reworking of how we see ourselves and relate to others, it is not unusual for tensions to escalate at times of change (Carter and McGoldrick, 1999).

The level of incapacitation can have a profound impact on identity and intimate relationships as well (Mattingly, 1998). For example, in advanced stages of Parkinson's disease, although the affected person may remain cognitively intact, problems in communicating tend to mean it is difficult to know what they are thinking, feeling or trying to say. In many cases it is difficult for the rest of the family to balance helping the affected person retain as much agency as possible with the need to rework their own lives to account for that person's altered functioning. Likewise, in some situations, symptom visibility has a profound effect on the affected person as well as their family and friends:

> Sheila felt able to accept the impact motor neurosis might have on her own life. However, as the condition progressed and her gait became increasingly clumsy, she was devastated by the fact that her daughter was embarrassed about being seen with her.

The actual nature of the treatment can have a significant effect on one's identity and interactions with others as well. Many consequences are short-lived, as with the side effects of a limited course of medication, while others are more long lasting, as when surgery to remove prostate cancer results in ongoing incontinence and impotence. In some cases the treatment challenges taken-for-granted ideas about personal boundaries and parenting, as when parents are required to apply forceful physiotherapy to the chest of children with cystic fibrosis. In other cases, it is difficult to distinguish the physiological from the psychological. For example, acting in a 'grumpy' way after a kidney or bone marrow transplant may relate to the side effects of drugs taken to minimize rejection. However, it may also be a psychological response to a potentially life-changing experience, issues quite unrelated to health, or a combination of all these factors.

Advances in technology are confronting individuals, families and health care professionals with ethical and relational dilemmas that were unknown before (McLamara, 2013). Soon after the death of her mother from breast cancer, Annabelle found out that she carried the BRCA gene. This meant that in addition to coming to terms with the loss of her much-loved mother, Annabelle faced having to decide whether to have a double mastectomy that would increase her chances of remaining disease-free, a bilateral oophorectomy (removal of the ovaries) by the age of 40, and the possibility that any future children would carry the gene as well. An additional complication was that her sisters did not want to be tested; however, if she went ahead with elective surgery, they would become more aware of their own health risks.

Advances in medical technology mean that organ transplants are more feasible: because the chances of a good match are higher when the transplant donor is a close relative, relatives are faced with balancing the benefits of donating a kidney or bone marrow to a child, sibling or partner with concerns about the risks to their own future health. An additional complication is that the success or failure of a transplant can have far-reaching emotional consequences for the individual, potential donor and the rest of the family (Franklin, Crombie and Boudville, 2003; Ummel, Achille and Mekkelholt, 2011):

> For example, when his older and more successful brother James was diagnosed with leukaemia, Leonard, who had left school early and was regarded as a failure by the rest of the family, agreed to donate some of his bone marrow to help him survive. However, although there was a close match in their tissue types, the transplant did not succeed and his brother died. There was nothing Leonard could have done to prevent this, but James's death felt like a confirmation of his position as a failure.

Advances in care also mean that it is more possible to keep people alive with life-supporting equipment than previously. Where the person who is dying is suffering, a decision may be taken to shift from curative to palliative care. However, as reflected in the controversy surrounding Falconer's Assisted Dying Bill (2014), withdrawing or withholding treatment touches on profound relational, ethical, clinical, legal and in many cases religious issues for the person concerned, their families and professionals.

Time frame in terms of the illness and family

At one point it was assumed that responses to medical conditions follow a set series of phases. However, this has shifted with increased recognition of the unpredictability of human responses, co-morbidity and variability in symptom progression. Nonetheless, certain patterns tend to be more common.

At the outset, there is often a period when the individual experiences unusual or ambiguous sensations but does not know how seriously to take them. If these sensations fail to abate or become more severe, the attention of that person and people close to them shifts to focusing more on the body: what were previously seen as sensations come to be seen as symptoms and decisions are taken about how to address this.

Diagnosis is usually the first time the professional, affected person and, particularly with young children and vulnerable adults, another family member meet. Some people prefer to seek medical help and process what they are told on their own before sharing this with others. However, the shock of hearing the diagnosis can affect the ability to process and remember. Consequently, it can be helpful for someone else to attend these consultations as well in order to listen and ask the questions one may not consider at a time of heightened emotional intensity.

Diagnosis tends to affect the boundary we construct between the outside world and ourselves. Although the boundaries we construct vary from family to family and culture to culture, at times of crisis they tend to become more permeable to allow health care professionals to undertake essential forms of assessment and life support. At this stage the affected person faces the challenge of forming an alliance with the medical team, following orders and learning how to deal with their symptoms and the consequences of treatment. In turn, families need to be flexible enough to support that person and the treatment required.

Where a child is hospitalized and there are two parents, one parent (usually, but not always, a mother) tends to assume primary responsibility for the ill child and the other for the rest of the family. The desire to ensure that the ill child receives the best possible care and the needs of other family members are respected means that dividing their attention in this way might be manageable for a short period. However, tensions can arise when this continues for longer as the 'system' focused on survival (mother, child and professionals) excludes the other parent and children: as this is in the interests of maximizing the ill child's survival, acknowledging the discomfort of feeling excluded tends to be difficult (Walker, 1983).

The boundary with the rest of the family, friends and others in the community may need to change as well. Teachers can play a pivotal role in supporting children when they, their parent or a sibling is ill, for example by helping children who have been absent to re-engage with their academic work and renegotiate relationships with peers. In some cases, families need to share aspects of their lives that they had chosen to keep private:

At junior school Stephen had been teased about the fact that his parents, Alice and Mary, were in a same-sex relationship. Consequently, on moving to senior school, they kept this information secret. However, when Alice was diagnosed with an advanced form of ovarian cancer, Stephen's parents decided to be more open with school to ensure their son received the best possible support as Alice's health deteriorated. As a result, Stephen was faced with coming to terms with the fact that his mother was dying at the same time as coming to terms with what the news about his parents' relationship meant to his teacher and school friends.

Following an initial period of assessment, diagnosis and treatment, many conditions enter a more chronic phase, during which relationships with medical professionals are less intense and families begin rebuilding their lives in a way that takes account of disruptions in family roles and altered expectations of the future. Released from the crisis, reality tends to set in, facing families with such dilemmas as how to balance the demands of the illness with other family needs and personal needs for intimacy and autonomy. In some cases, couples are able to 'be there' for one another during crisis phases but find it more difficult when faced with the return to some semblance of 'normality'.

Advances in care can mean that treatment results in cure, at which point the 'survivor' and family are faced with restoring aspects of their lives that were integral to self and family before. Here, too, responses are far from uniform: whilst some people are able to do so with relatively little difficulty, or re-examine the premises on which their lives are based and free themselves to live more fully, for others life remains dominated by loss, alienation and a sense of foreboding (Little et al., 2002). Similarly, where the person's condition deteriorates further, some people seek as much intimacy as possible, while others become more distant or go into overdrive as if trying to deny reality. Nonetheless, what appears to be denial may not be a 'real' denial but unwillingness to acknowledge how one feels at this point in time and in the presence of these particular people (Shotter, 1994).

It is often assumed that older people do not want to talk about death. However, older adults are often less fearful than people who are younger and welcome the opportunity to talk about death (Anderson, 1997). For example, in a study of 200 older adults (with a mean age 70) who were in advanced stages of cancer and in their final few weeks of life, 9.5% denied awareness of both their terminal prognosis and foreshortened life expectancy, 17% were partially aware but the majority (73.5%) were fully aware of their position. As importantly, depression appears to be almost three times greater among terminally ill people who did not acknowledge their prognosis, as compared with those who partially or completely acknowledged their situation (Chochinov et al., 1999). This attests to the importance of engaging with older adults' anticipations of death. Indeed, the person who is dying is often more ready to acknowledge reality than others in the family.

Some thoughts and feelings can seem too frightening or shameful to acknowledge to oneself, let alone others, which is why it is not unusual to slip into and out of denial over the course of the illness or even during a single conversation. However, failing to acknowledge the end is near can isolate loved ones from one another, leading to tensions and regrets that complicate experiences of mourning. Consequently, even if the dying person is no longer able to speak, it can be extremely helpful to encourage them and their loved ones to reach out to one another as a touch, a smile or moment of eye contact can be enormously sustaining to the dying as well as their survivors. However, it is important to recognize that the emphasis Western medical practice places on the person's right to know that their condition is terminal is relatively new. It is also important to recognize that speaking more openly about death is antithetical to people from societies where holding back and speaking in an indirect way reflects a different appreciation of caring for those who are vulnerable (Candib, 2002).

If the dying person held the family together, their death is likely to force the rest of the family to rethink relationships with one another. Where relationships have been fraught, the emotional intensity surrounding anticipations of death can create a different understanding of one another and of the past. In other cases, the years of anger, guilt, regret and blame overshadow the possibilities of reaching a more comfortable resolution before parting.

Freud (1917) proposed that when we love, we incorporate aspects of the loved one into our ego. This may explain why when someone we love dies it can feel as if a part of ourselves has died. At times of grief some people draw strength and solace from institutionalized religion, some from a less traditional and more personal sense of spirituality, while others see spirituality as largely irrelevant to their lives. As discussed in greater detail in Chapter 4, culture can have a profound effect on experiences of grief and mourning: being unable to carry out prescribed religious and cultural rituals one holds dear can interfere with the possibility of mourning. Nonetheless, our lives do not operate according to set cultural religious patterns but 'more or less patterns' that evolve in response to altered circumstances (Krause, 2002). Some people lose whatever faith they had in the face of death. Because our deepest convictions are informed by relationships with the people we are most connected to, one person's crisis of faith can have far-ranging implications for the rest of the family as well (Roehlkepartian et al., 2006; Walsh and McGoldrick, 2004). Consequently, there may be times when the dying and their relatives value the space to reflect on their understanding of spirituality and the possibility of an afterlife.

Positions in the life cycle

Most families move through periods of greater or less closeness as members move through the life cycle. For example, during early child-rearing years, the preoccupation of the family tends to focus inwards. As children reach adolescence, there is usually a shift towards greater engagement with relationships external to the family. This tends to shift once more as parents and other relatives become older and increasingly frail (Combrinck-Graham, 1985).

Experiences of illness involve a similar shift in focus. For example, when someone is seriously ill, the attention of the family tends to focus inwards. Where this inward pull coincides with age-related patterns, there may be less disruption to anticipated family roles. However, there is a greater risk of the family continuing to focus inwards despite subsequent changes in health (and positions in the life cycle). In contrast, where the pull of the illness is at odds with the anticipated life cycle, it can be difficult to balance age-related aspirations with the constraints posed by the illness and treatment regime.

For example, in Western societies, adolescence tends to be a time when young people become increasingly independent and questioning of authority. This is less possible when an adolescent has a life-threatening condition that requires repeated medical appointments, and adherence to a strict regime of treatment (as with diabetes, renal failure and HIV/AIDS), as the young person may need to rely more on parents, and parents are more vigilant in monitoring their health and levels of activity than usual at this age. Many families are able to find ways of managing this dissonance between anticipated and lived experience. However, tensions can arise which mean that even when the young person wants and needs to look to their parents for support, doing so feels uncomfortable or even shameful.

In many Eastern, African and Asian societies, becoming a couple involves moving in with one's parents-in-law or bringing a wife into one's family home. In contrast in Western societies, this tends to be a time when couples establish a greater independence from their family of origin. In both situations most people reach an unstated agreement on the amount of support they want and are prepared to give to one another. However, at times of illness, this usually needs to be extended to maximize the chances of survival and adjust to the shifts in power and dependency that tend to develop when one partner is healthy and the other seriously ill (Altschuler, 2011). The emotional intensity surrounding situations of illness can lead to increased intimacy. However, particularly when the relationship is relatively new and there are financial and other worries, the ill partner may be drawn into a closer relationship with their family of origin, creating tensions that are difficult to acknowledge or address. Moreover, many young adults find it difficult to prioritize their own health over the needs of older members of the family. This is particularly difficult when doing so goes against the grain of personal, family, gendered and cultural understandings of intergenerational care (Chao and Tseng, 2002).

Although many of the challenges older adults face at times of illness are similar to those who are younger, some are different. For example, the shame associated with breaching certain social norms means that it is not unusual to feel ashamed of the loss of control, helplessness and incapacitation associated with many medical conditions, whatever one's age. However, the neurological impairments that cause memory loss and behaviours that would otherwise be seen as breaching social norms are more common in later life, as with Alzheimer's disease and vascular dementia (Curtis and Dixon, 2005; Surbone et al., 2006).

In later life, there is also a greater chance one's partner will have died or is too frail to provide the support that is needed. Consequently, when one partner requires residential care, the healthier partner has to decide whether to join them, live alone or move in with one of their children. An added complication is that where adult children are still responsible for caring for their own children, it can be extremely stressful balancing caring for one's parent and children, as reflected in the terms 'sandwich' or 'pivot' generation (Mooney and Statham, 2002). Where there is more than one adult child, differences in caring responsibilities can evoke feelings that relate to far earlier negotiation of sibling differences (Kramer, Boelk and Auer, 2006). However, it is important to recognize that the current obsession with independence fails to take account of the extent to which long-term mutual dependence is integral to the human condition (Segal, 2013). Caring for a parent in later life, or being cared for by an adult child, can be deeply satisfying, and where relationships have been difficult, can lead to a different appreciation of one another.

There is growing evidence of inequalities in the health and health care provided to older adults compared to those who are younger, as shown, for example, by a recent survey carried out by Oliver, Foot and Humphreys (2014). Although the number of winter deaths in the UK in 2012–2013 increased by 29% compared with the previous winter, most of what are described as 'excess deaths' were people aged 75 and over (Office for National Statistics, 2014). Similarly, some studies have found that a high percentage of older women diagnosed with certain forms of breast cancer ('triple negative') receive less chemotherapy than those who are younger and that, although colorectal cancer is more common amongst older people, the treatment is not as good for those who are younger (Lawler et al.,

2014). An added complication is that older adults are also more likely to suffer in silence, have less understanding of how the health system works and where to go with their complaints. Although the increased frequency of co-morbidities in later life may very well determine the prognosis and overall survival, influencing decisions of treatment, these studies illustrate the importance of paying more attention to the illness experiences and care of the elderly.

Children's experiences of illness

Considerable controversy surrounds the long-term consequences of childhood physical illness. A wide body of research suggests that children who have had a life-limiting illness or whose siblings or parents have been seriously ill show higher levels of emotional and behavioural problems than the norm for short, and in some cases for longer periods of time. This includes becoming hyper-alert to danger, and developing problems in concentrating and memory. Other studies have found it impossible to distinguish these groups of children and/or that they perform better than the norm, attesting to the importance of understanding the factors contributing to risk and resiliency (Cantrell, 2011; Michel et al., 2010; Romer, Barkmann and Thomalla, 2002).

Analysis of the responses to a wide range of adverse situations including illness, divorce and political conflict (Alayarian, 2015; Brom and Kleber, 2009; Pat-Horenczyk et al., 2009), indicate that children are more resilient and less likely to develop long-term problems when they have access to someone who can help them make sense of their experience and hold their needs in mind; when there are opportunities to enhance self-esteem and have their input recognized; when daily routines are as unchanged as possible, they know what to do and who to call in emergencies; and when the family is supportive, optimistic and communicates openly.

In addition, research and clinical experience suggest that children who are ill tend to cope best when the diagnosis is early, the treatment relatively short and successful. Age informs responses to illness as well: the child's age at the time of diagnosis gives some indication of their capacity to separate from parents (and other caretakers) and whether parents had an opportunity to establish confidence in their parenting before the onset of illness. Conditions that involve deficits in social communication and imitation are particularly challenging, impacting on the possibility of developing attachment with one's children, and affecting parental confidence in their capacity to care for their child (Helps and Shepherd, 2014; Solomon, 2012).

When younger children are admitted to hospital and undergo surgery, the protection and containment of adults who are sensitive to, and can meet, their needs is of paramount importance. Without appropriate support, they are unlikely to be able to comprehend or deal with the blinding lights, surgical instruments and drug-induced altered states they are confronted with. Consequently, other than in emergencies it is important to ensure interventions such as injections do not take place when children are terrified and that they do not wake up alone in the recovery room. Likewise, it is important to prepare the child for what will happen by telling the truth without unnecessary details, if possible by meeting the staff concerned, and through play, for example by using toy medical kits or dressing a doll or stuffed animal in a gown to 'play hospital'. As Levine and Kline (2007) suggest, this could involve making up a story with a child who requires a full anaesthetic about an animal who goes to sleep very quickly and wakes up slowly to find their mummy, daddy and/or nurse ready to give them something good to eat.

Age informs children's ability to process what they see and hear, and how much they are likely to be told. Most parents and professionals have an understandable desire to 'filter' what children are told. As mentioned earlier, in some cultures holding back and speaking in an indirect way is seen as more appropriate when people are particularly vulnerable. Although it is important to respect parents' positions, it can be helpful to share that where there is a lack of fit between what is seen and heard children develop their own understanding, and that these understandings are more frightening than the reality they face. Even if one tries to protect children from hearing worrying news (for example, that a child being treated with the same condition has relapsed or died), it is not unusual for them to learn this by overhearing conversations on the ward or waiting for an outpatient appointment: indeed, children's drawings and dreams often reflect a preoccupation with health and bodily mutilation even if they do not 'know' someone is ill (Gabriels et al., 2000):

For example, 6-year-old Samuel had never been told that his mother had cancer. The family were referred for therapy because he had become increasingly aggressive at school. On asking his mother if she had any idea what might have changed for him, she said she did not think anything had. While his mother was talking, Samuel drew a picture of a woman and scratched a big hole on the left side of her body, the side of her body where her breast had been removed.

Likewise, 5-year-old Melissa had not been told that Peter, her 10-year-old brother, had been diagnosed with Duchenne muscular dystrophy (DMD). However, his altered gait, frequent hospital appointments and their parents' whispered conversations meant she sensed something was wrong and dreamt

Peter was dying. Although Peter knew far more than Melissa, his parents' attempts to underplay the likely progression of DMD meant that he was left to make sense of the fear of becoming wheelchair bound and death on his own. The symbolic importance of parent–child relationships means that Melissa and Peter's experience was bound up with that of their parents: it was only after Peter became aggressive at school that his parents felt ready to confront the social and academic difficulties Peter was experiencing and the impact his deteriorating health was having on his sister and their relationship with one another.

Most children learn death is final between the ages of 5 and 8. However, children like Samuel Peter and Melissa who are exposed to life-limiting illness and the threat of death develop this understanding earlier (Slaughter and Griffiths, 2007). While adults tend to oscillate between periods of sadness and being able to get on with their lives, this is more pronounced with children: even when they have fully recovered and being ill seems to be a thing of the past, feelings of loss can re-emerge, particularly at significant times in their lives (Packman et al., 2006).

Until relatively recently, little attention was paid to the positions of siblings of children with a life-limiting and disabling condition. This is not particular to illness but reflects a wider neglect of siblings within the psychological literature (Edwards et al., 2006). This is an unfortunate omission because, as Mitchell (2003) suggests, siblings are the people who at one level are most like us, but at another stand in our place: consequently, a sister or brother's illness may signify a threat to the healthy child's sense of security and an actualization of the fantasy of replacing the other in the eyes of their parents. However, sibling relationships are not necessarily confined to experiences of rivalry and competition (Mauthner, 2003): they have the potential for a deep sense of companionship, which can be enormously sustaining at times of illness.

Here too research yields conflicting findings. Some studies indicate that social withdrawal, anxiety, jealousy, enuresis and academic underachievement are more pronounced amongst siblings of ill children, and/or that that their anxiety and low self-esteem mirrors or even surpasses that of the ill child. Others indicate that siblings who feel supported do not go on to develop more problems, and/or that living with an ill sibling can increase one's sense of compassion and sensitivity towards others (O'Brien, Duffy and Nicoll, 2009; Sharpe and Rossiter, 2002; Woodgate, 2006). Nonetheless, for many children, having a seriously ill sibling represents 'a different way of living in a family' (Woodgate, 2006, p. 26). For example, siblings are more likely to be faced with untimely and unexplained separation from parents and disruptions to daily routines. Many experience considerable worries about their own health and are ambivalent about succeeding in areas that are no longer open to their sister or brother. This is even more difficult when a sibling dies, particularly where parents' grief mean it is difficult to celebrate the achievements of their surviving child or engage with their distress.

It is inevitable that there will be times when illness consumes all aspects of family life. However, it is important to ensure someone (ideally a parent, but if not, another trusted adult) is able to take account of the ill and unaffected children's fears, worries and questions, and assist them in making sense of their similarities and differences in experience (Buchbinder, Casillias and Zelzter, 2011; Foster, Gilmer and Venatta, 2012; Woodgate, 2005). It can also be helpful to offer siblings an opportunity to meet other children who know what it is like to live with a seriously ill brother or sister or the death of a sibling (Barrera, Chung and Fleming, 2004).

Until recently, relatively little research and clinical attention focused on the impact of parental illness on children as well. This is starting to shift, as reflected in the growing numbers of studies aimed at identifying factors that increase risks and resilience, and projects focused on child carers (Annunziato, Rakatomihanmina and Rubacka, 2007; Diareme et al., 2007; Thastum et al., 2008). As with studies of childhood illness, age appears to be an important factor: for example, a large-scale study of children from 6 to late adolescence found that the concerns of younger children tend to revolve around guilt, worry about the possibility of the parent dying and fears of becoming ill themselves. Although adolescents expressed similar worries, they placed greater emphasis on the burdens of being expected to assume greater responsibility for household chores and caring for younger siblings. Across the age range, where the relationship was particularly conflicted, children were more likely to feel they were to blame for their parents' illness (Romer et al., 2002). There is also evidence that children (particularly girls) show more symptoms of distress when they are the same gender as the ill parent (Davey, Askew and Godette, 2003). Although some studies indicate distress levels are higher when the prognosis is poorer and the duration of the disease is longer, others suggest subjective perceptions are more predictive of distress than the objective characteristics of disease (Visser et al., 2005).

As with adults, individual characteristics and subjective experience inform how children respond in these situations. However, as reflected above, children tend to cope best when it is possible to maintain as much routine as possible, to have access to a person they can trust who can help them make sense of their experience (rather than the experience of their parents or siblings), to engage in activities that build self-esteem and opportunities to experience agency.

Parenting in the face of illness

All parents will have been through times when other aspects of life have to be put on hold to care for an ill child. In most cases, the experience is brief and we return to our former lives relatively unaffected. However, this is less possible when a child has a life-limiting and debilitating condition. For example, parents are likely to be faced with such challenges as educating themselves about the condition and treatment options, collaborating with the health care professionals, explaining the condition to the affected child without exposing them to unnecessary anxiety, and if their condition deteriorates, helping them deal with the feelings of panic and despair that tend to set in at such times.

Where there are other children, parents are also faced with explaining the condition to them, trying to schedule time with each child to ensure they feel treasured, helping them deal with the differences in their positions, inspiring hope and maintaining as much of their everyday routine as possible. Where the treatment reduces the child's immunity or the condition is contagious, parents are also faced with explaining what level of contact is safe and keeping others informed while respecting the child's need for privacy.

Possibly the most painful challenge parents face is relinquishing the dream of bringing up a 'normal' child. When the diagnosis is affirmed at birth, as with many hereditary and birth trauma disorders, feelings of grief can interfere with parents' ability to bond with the child. Weingarten describes the experience of finding out her baby had a rare genetic disorder as 'falling in love while living in terror' (Weingarten and Worthern, 1997, p. 47). Key points in the life cycle can re-evoke earlier feelings of grief. Where the condition affects the child's life expectancy, parents are also faced with the loss of an imagined future and possibility of grandchildren. However, because no one has died, feelings of grief are 'disenfranchised' (Doka, 1999), and therefore difficult to acknowledge.

Watching one's child suffer may be not only deeply distressing, but also traumatic (Barakat et al., 2000; Stoppelbein and Greening, 2007). As discussed earlier, current experiences of trauma have the potential to re-evoke feelings related to the past. Consequently, parents can find themselves overwhelmed by feelings related to previous situations of powerlessness, abuse and abandonment. In the context of a busy paediatric unit where their child is critically ill or dying, it is important to help parents remain focused on the present and being there for their child. However, in some situations this is only possible once parents have had an opportunity to disentangle feelings related to the past from the present.

Even if parents' distress does not reach this level, watching one's child suffer can trigger feelings of loss and powerlessness. Although we will all have been through experiences that confront us with how powerless we are, this is more likely when a child is seriously ill or disabled. Some parents are faced with this fairly early on, when an infant child cannot feed, is inconsolable and struggles to breathe. Others are faced with powerlessness later, as when Peter (discussed earlier) was diagnosed with Duchenne muscular dystrophy at the age of 10 or in later life when an adult child is ill or disabled and parents are too frail to help care for them.

Experiences of powerlessness are not necessarily confined to the real. As discussed earlier, faced with situations of loss and powerlessness, it is not unusual to blame others, or blame oneself (Benjamin, 1998; Klein, 1975). Parents are vulnerable to self-blame or being blamed by others because they tend to be seen as children's main source of protection. This is particularly difficult when parents are required to play a significant role in their child's treatment and despite their best efforts their health deteriorates. In some cases parents are expected to act in ways that contradict deeply held beliefs of what good parenting entails, for example by performing procedures that cause pain or discomfort (pummelling the chest of a child with cystic fibrosis to prevent mucus in the chest blocking the airways), having to be more watchful of children with diabetes or renal failure, or having discussions about sexual contact with the child infected with the HIV virus that feel inappropriate for their age.

Finding the right balance between protection and allowing age-appropriate independence can be extremely difficult. While acting in an overly restrictive way can push children into becoming overly anxious about their health or so frustrated that they rebel against the treatment, failing to monitor one's child's diet, intake of medicine and level of activity can mean they are less protected; it also means that as their health deteriorates the child can be seen as responsible.

Over the past 40 years, shifts in gendered expectations and patterns of employment mean that, particularly in the West, the roles of mothers and fathers are more fluid than previously. Despite these changes, mothers (and/or other female members of the family and community) tend to assume a greater level of responsibility for caring for children (Herbert and Carpenter, 2007). It has often been noted that mothers and fathers tend to view their child's prospects differently. Whilst other factors may be implicated, Sallfors and Hallberg's (2003) study of parents of children with juvenile arthritis suggests that mothers tended to be more pessimistic because they carry primary responsibility for that child and are therefore more in touch with their child's emotional and practical needs than the father.

Some studies suggest that parenting a seriously ill child has a negative effect on marital satisfaction and sexual relationships. Others have found no difference, that the experience leads to an increased sense of trust and capacity to communicate and solve problems, or that the rates of divorce are no higher than the norm (Gerhardt et al., 2003; Lavee and May-Dan, 2003). Nevertheless, the experience can be extremely challenging: having to accompany one's child to medical appointments and caring for them when they are too ill to attend school interferes with the possibilities of working and maintaining one's usual social activities, facing couples with greater financial difficulties and the loss of self-esteem and companionship interactions with colleagues and friends can provide. As a result, couples may turn to one another for support far more than before, leading to a deeper sense of intimacy and trust in one another. Looking to one another for support is particularly difficult when the relationship has always been hostile and one or both parents' earlier experiences of intimacy have been abusive. However, even where relationships are more supportive, being confronted with one another's grief can feel intolerable.

In some cases, the need to maximize the child's chances of survival means parents are faced with significant shifts in patterns of power and care. This tends to occur when one parent (more usually a mother) spends more time at the hospital and has greater contact with the medical team. Becoming the 'family expert' can mean one is more vulnerable to self-blame and the criticism of others if things go wrong. However, where that parent adopted a more subservient role before, becoming the expert on one's child's condition can lead to an increase in agency and self-esteem. Likewise, if the parent taking primary care of the rest of the children spent relatively little time with them on their own before, engaging on a more ongoing basis can result in a shift in their relationship with their children, altering understandings of themselves and the roles their partner played.

One of the other issues to bear in mind is that caring for an ill child can confront parents with differences they were unaware of before: for example, one parent may find it helpful to express their greatest worries but the other finds this intolerable and prefers to cope by underplaying the seriousness of the child's condition. Likewise, parents may disagree about whether it is better to confront medical professionals when they feel the quality of care their child receives is inadequate, or to avoid acting in ways that might alienate the staff. A certain level of difference can be helpful: one parent's optimism can go a long way towards balancing the pessimism of the other. Indeed, arguing can be a way of breathing life into a relationship when one feels ground down by grief and powerlessness. However, maintaining polarized positions can limit partners' ability to recognize what is shared and reach decisions about their ill child and other aspects of family life.

With the exception of palliative care and HIV/AIDS services, until recently very few hospitals offered parents with a life-limiting illness additional support in thinking about the impact of their condition on parenting. For example, Barnes et al. (2000) found that mothers diagnosed with breast cancer were rarely asked about their children and how they would tell them about the diagnosis, or offered guidance on the consequences this may have for their children. The reasons for this omission could include the fact that there is no one professional who holds an overall responsibility for their psychological and physical wellbeing, that medical professionals have limited time with adult patients, and professionals' concerns that talking about their children might increase parents' distress and affect their recovery. However, in view of the importance attached to providing parents with practical and emotional support when a child is ill, this omission suggests a taboo against confronting the reality that despite their best efforts, parents may not be able to protect their children from harmful situations. Nevertheless, rather than helping, failing to engage with parents' concerns about their children means they are left to deal with these concerns without the support and knowledge of professionals who have worked with others in a similar position.

Although prioritizing the needs of one's children is seen as integral to being a good parent, this can be difficult when one has a life-limiting condition. Gender does not prescribe all aspects of identity and behaviour. However, because women's sense of identity tends to be more bound up with caring for children and other vulnerable family members than is true of men, prioritizing one's own health may be more difficult for mothers than fathers (Weingarten, 1994):

> Melanie had been diagnosed with an aggressive form of breast cancer that required surgery, radiotherapy and chemotherapy. While on chemotherapy, there were times when Melanie felt exhausted and feared she might say or do something she would regret. As a result she put her children to bed far earlier than they needed. Although respecting her own health and energy levels meant she was more able to be there for them at other times, this required a significant shift in expectations of her role as a mother.

Many parents feel extremely guilty about the effect their illness has on their children. Feelings of guilt may relate to situations when they are less available to their children, as when hospital medical appointments mean it is impossible to take one's children to school, oversee homework or participate in bedtime rituals. Likewise, there may be times when pain, weariness and nausea mean that parents' primary preoccupation is with their body rather than the people with whom they are most intimately connected. In some cases, children are required to assume responsibility for aspects of their parents' care, which makes it more difficult to set realistic boundaries. Understandably, the potential to see oneself as harmful is heightened when the condition has a genetic component or the disease has been transmitted to a child:

Although Busiswe could accept the impact HIV/AIDS was likely to have on her own life, it was far more difficult to come to terms with the knowledge that the virus had been transmitted to her son: feelings of guilt and shame added to the difficulties of telling her son about his status and helping him think about what to say to his friends.

If parents live together, the healthier partner is often able to step in at times when the other is physically or emotionally unavailable. However, there are likely to be times when the healthy partner's own anxiety, fear and regret mean both parents are 'emotionally absent' even if they are physically present (Boss, 2006). An added challenge is that it is often difficult to know how much to take on without undermining the other parent, particularly when the condition is terminal. In some cases, the desire to protect one's terminally ill partner from facing the fact that they will not be able to see their children become adults and parents themselves results in avoiding discussions about the future. However, instead of helping, avoiding such discussions can build a wall at a time when parents are likely to need one another most. Where possible, sharing ideas about what one's children are likely to need, hopes for their future and how to help them hold on to memories of being together that are not only about illness, (for example, through compiling a memory box) can go a long way towards ensuring children will be cared for as one had hoped. This may include discussions about pain control and how to ensure that medication one takes does not affect the possibilities of remaining connected with one's children. However, conversations about the future are less feasible when the condition affects mental functioning and personality:

Adam had been diagnosed with leukodystrophy, a progressive degenerating condition that meant he began acting in an increasingly disinhibited and aggressive way. Although he wanted to be more engaged with his children, uncontrolled outbursts of rage meant his partner could not trust him to be alone with them.

In other situations the diagnosis of a life-threatening condition frees parents to separate. Being told she had an invasive form of breast cancer helped Sally recognize how damaging the relationship with her partner Mike had been to herself and her children and asked him to leave. This meant that her 6- and 8-year-old daughters were faced with the news that their mother was seriously ill at the same time as hearing their parents were separating. However, the decision to separate also meant they were less caught up with battles between their parents, and that, particularly when their mother was recovering from chemotherapy, they were able to draw on the support of their father far more than seemed feasible before.

Where parents seem unable to understand what their children are going through, it can be helpful to work towards increasing their curiosity about their children's experience. In this case, Sally had tried to underplay how serious her condition was: although she told her children she was ill she had avoided using the term cancer for fear that if they said this to their friends they would be told she was dying. Asking Sally to imagine what changes her daughters had noticed and how she might feel or respond if she was in their position helped her recognize that they were more worried than she wanted to acknowledge, and decide to bring them to a session with her and their father.

At this session the girls' questions and drawings suggested that they were afraid their mother would die and extremely distressed about their parents' decision to separate. As such, the session became a forum for talking about their mother's illness and their parents' decision to separate. This included trying to disentangle difficulties that were an almost inevitable consequence of illness from other family issues. When Nathalie, the younger of the two, asked her parents if they 'couldn't at least try' to stay together, their parents explained that this was their decision and that even though they no longer loved one another, this did not mean they loved their children any less. Because children often blame themselves when a parent is ill or separate, it was also important to help them understand that neither situation was their fault.

Experiences of illness in adulthood

As discussed earlier, some people seem able to adjust to the disjunctions illness and treatment pose to their sense of self and relationships with relatively little difficulty, but this is more difficult for others. Most indexes of distress tend to reduce following the initial diagnosis and treatment period. However, concerns about body image, sexuality and the impact of illness on family, couple and parenting relationships can persist well after successful treatment (Halford, Scott and Smythe, 2000; Kim et al., 2012; Little et al., 2002; Witty et al., 2014). Indeed, in a survey of 862 long-term survivors of non-Hodgkin lymphoma, a third reported continuing or worsening symptoms of PTSD (Smith et al., 2011).

The level of distress one experiences is influenced by the severity of the condition and physical limitations. However, it is also influenced by the perceptions of the individual and the people with whom they are most connected. Indeed, fears of illness and death can take over as much when chances of survival are higher as when survival rates are poorer (Lee and Dwyer, 1995).

It has long been recognized that we are more able to offset the stresses and challenges we face when we have access to a relationship in which it is possible to feel listened to and understood (Helgeson, Cohen and Fritz, 1998). Nonetheless a sizeable proportion of people who are ill and disabled live alone, and many will have chosen to do so. In common with people living with a partner, close family or friends, those who live alone are likely to experience similar anxieties about the effects that illness and medical treatment might have on their lives, relationships and prospects of employment. What is different is that people who had hoped to develop a permanent relationship may feel that disability, disfigurement and/or the risks associated with becoming pregnant preclude this. Moreover, the loss of self-esteem that so often sets in when one is vulnerable can mean that one avoids social situations, limiting the possibilities of establishing new relationships.

Even if one has a wide circle of supportive family and friends, it is often more difficult to call on taken-for-granted support in containing one's worries and attending to basic needs like eating, washing, housework, or asking others to collect medication from the pharmacy. Concerns about burdening others mean some people avoid asking for help until this is absolutely imperative or too late, which may explain why people who live alone are less likely to remain at home when they develop a severely debilitating condition, particularly when older (Wenger, Davies, Shahatahmasebi and Scott, 1996). In some situations, the need for additional care forces people to become more dependent on their family of origin. As helpful as this may be, particularly where living alone has felt the only way of prioritizing one's own needs, this enforced dependency can feel intolerable. In other cases, friends and relatives share in caring for the ill person in their own home. However, because informal circles of care are rarely recognized by the palliative and other health care services, they rarely receive the psychosocial support they need when the responsibility feels too stressful to bear, or when they, the dying person and their relatives disagree on what is needed. As in all situations where someone is dying, this is particularly difficult when the terminally ill person lacks mental capacity, has not written an advanced care plan or shared their wishes with others.

In contrast, where ill people are in an ongoing relationship, many people turn to their partner for support. This is not always the case: as reflected in discussing Sally, the woman who asked her partner to leave after she was diagnosed with an aggressive form of breast cancer, ending a destructive relationship may feel like the only way of prioritizing one's own needs and maximizing the chances of survival.

Understandably in most clinical settings, primary emphasis is placed on supporting the person who is ill. However, partners can experience as much or even greater levels of anxiety and distress in coming to terms with the practical demands and threatened loss than their ill partner (Fisher, 2006; Hagedoorn et al., 2008; Weingarten, 2013). Although there are obviously many differences between the ill person and their partner, in a study exploring couple's views about the effects of long-term illness on their relationship, both partners drew attention to difficulties in communicating, uncertainty about how to respond to one another, the desire to be understood and worries about driving the other way (Ardenne, 2004).

It is obviously unrealistic to imagine that couples (and other family members) might want or feel able to express their feelings or confront loss on an ongoing basis. Indeed, there appear to be gendered differences in the extent to which men and women feel comfortable with expressing how they feel in words (Weingarten, 1991). However, moments of intimacy that allow for a shared understanding of one another's experience (even if this is different) can go a long way towards maintaining some sense of 'we' in a context that is dominated by difference, loss, powerlessness and isolation. Research focused on couples facing a range of acute, chronic and terminal conditions including cancer (Kayser, Watson and Andrade, 2007), heart attacks (Figueiras and Weinman, 2003), rheumatoid and osteoarthritis (Cremeans-Smith et al., 2003) and chronic pain (Cano, Johansen and Geisser, 2004) indicate that the ability to view at least some aspects of the illness experience in terms of 'we' has a positive impact on couple relationships, adjustment to the condition and the lifestyle changes required.

Although it can be helpful to set aside thoughts about ill health for some of the time (Fagundes, Berg and Wiebe, 2012), couples who engage with, rather than avoid, illness-related challenges are more able to collaborate, hear and respond to one another's distress (Kayser, Watson and Andrade, 2007); indeed, research suggests that where partners are responsive to one another and can tolerate difference, the shift to one partner becoming more of a carer and to the other becoming cared for need not affect overall satisfaction with their relationship (Manne et al., 2004).

Nevertheless, adjusting to the challenges illness and treatment present can push even the most supportive couples over the edge. Most of us vary in how much we want to know, acknowledge and disclose to our loved ones, how we balance the desire for connection with individuality, and the desire for openness with privacy (Migerode and Hooghe, 2012). The difficulty is that whilst speaking openly carries the risk of driving people away, failing to do so limits the possibility of maintaining that authentic sense of connection one is striving for (Alvarez, 1999; Rathbone, 2009).

However the intense and in some cases shameful emotions differences in health status, power and dependency evoke can make it difficult to know what to acknowledge to oneself, let alone others. While underplaying differences may appear to maintain some sense of continuity, paradoxically it tends to create an artificiality that limits the possibility of maintaining that sense of continuity both parties are striving for (Alvarez, 1999). Unacknowledged, these feelings may find expression in guilt about being able bodied, resentment about the burden of care, neglecting one's own needs in the case of the healthy partner, and for the partner who is ill, resentment about the health and freedom of the other. Conversely, acknowledging differences allows for greater openness. However, underplaying what is shared can mean suffering, dependency and caring responsibilities become the primary ways of seeing one another. Moreover, where the relationship was unsupportive before, and one or both partners feel they are to blame, differences in health status can be used to make claims that relate to other aspects of their relationship.

One of the other challenges is that although a satisfactory sexual relationship can offer a chance to feel 'normal', this is less feasible when one is overwhelmed by pain, fatigue, anxiety and grief, one's body image is significantly altered and the condition or surgery results in impotence. It is also more complicated when dependency and fear of hurting the other person mean it feels impossible to refuse unwanted sexual advances.

With the exception of HIV/AIDS, very few studies exploring the impact of illness on couples focus on same-sex relationships. Many of the issues discussed in relation to heterosexual couples are equally applicable to those in a same-sex relationship. However, research and clinical experience suggests that many same-sex couples are exposed to anti-gay prejudice over the course of their treatment and feel professionals do not understand the unique challenges they and their families face (Albarran and Salmon, 2000; Blank et al., 2009; Fobair et al., 2001; Green and Mitchell, 2002; McCann, 2014). Moreover, in some societies same-sex relationships do not have the legal and social recognition that helps to ensure parents and other family members acknowledge and support their relationship. Furthermore, confusions about the origins of being gay and theories blaming parent–child relationships mean that guilt, stigma, anger and disappointment lead to distancing oneself from family, keeping this aspect of one's life secret and/or investing all one's energy into the couple relationship.

Where anti-gay prejudice means one or both partners avoided disclosing that they are gay to their family and colleagues, becoming ill and requiring additional practical and emotional support can force one to speak more openly. In these situations, the individual, their family and colleagues are faced with coming to terms with illness at the same time as coming to terms with what being gay means for them and their relationship with one another. Where families have known and disapproved of their child (or sibling's) sexuality, it is not unusual to feel caught in a battle between one's family and partner. However, this is not necessarily the case: seeing how supportive one's child's partner is can lead to greater acceptance of one's son or daughter, their couple relationship and of oneself (Walker, 1991).

Where disclosing to family and/or friends and colleagues has been extremely difficult, couples may benefit from an opportunity to reflect on the impact of this for their relationship with one another and others, and what they want and need from one another now. In some cases, exploring how they might feel if they were in the position of the person whose views they find most upsetting can lead to a different understanding and what is needed for anything to change.

In other cases, this feels too difficult or even dangerous. With this in mind, it can be helpful to explore who each partner sees as belonging to their circle of care. For example, in a study based on interviews with gay HIV-positive men attending an HIV clinic in London, many said they regarded friends and partners as their primary social support system rather than their biological family (Bor, du Plessis and Russell, 2004).

Recommendations for practice

Confronted with a life-limiting illness, disability and the threat of death, many people are able to turn to family and friends for the practical and emotional support needed at times of particular difficulty. Others prefer to cope on their own. However, the stresses and strains of living with ongoing uncertainty, shifts in patterns of power and dependency and practical demands mean that most people would benefit from an opportunity to reflect on the impact of illness on themselves and their loved ones as a matter of course, rather than waiting for problems to escalate.

In the context of a busy clinic or hospital ward organized around medical intervention and trying to 'fix', it is easy to forget the healing power of 'being there' (Meyerstein, 2015), of listening to the stories people tell, and engaging with their pain, hopes and fears of abandonment. Listening shapes the experience of speaking: so it is important to listen in a way that allows people to tell their story (Mann and Russell, 2002). Reflecting on her experience of caring for her partner, a man with motor neurone disease (MND), Rathbone said she often felt as if they were being 'chaperoned' through MND by 'experts', and wished professionals had been more ready to enquire 'about our hopes for conversations, connection and community (realistic or otherwise) which have sometimes been straightforward and practical and other times harder to articulate' (Rathbone, 2009, pp. 18–19).

Engaging with people in a similar position

As evidenced by the proliferation of self-help organizations and online blogs and discussion groups offering information and support to people living with a life-limiting and debilitating condition, it can be extremely helpful to connect and share experiences with others who are in a similar position. Although each person's situation and responses are different, people who have been through similar experiences are likely to have some understanding of how lonely, exhausting and private experiences of illness and caregiving can be. In hospital settings, this tends to happen on an informal basis, on the ward or while waiting for an outpatient appointment. However, there is rarely enough time or privacy to address more problematic concerns experiences of illness and disability tend to present in these sorts of settings. As such, it can be helpful to meet in more structured group meetings to discuss illness-related dilemmas, share information and learn from one another.

At one point, there was a hope that group therapy would increase the likelihood of survival, for example in relation to cancer. Spiegel, Bloom, Kraemer and Gottheil (1989) found that group therapy helped breast cancer patients live longer. However, subsequent research suggests that this is not necessarily the case (Spiegel et al., 2007). Nonetheless, there is considerable evidence that group therapy can help people cope better with a wide range of life-limiting conditions, even though there is not sufficient evidence to suggest that this will prolong life. For example, Kissane et al. (2007) found that group therapy helped with depression, reduced hopelessness and helplessness, reduced trauma symptoms and improved social functioning amongst the 227 women with breast cancer that they studied. Similarly, Spector, Gardner and Orrelle (2011) found that group therapy had a positive impact on the way in which people with dementia and their carers coped with the condition. Some studies suggest that group sessions tend to be particularly effective when they include some psycho-educational input and are led by a professional who has an understanding of group dynamics as well as experience of working with people facing illness (Broome and Stuart, 2006).

Meeting with others in a similar position can be extremely helpful for children with a chronic condition: it provides children with opportunities for modelling, problem solving, helping others and relating to peers who share similar circumstances. This is particularly important as because social adjustment is an area of particular vulnerability for many children with chronic illnesses and peer relationships may affect adaptation to the disease (La Plante, Lobato and Engel, 2001). Likewise, siblings have a great deal to gain from engaging with other children who have a chronically ill sibling (Barrera, Chung and Fleming, 2004). As parents' understanding and responses have a significant effect on the experience of children, where ill children or siblings of ill children are seen in a group it can be helpful for parents to meet with other parents who are in a similar position even if only at the start and end of this work. Whilst it is important to respect confidentiality, these meetings offer a forum for alerting parents to aspects of the child's experience that they are unaware of.

Individual, couple or family counselling

Some people require more intensive psychological support on their own, with their partner and/or family. In these situations it is important to discuss the idea of seeing a therapist or counsellor carefully before referring someone on, to ensure they do not feel they are being abandoned or pathologized. Working with people facing illness involves listening to what people say, engaging with their experience and helping them reflect on the meaning of the illness for themselves and their loved ones. However, one story can never embrace all aspects of our experience; as such, other stories are always possible. Consequently, where people are struggling, it can be helpful to introduce questions and comments aimed at bringing alternate stories and understandings to the fore.

Uncovering these alternate and less acknowledged stories involves a process of 'double listening': instead of purely listening to stories with a view to gathering information or noting symptoms, we need to 'listen out' for stories, for stories that are absent, underplayed or implicit in what is said (White and Epston, 1990). It also means listening out for how these stories are told: for example, some people treat their experience of illness with enormous seriousness, some use humour in what may be an attempt to deny or minimize the consequences of the illness, and others oscillate between these two positions. Noticing differences like these offers some guidance on how to ensure that what we say fits with the ways in which people respond to and conceptualize their experience.

For example, where a parent who has a life-limiting illness has not told their children they are ill but is worried about them, it can be helpful to ask what effect they think their diagnosis is having on their children, what their children might need from them now, how they know their children are worried or sad, and what they themselves would like to ask of others to get through difficult times. Similarly, where an adult with a chronic condition is struggling but is reluctant to turn to their partner for support, it can be helpful to 'figuratively' bring them into the session by asking such questions as what they might say if they were actually present, how they can tell when their partner is worried, how their partner knows when their support is needed and how they resolve difficulties when blow-ups occur.

Where accounts of experience are dominated by illness, it can be helpful to encourage people to reflect on other aspects of their lives; similarly where most of what is said focuses on other aspects of life, it can be helpful to ask if they would also like to discuss the illness and its potential consequences for themselves and others. As reflected in Chow's (2015) study of stroke survivors, where people are trapped in 'problem-saturated' identities and accounts are dominated by powerlessness and self-blame, asking what they have found sustaining at other times of difficulty and, where appropriate, drawing attention to exceptions to the problem-dominated story can go a long way towards helping people reconnect with their strengths, values, and the wisdom they developed during their earlier years, re-authoring and rebuilding their lives within the limits of debilitating challenges. Figure 3.1 depicts the four main issues to bear in mind in considering the balance between risk and resilience in relation to illness as well as migration (Burnham, 2015):

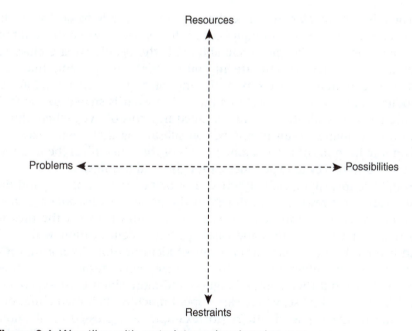

Figure 3.1 Wrestling with restraints and embracing resources

The term 'problems' refers to the range of reasons people seek health care (including dilemmas, fear and uncertainty) or refuse the health care on offer (for example, immunizations and other preventative services), whereas 'possibilities' represent what people are hoping for: their desires, aspirations and future dreams. 'Resources' refer to personal and family strengths, to what keeps one going, helps one resist the pull of problems and generate solutions. In contrast, the term 'restraints' refers to what holds one back, to anything that gets in the way and to obstacles to change (Burnham, 2015).

Comments and questions aimed at normalizing common responses to illness-related challenges can help in creating a less pathologizing frame for understanding oneself and others. This is particularly important because by the time people turn to a counsellor and therapist, they have often reached a point where they believe there is something wrong with them, that they or something about them is problematic. Where problems related to illness have become internalized, externalizing questions can help in separating the person from the problem (White and Epston, 1990). This includes asking questions in which we change the adjectives that people use to describe themselves into nouns, for example by responding to statements such as 'I am depressed' by asking 'how long has this depression been influencing you?' and exploring how the problem (the illness or illness-related anxieties) affects their thoughts, feelings and interactions with others.

There is considerable evidence that we are more able to deal with the practical and emotional consequences of illness when we embrace rather than avoid these challenges, preferably with the people we are close to. Consequently, where people are in couple relationships, and much of what is said is framed in terms of 'I', 'me' or 'my', it can be helpful to introduce comments and questions that bring what is shared to the fore. Alternately, where all that is said is framed in terms of 'we', where illness and caring demands result in one person subsuming their own needs and responding in terms of the imagined needs of the other, it can be useful to ask about differences in experiences, thoughts and feelings.

Family scripts (Byng-Hall, 1995) and prior experiences of loss and difficulty can affect responses to illness in the present. Consequently, there are times when it is important to explore the links between the present and past. For example, in some cases, parents' identification with their child is bound up with far earlier forms of identification. Exploring these connections can allow parents to recognize when responses to their child are less about their son or daughter and more about their experience at a similar age. Likewise, where carers spent much of their own childhood attending to the needs of others (for example, a depressed or alcoholic parent, or having to put their own needs on hold to ensure their disabled or ill siblings received the care they needed), exploring the links between the past and present can lead to a wider understanding of one's current struggles, including struggles to balance caring for others with caring for oneself.

However, this may not be possible or advisable: where people are afraid that reflecting on the past might increase their levels of stress, limiting the ability to deal with the challenges they are facing in the present, they may be wary of opening up distressing memories of the past. Similarly, where the past has been extremely traumatic, memories of the past may have been blocked out. As such, it is important to help people take one step at a time and cope with what is immediately at hand. Nonetheless, particularly when working with refugees and asylum seekers, it is important to bear in mind that responses to the present, including seeing a loved one struggling to breathe or withdrawing because they are in so much pain, may be influenced by conscious and unconscious memories of the past.

Working with children

When the child or someone close to them is ill or dying, it is important to create an environment in which children feel listened to rather than judged, where it is possible to communicate through play rather than having to rely purely on words, and where the focus is not only on troubles. Having play materials on hand, for example dolls, toy animals, puppets, soft objects like a teddy bear and drawing materials, helps to reduce the fear and anxiety that tends to be associated with doctors and hospitals, enabling us to engage with some of the thoughts and fantasies expressed through their play.

Drawing materials are particularly helpful as they can be used to explain where the illness is located, how it developed and ask questions about what they have been told. Likewise, children's own drawings can offer insights into their understanding of illness. Where children and their parents seem stuck in crisis mode, asking children to draw a picture of their home 'before' and 'after' illness (or migration) occurred opens up the possibility of thinking about what needs to happen before children feel ready or are allowed to resume aspects of their pre-illness (or pre-migration) lives.

The powerlessness and shame that tends to surround problems that feel close to home can mean that it is difficult to separate oneself from the illness and its consequences. With this in mind, it can be helpful to externalize or objectify the illness and/or its consequences. This could involve asking the child (and/or the rest of their family) to name the problem, draw it and speculate about its characteristics and motives. This process is reflected in White and Epston's (1990) description of their work with a boy who had started to soil himself. Naming encopresis 'sneaky poo' enabled the family to talk about the problem as if it lay outside of this child, helping him and his family engage with it in a more playful and positive way. Discussing how the 'sneaky poo', an invisible entity, seemed to creep up unawares, making this young boy soil his pants, helped to reduce the powerlessness and shame he and his parents felt and work together to reduce the likelihood of the problem reoccurring.

As suggested above, it is sometimes preferable to start by addressing children's concerns at one step removed. For example, Fredman, Christie and Bear (2007) used a toy bear (the author named 'Bear') in working with a 10-year-old girl who was refusing to have any more surgery. As she would not explain why she was refusing surgery to her parents or medical team, she was asked if Bear could express her views and if she would let the therapists know when the bear got things wrong. Listening to Bear and commenting on what 'it' said helped to keep her engaged. As importantly, it helped her parents hear her and recognize that their daughter was not actually refusing surgery: she 'just' wanted them to know how difficult the idea of more surgery was for her.

A useful way of helping children and parents communicate about issues that are troubling is to ask members of the family to choose an animal counterpart to represent themselves and others, and use these images to construct a story (Arad, 2004). Although families are not asked to focus on illness, their stories tend to reflect illness-related preoccupations. As outlined above, discussions about what is said need to begin with the animals in the stories before moving on to the people they might represent. Similarly, games like asking children to write or draw their worries and place them in a 'worry box' can go a long way towards helping them contain feelings that have become uncontainable.

Activity sheets offer another way of helping children make sense of their experience, for example activity sheets headed with such statements as 'who is in my family' and 'things that make me sad/happy', columns marked 'life at home before (or after) X became ill' and diagrams of faces, animals or what has been called a 'jelly bean tree': a sheet of paper with jelly bean characters sitting at the top or bottom, climbing up and hanging on by their fingernails, depicting different sorts of emotions and connections to others. The worksheets and games mentioned above are available on the Internet and in books. However, there may be times when it is more helpful to design something with the particular needs of that child in mind. As play offers children the space to work through their own experience, opportunities for less structured play and drawing are invaluable in helping children make sense of their experience.

When children are seen with their parents, it is important to avoid these sessions becoming adult sessions and ensure that everything that is said fits with the child's level of understanding. Where parents' own anxieties, frustrations and fears mean it is difficult to relate to their children, rather than acting as a 'better parent' it is important to focus on enhancing parents' sensitivity to their children, and help them regain or establish confidence in their capacity to engage with their children, for example by noticing, imagining what they are feeling and are trying to show, and reflecting on their own responses at such times (Helps and Shepherd, 2014; Wilson, 2005). These ideas are equally pertinent to working with parents who are so locked into fears and anxieties related to migration that they cannot engage with their children's distress.

Personal–professional resonances

Helping to ease the suffering of people who are ill or dying can be enormously rewarding. Jung (1954) coined the term 'wounded healer' in arguing that many of us are driven to caring for others in an attempt to heal ourselves. However, despite our best efforts and the efforts of other professionals, the ill person and their family, some of the people we work with die or become increasingly disabled. As such, work with illness can confront us with our own sense of mortality and powerlessness, giving rise to feelings that are difficult to manage or understand. At these times it is important to acknowledge and tolerate the strength of our feeling, and those of the people with whom we are working, and remain present, interested and alert enough to understand the complexities inherent in their accounts of experience. This is not only relevant to working with adults: the chances of being confronted with personal resonance, re-evoking feelings and memories that relate to our own childhood, is particularly strong when working with children; consequently, there may be times when instead of empathizing, we find their behaviour irritating, aggressive and difficult to manage (Wilson, 2005).

Unconscious phenomena mean we can never be fully aware of the ways in which our own thoughts and feelings inform interactions with others. However, these thoughts and feelings can have a profound effect on the ways in which we relate to others. As such, it is important to disentangle the professional from the personal by increasing our awareness of what psychoanalysts call 'transference' and 'counter-transference' phenomena (Freud, 1912). Transference refers to situations when our thoughts and responses seem to be a reflection of issues that relate more to the people with whom we work than ourselves. Reflecting on the possibility of a link can alert us to concerns that people are unable or reluctant to raise, and situations where tensions between the staff might be a reflection of tensions that relate to the person or family they are working with.

In contrast, counter-transference refers to situations when our views are less about other people's experience than our own. As such, reflecting on the links with our own experiences can alert us to the ways in which blind spots (including those in relation to prejudice, cultural differences, sexual orientation, the consequences of migration or an unsupportive partner) limit our ability to engage with the suffering of others. Reflecting on these links can also alert us to situations where the stresses we experience are not only about external demands, but our own unattainable goals.

4

CULTURAL DIVERSITY, LANGUAGE BARRIERS AND PREJUDICE

As Britain's Asian, West Indian and African populations have grown, and the influx of people from EU countries has increased, many health care professionals, particularly those in inner city areas, are working with populations in which a greater proportion of people belong to ethnic minority groups. Consequently it is no longer a question of whether or not Britain is a multicultural society: it is a question of how we engage with the tensions and opportunities that arise from living in a society in which people have different cultural backgrounds (Rober and de Haene, 2014) and, in some cases, diverse constructions of health, illness and health care.

There will always be differences between the experience and understanding of 'insiders' and outsiders' to any particular cultural grouping. However, it is important to ensure we have sufficient 'cultural competence' to be able to engage sensitively and effectively with the people with whom we work. 'Cultural competence' was first used by Cross (1988) but it was not until about a decade later that greater emphasis was placed on applying this concept to health care and the training health care professionals (Betancourt, Green and Carrillo, 2000; Kai, Beavan and Faull, 2011; Papadopoulos, Tilke and Taylor, 1998; Srivastana, 2007).

Cultural competence refers to four aspects of experience: awareness of one's own cultural worldview, attitude towards cultural differences, knowledge of different cultural practices and worldviews, and skills in working across cultures. Whilst the concept of cultural competence offers a valuable framework for thinking about cross-cultural work, it suggests that professionals need to learn what it is important about others as though our own cultural beliefs and traditions do not have a similarly powerful influence on our responses, and ideas about what is right. With this in mind, Falicov (2013) suggests using 'cultural humility' or 'cultural attunement', terms that rebalance the power dimension in the clinical encounter and incorporate a commitment to self-evaluation and engagement with the other on the part of the practitioner to ensure treatment is more synchronized with the ethnic cultures and social context of the people with whom we work. However whichever term we adopt, it is important to understand what we mean by 'culture'.

Understanding what we mean by 'culture'

Interpretations of culture and its impact on experience, thoughts and values have varied over time and across different contexts. Until recently, Western theorists saw culture as a complex whole encompassing a list of characteristics such as knowledge, beliefs, morals, customs and visible markers. However, increased recognition of the fluidity of culture means that the term has been extended to describe the primarily symbolic, ideational and intangible aspects of human societies that inform the ways in which meaning is produced and exchanged (Hall, 1993). In turn, ethnicity refers to the groupings that share these cultural beliefs, values and practices. While some aspects of culture are explicit (such as traditional dress, social rituals and cuisine), others (such as patterns of family relationships, emotional orientation, sense of embodiment, agency, and linguistic and social history) are more implicit, rarely shared with outsiders and often unconscious. Many aspects of culture, including cultural meanings, are transmitted from one generation to the next through the practices of daily life. Nevertheless, individual variations and particular experiences, including experiences of the wider society, mean that our lives do not operate according to set cultural patterns but 'more or less patterns' (Krause, 2002). Although there is some continuity across the generations, understandings and experiences of culture are informed by particular forms of social and emotional engagement (Maitra and Krause, 2015).

Until recently, most studies of the clinical ramifications of culture focused on comparisons between minority and majority groups, with the implicit assumption that the health care beliefs and practices of the majority group represent the norm. This is shifting, with increased recognition that all ethnic groups, including majority ethnic groups, draw on cultural norms and beliefs in trying to make sense of all aspects of experience including illness. Indeed, prioritizing culture to the exclusion of other aspects of experience fails to take account of the ways in which socio-economics, gender, age, location, family circumstances, prior experiences of trauma, migration status, sexual orientation, religion, skin colour and personal philosophy inform illness and health care. Likewise, it fails to take account of the similarities that exist across ethnic groups, how differences amongst members of the same ethnic group experiences of culture vary from one region or social group to another, and the influence of other 'micro-cultures', including work, family and religious groupings. Similarly, it fails to take account of the 'bifurcation' of cultural identities, as with someone like myself whose identity, or identities, draw on my positioning as Jewish, British, South African and white; as an immigrant, psychologist and family psychotherapist; and as a mother, sister and daughter.

It is also important to take account of the fluidity of cultural experiences, and of the ways in which family forms, patterns of care, traditional beliefs and practices change in response to altered circumstances. For example, Chinese cultures are generally assumed to be more accepting of illness than in the West, to view dementia as an expected part of ageing and see the responsibility of caring for vulnerable relatives as resting with members of their family. However, increased longevity, the rising number of people with degenerative and disabling conditions, and the reduction in the length of hospital stays mean that, in common with other families, many Chinese families find the experience of assuming primary responsibility for caring for elderly and vulnerable relatives more difficult to sustain and are less willing to take this on than before (Helman, 2007). Similarly, although earlier studies of South Asian families living in London found that grandmothers and other female kin played a major role in supporting young mothers to care for their children (Bhopal, 1998; Marshall, Woollett and Dosanjh, 1998), this is changing as extended family networks become less common than before (Phoenix and Husain, 2007).

It is also important to take account of the fact that we vary in the extent to which traditional beliefs and practices are maintained following migration. Although many continue to retain a strong identification with their cultural heritage, in some situations this is 'reified', as reflected in reification of gendered roles amongst Italian immigrants attending an Italian cultural centre in London (Fortier, 2000). In other situations, 'bicultural encounters' (exposure to alternative value systems and practices) result in a merging of beliefs and practices (Phinney and Ong, 2007). However, this is less possible when living in a society that is hostile to one's beliefs, traditions and if one is identified with a group that is seen to occupy a socially inferior position, as is the case for many minority ethnic groups living in multicultural societies where the values of the majority white population are regarded as the norm (Kymlicka, 2001).

Essentializing culture, racism and othering

All cultural systems operate under constraints. However, minority cultures are subject to scrutiny in a way that majority cultures are not, a scrutiny that often carries racist overtones that fix and essentialize certain cultures and people (Malik and Mandin, 2012). Essentializing involves assuming differences can be explained by inherent, biological and 'natural' characteristics shared by members of a group, without taking account of individual differences. In these situations, the pressure to bridge gaps in understanding, abide by the principles and practices and manage the prejudices of the more powerful majority can result in rapid assimilation, disowning or minimizing identifications with traditional beliefs and life-styles, confronting families with challenging transformations, for example in gendered and intergenerational roles. This pressure can have the reverse effect as well, of closing ranks, looking to one another for support, elaborating cultural distinctiveness, or to oscillating between these two positions (Falicov, 2013; Fortier, 2000).

To make sense of cultural constraints and pressures, it is important to take account of the overlapping and often inconsistent ways in which culture, ethnicity, religion and 'race'[18] are used (Doron and Broom, 2011). For example, it is often difficult to differentiate between markers of religion, culture and the unquestioning assumptions about values and belonging associated with these markings. This is reflected in the use of attendance at a mosque and the wearing of a 'burkha' or 'niqab'[19] as markers of being Muslim and identification with Muslim cultural values, without taking account of the range of values women identified as Muslim ascribe to. The same is true of using attendance at a synagogue and wearing a 'kippah'[20] as indicators of being Jewish, and assuming all people who identify themselves as Jewish believe, think and act similarly. Indeed, culture is often seen as emblematic of all that is good and true of ourselves rather others, and in so doing provides the grounding for racism and other forms of discrimination to flourish (Maitra and Krause, 2015).

Geneticists have long argued that the boundaries used to mark 'race' do not reflect clear biological differences. Nonetheless, 'race' tends to be treated as if it is inherited and with discernable biological and physical markers. Although 'race' is socially and politically constructed through law, public policy and social practices, it produces real effects on the people racialized as 'black' or 'white'. Racialized discourses do not determine how we respond or think; however, they inform the range of issues we draw on in deciding how to respond or think, including who defines ethnic or racialized groupings and where the boundaries between different groupings are drawn (Bonilla-Silva, 2006; Graves, 2002; Phoenix, 2004). While racism may be based on skin colour and physical characteristics, prejudice is commonly based on beliefs and ideas, practices and traditions, group and individual identification and points of connection and disconnection (Maitra and Krause, 2015).

The concept of othering offers insight into the ways in which racialized and other discriminatory boundaries are constructed and maintained. Said (1978) argued that Western colonialism depends on its own identity and superior position by defining and categorizing a subjugated exoticized oriental 'other'. Similarly Derrida (1988) proposes that identity cannot be established without forming, if only by implication, the group of those who do not belong. Essentially, 'othering' is about maintaining positions of power and control: it defines which voice is expert and which is not, which representation is permissible and which is not, dismissing the other's personhood and framing them as less worthy of dignity (Byrne, 2000; Wilkinson and Kitzinger, 1996). The importance of claiming greater ownership over what is and is not permitted and the way definitions of identity are constructed and maintained by those in a more powerful position (the white majority) is reflected in calls to shift from using the term West African to Afro-Caribbean and subsequently to African Caribbean, and to substitute Bengali, a term which is based on language, for the previously used term Bangladeshi, which implies nationality and could therefore be seen as incompatible with British nationality (Phoenix and Husain, 2007).

'Othering' is particularly relevant to understanding the risks of attributing all differences to culture. For example, it may account for why, where people are experienced as problematic and the incidence and/or death rate of the grouping with which they are identified is higher than the norm, health problems tend to be attributed to cultural factors rather than challenges that arise from migration, racism, socio-economics and difficulties in accessing health care. As importantly, othering may be a way of dealing with the powerlessness and frustrations health care professionals experience when cultural and language barriers mean it is more difficult to understand and be understood, medical examinations take longer, accurate diagnosis is more problematic and compliance is worse.

Diversities in constructions of disease, illness and treatment

As with culture, understandings of disease and illness change over time and vary from one context to another. Although the terms disease and illness are often used interchangeably, in Western contexts disease is generally used to refer to objective abnormalities in the structure and function of bodily organs that relate to natural scientific phenomenon. Consequently, treatment focuses primarily on combating microorganisms, surgery and may involve the use of sophisticated technology. In contrast, illness refers to the more subjective aspects of disease, to personal and interpersonal reactions to disease and discomfort.

The boundaries between disease and illness are not always that clear. For example, it is possible to have a life-limiting disease without feeling ill, as in the case of undetected cancer. Likewise, comparable degrees of organ pathology can give rise to markedly different reports of pain. While doctors tend to focus most of their attention on identifying and treating disease, patients and their families are usually more concerned with the personal, social and disabling experiences that result from disease. Differences in preoccupation can lead to misunderstandings and dissatisfactions, regardless of cultural differences.

However there is a greater chance of misunderstandings and dissatisfactions arising when the providers and recipients of health care have different cultural backgrounds and different views about health, illness and treatment, as for example when Western practitioners work with people from cultures that place a higher value on acceptance of illness and death, prayer and more spiritual forms of intervention than in the West (Kreuter and McClure, 2004; Papadopoulos and Lay, 2006), where illness is attributed to an excess or deficiency in bodily fluids (yellow bile, black bile, phlegm and blood), the balance between 'Hot' and 'Cold' food (qualities that may not relate to the actual food temperature) and/or supernatural phenomena, such as the Evil Eye (Helman, 2007; Kleinman, 2006). Misunderstandings and dissatisfaction are also more likely in working with people from cultures which place greater trust in verbally transmitted information but are expected to rely on written information, on reading letters and leaflets (Manderson and Allotey, 2003). Likewise, consultations are more likely to be seen as unsatisfactory where the patient is from a society where preventative medicine is less prevalent than in the West and one is not given an injection or additional tablets (Galanti, 2015).

Although culture does not determine how we act, it predisposes us to certain points of view and actions rather than others. For example, research and clinical studies suggest that culture can have a profound influence on perceptions of the cause of disease (Kleinman, 2006; Tellez-Giron, 2007); on identifying whether one requires medical attention (Dixon-Woods et al., 2006; Kreuter and McClure, 2004); the uptake of screening and compliance with treatment (Papadopolous and Lay, 2006); how, when and to whom one should communicate physical and emotional problems (Ahmed, 2004; Friedlmeier, Corapci and Cole, 2011; Martinson and Yee, 2003); experiences of and responses to pain (Campbell and Edwards, 2012); expectations of outside support and interactions with health care professionals (Helman, 2007); gendered and age-related expectations of caring (Thibodeaux and Deatrick, 2007); expectations of family in situations of illness (Flores, 2000; Munet-Vilaro, 2004); whether decisions about health care should rest with the family or the individual in question (Kleinman, 2006); anticipations of and responses to death (Ekblad, Marttila and Emilsson, 2000); the meaning ascribed to dying in a hospital or hospice rather than at home; the process of burial and whether mourning is a primarily public or private experience; gendered roles in marking death; the importance of burying deceased migrants in the country in which they were born (Gunaratnam, 2013; McGoldrick et al., 2004); and expressions of emotional distress (Takeuchi et al., 2002).

For example, Kleinman (1980) found that from a very young age, Taiwanese children learn that their own feelings, both positive and negative, should not be expressed openly as this might endanger close interpersonal relationships whose harmony is more important than their own psychological status. As a result, powerful emotions tend to be dealt with through minimization, dissociation and somatization. This finding has been replicated in subsequent research indicating that where people are from cultures where acknowledging distress is seen as dangerous and might bring shame to the family there is an increased tendency to somatize rather than verbalize emotional distress; this is reflected in the underplaying of emotional distress and presentation of medically unexplained symptoms amongst Kurdish women living in Sweden, Turkish women in the Netherlands (Bengi-Arslan, Verhulst and Crijnen, 2002) and my own clinical work in the UK.

Indeed, many societies place less of a boundary between the physical, emotional and spiritual than is true of most Western societies: in her study of a condition people from the Punjab call a 'sinking heart', Krause (1989) found that people attributed their symptoms to external physical factors such as heat, weakness from hunger and physical exhaustion, and social and emotional difficulties arising from interpersonal relationships, as well as moral dilemmas concerning socially acceptable behaviour. Although Western notions of depression, heart disease and/or personality disorders might account for these symptoms, as Krause suggests it can be difficult to know how to diagnose or treat symptoms of a 'sinking heart' as the condition draws on Punjabi ideas about the heart, person and selfhood.

However, even if these symptoms reflect a combination of psychological and physical distress, it is important to recognize they are are real. This is particularly relevant in trying to address conditions like chronic fatigue syndrome (a disorder characterized by extreme fatigue that cannot be explained by any underlying medical condition), fibromyalgia (characterized by symptoms of pain for which the cause cannot be established) and other medically unexplained symptoms: where people feel their symptoms are regarded with suspicion there is a tendency to edit out what one assumes others would think wrong, inappropriate or irrelevant.

I was asked to see Doris, a woman from Uganda who had been suffering from chronic head pains for which no organic cause could be found. Whilst the health care professionals felt these pains related to traumatic experiences in her country of origin and subsequent to moving to the UK, Doris thought they were an indication of a disease or physical imbalance the doctors had yet to identify. With this in mind, an important aspect of our initial work focused on the challenges of managing chronic pain for which no medical explanation or cure could be found, and the experience of being disbelieved.

At first Doris was reluctant to consider the possibility of a link with previous experiences of trauma and abandonment. It was only after I had seen her several times and greater trust had been established that, on asking her about the treatment she would have received had she been in Uganda, Doris said her pains were caused by a jealous cousin and could only be cured by a traditional healer empowered to defuse this. This led to exploring the other forms of treatments she had tried, which led to Doris saying she had asked someone to see a faith healer in Uganda on her behalf. She also spoke about her faith in Christianity and the sustaining influence of prayer. Discussing these aspects of her life seemed to free Doris to speak more openly about her past, including childhood memories about being abandoned by her parents, living with relatives and being made to feel unwelcome by the cousin she felt was trying to harm her.

Malik, a Pakistani-born family psychotherapist, refers to this tendency to 'edit out' issues one assumes others would not believe or understand in discussing her work with a Pakistani family whom she saw with a white British-born colleague. It was only when her colleague was unable to attend a session that the family said they thought their difficulties were caused by a djinn, which, according to Islamic faith, is a supernatural force that can possess human beings and cause disease and accidents (quoted in Maitra and Krause, 2015).

However, it is important to recognize that as practitioners we may edit out what we see and hear as well: when faced with people who seem to be presenting with symptoms that do not fit within the parameters of Western medicine, for example with total body pain, the difficulties of transcending cultural and language barriers may mean we stop taking account of the various distinct areas that are painful.

Causality, blame and preventative medicine

Across all cultures, one of the first reactions to realizing that we, or someone else, is ill is trying to understand why this has happened. These explanations are central to sustaining hope through times of difficulty and reaching decisions about future action (Radley, 1994). In contemporary Western societies, constructions of causality tend to focus on biomedical factors. However, as important as biomedical explanations are, they fail to answer the almost inevitable personal and existential questions of 'why me?' and 'why now?'

Amongst the more usual responses in trying to understand 'why' in the face of uncertainty and powerlessness are to project responsibility for what is hated and feared onto someone else or an entirely different situation, or to blame oneself (Benjamin, 1998; Klein, 1975). Blame tends to be heightened when the condition is associated with considerable fear (Sontag, 1991).

It is interesting to note that despite extensive evidence of the role genetic, biomedical and environmental factors play in the development of disease in most Western societies there is a strong belief in the ability to control one's own health. This is reflected in the importance attached to maintaining a 'fighting spirit' in the face of cancer (Greer, 2000). Whilst I would not want to dispute the fact that mental attitude and abiding by a particular dietary and exercise regime can affect one's health, much of the evidence for 'fighting spirit' relies on anecdotal accounts.

Moreover, if a recurrence of the condition occurs, the idea that remaining healthy is a matter of having 'fighting spirit' implies that the affected person is responsible for the recurrence (Watson et al., 2000). In addition, the idea of a fighting spirit is likely to be less relevant to people from cultures where greater importance is attached to fatalism. For example, in a study of 132 Hindu women undergoing treatment for cervical cancer, those who believed cancer was caused by God's will were more effective in dealing with the crisis and their psychological recovery was better than those who blamed themselves by linking cancer to their own mental stress, family circumstances and bodily weakness (Kholi and Dalal, 1998). Likewise, in his study of bereaved Latino families living in the USA, Tellez-Giron (2007) found that believing terminal illness is punishment for something one has done or failed to do (a belief prevalent amongst many other cultures too) increases difficulties in coming to terms with death.

Constructions of causality influence the uptake of preventative services as well. For example, in analysing the health practices of travellers, refugees, asylum seekers and people from minority ethnic groups, Papadopolous and Lay (2006) found that those with a more fatalistic attitude to illness were less likely to engage with screening and immunization programmes than a comparable group of UK-born people. Similarly, in a study of the views of South Asian women with breast cancer, Karbani, Lim and Hewison (2011) found that believing cancer can be caused by one's own actions, is contagious and affects one's child's marriage prospects influenced the likelihood of acknowledging the risks of breast cancer and uptake of screening, delaying the possibilities of diagnosis and commencement of treatment.

The impact of constructions of causality on readiness to use preventative services might explain why the mortality rates for cancer are higher amongst minority ethnic people than the majority white population in the UK, even where the incidence of cancer is lower (Ben-Shlomo et al., 2008; National Cancer Intelligence Network and Cancer Research UK, 2009; Webb et al., 2004). Nevertheless, it is important to take account of the intersection between culture, discrimination and other aspects of experience. The tendency to delay seeking help is more common amongst people from black and minority ethnic groups; as such these differences may relate to racialization and difficulties in accessing culturally appropriate services (Karbani, Lim and Hewison, 2011; National Cancer Intelligence Network and Cancer Research UK, 2009).

Cultural beliefs appear to influence readiness to seek health care when faced with other conditions as well. For example, where dementia is seen as a form of punishment for actions related to one's present and past life, people tend to seek medical care later, often waiting until a crisis point (Azam, 2007). Once again, because this is more common amongst people from black and minority ethnic groups, it is difficult to separate self-blame and the fear of being diagnosed with dementia from anticipations and experiences of discrimination.

Interactions with health care professionals

Although views and practices of everyone who identifies or is identified with a particular cultural group are far from homogenous, cultural factors inform assumptions of what interactions between the providers and recipients of health care should entail. For example, establishing a collaborative relationship with patients and their families is currently seen as best practice in the West. However, this might feel confusing or even inappropriate for people from societies in which the authority of the doctor is never questioned, as in many Russian and Middle Eastern societies.

Likewise, where people are from cultures where families see themselves as responsible for ensuring the patient gets the best possible care, behaviours Western professionals view as overly demanding or even aggressive (for example, families wanting to stay with the patient to ensure they are not left alone) are likely to reflect a different appreciation of the roles that family and health care professionals should play. For example, a paediatrician who grew up in a Jewish immigrant family said he had always assumed that eating home cooked food and having a family member present almost all the time a family member is in hospital was the norm. Consequently, when he began his medical training he could not understand why native-born British families did not support loved ones in this way.

Where interactions with health care professionals and folk healers have been more personal than is usual in Western medical settings, people may resist disclosing personal information if they do not understand why this is requested. Taboos against disclosing personal information to strangers can mean that discussions about wider aspects of one's life are viewed with suspicion; people may need to know more about the health care professional before being able to take on board what is said. Consequently, interactions aimed at establishing trust may be experienced as cold, overly intrusive or inappropriate (Kagawa-Singer and Blackhall, 2001; Mitchell and Mitchell, 2009).

End-of-life care presents a unique set of challenges where expectations of professional–patient relationships are discordant, as exemplified in attitudes to 'truth telling' (Candib, 2002; Gunaratnam, 2013; Mitchell and Mitchell, 2009). Until relatively recently, it was common practice in the West to avoid sharing 'bad news' (for example, that someone is terminally ill) with people who were particularly vulnerable. This practice was based on the understanding that sharing bad news might reduce the patients' ability to maintain hope, optimism and belief in their treatment, hastening the possibility of death. Growing recognition of the disadvantages of withholding such information (for example, that it robs the dying person of the chance of putting their affairs in order and isolates families at a time when they are most likely to need one another's support) means that, currently, Western practice favours being far more open.

However, in many other societies, speaking openly and sharing 'bad news' with someone who is vulnerable continues to be seen as inappropriate, uncaring or even damaging (Kagawa-Singer and Blackhall, 2001): although communicating more indirectly is seen as withholding from a current Western perspective, it may reflect a different appreciation of the care and sensitivity that is needed when someone is ill and faces the possibility of death. This tends to be true of many people from South American, Chinese and Middle Eastern societies (Tse, Chong and Fok, 2003). The emphasis Western medical practice places on the individual's right to information and to reach their own decisions about care is likely to be seen as inappropriate or uncaring where the rest of the family are expected to contribute to, or take full responsibility for, these decisions. Similarly, where people are from cultures where older people are accorded greater respect than is usual in the West (as in the Arab Muslim world) and an older relative (often an older brother) is expected to act as the main decision maker and spokesperson, older relatives are likely to feel affronted if they are not consulted, particularly where the condition is terminal (Fedorocicz and Walczyk, 2006; Tellez-Giron, 2007).

Expectations of the family

Across all cultures, the family is central to experiences of illness and health care, influencing decisions about when to seek medical attention, providing care and negotiating the emotional consequences of illness and the threat of death (Rolland, 1994). The family is also central to experiences of culture and ethnic identity: it links us with preceding and succeeding generations and provides the markers of successful development. However, although many immigrants draw on family experiences to find the strength to move on and make meaning of their lives following the disruptions associated with migration, the family is often the main arena for expressing and negotiating cross-cultural tensions and conflicts in identity (Phinney and Ong, 2007).

As discussed earlier, in working cross-culturally, one potential source of tension is that while Western industrialized societies view individuation and autonomy as integral to psychological development and emotional wellbeing, more collective societies prioritize a greater sense of interdependency with family and the wider community, as is true of many Muslim Arab, Asian and African societies. Consequently, whilst remaining closely connected with one's family may seem problematic when viewed from a Western perspective (as reflected in the pathologizing terms 'enmeshed' and 'overly involved'), where a higher value is placed on connectedness (for example, where children are brought up as part of an extended family with the mother- or brother-in-law playing a significant role) the drive towards independence is more likely to be seen as problematic.

Likewise, where greater emphasis is placed on interdependency the desire to maintain harmony and avoid conflict can mean people do not ask questions or provide information that contradicts the health professionals' view even if they do not agree and do not intend to act on what they are told. In some cases, the links between the individual, family and culture extend to ancestors, as in traditional Chinese culture (Lee and Chan, 2004). However, as with Jane and her family, it is important to take account of the intersection between cultural beliefs and other aspects of experience, including particular family dynamics:

> Jane, a white British-born young mother, sought help as she was finding it difficult dealing with her 4-year-old son's grief following the sudden death of his father, Chinese-born Chang, as she felt overwhelmed by her own feelings of grief. What she found particularly difficult and confusing was her parents-in-law's reluctance to have anything to do with their grandson. Conversations with a Chinese colleague helped me understand that although Chinese cultures tend to be more accepting of death than is usual in the West this is more

complicated when the deceased is a child. This is particularly difficult when the deceased is an only child like Chang: because children are required to perform certain rituals at their parent's funeral, their death poses a threat to the wellbeing of the surviving parents as well as the wider community. Over the course of our work, it became apparent there had been long-standing disagreements between Chang and his parents, including their disapproval of his choice of career and decision to 'marry out'. However, what was different now was that she needed their support and wanted her son to engage with the only people who could share stories of what his father was like when he was her son's age.

In working cross-culturally there may be cultural differences in constructions of what good parenting entails. While Western psychological theories prioritize the dyadic relationship between a child and one caregiver (Bowlby, 1969/1999), in many other societies the extended family and other affiliates are more central to the child's upbringing. For example, in many parts of Africa practicalities mean children spend far more time away from parents than is usual in the West: this has the effect of strengthening family ties and spreading the costs and benefits of children (Skovdal and Daniel, 2012).

Approaches to parenting styles are not simply transferred from parents to children, and in the case of migrants from one's country of origin to the country of settlement, but are informed by the wider socio-economic and political context in which one lives (O'Conner and Scott, 2007; Phoenix and Husain, 2007). Studies of cultural differences in parenting suggest that authoritative styles of parenting (being supportive and setting clear expectations with moderate limits) are more effective than authoritarian (monitoring children more tightly), permissive ('indulgent') and withdrawn ('uninvolved') styles of parenting (Darling, 1999). However, studies that take account of ethnicity, social class and gender produce outcomes that run counter to these conclusions. Moreover, first-generation Chinese children whose parents adopt an authoritarian approach have been found to do as well as those whose parents act in a more authoritative way (McLoyd et al., 2000).

It is also important to take account of how assessments of good parenting are reached. For example, researchers with an insider knowledge of the cultural grouping they are studying rate parent–child interactions differently to those who are outsiders: Russell, Crockett and Chao (2010) found that interactions between Chinese parents and children that 'outsiders' rated as authoritarian and lacking in warmth were rated differently by researchers with an insider understanding of the value of giving children clear concrete guidelines, and providing practical and instrumental support rather than purely verbal expressions of support. Similarly, researchers with an inside experience of Latino culture rated interactions between Latino parents and children normal which white middle class American researchers rated as overprotective (Falicov, 2013). Although there are few comparable studies in the UK, those that have been conducted present similar findings (Phoenix and Husain, 2007).

Of particular relevance to situations of illness is that whilst current Western practice favours being open with children about their health, encouraging children to ask questions and express how they feel, parents from cultures where parents and other older relatives are expected to ask questions on behalf of children, and where emotional expression is considered harmful to health and maintaining harmonious relationships, are likely to view this approach with scepticism (Gray et al., 2014; Thibodeaux and Deatrick, 2007). For example, in their study of the views of parents living in mainland China on parenting a child with cancer, the parents Martinson and Yee (2003) interviewed thought bad news and sadness should not be discussed with their children and tended to withhold the diagnosis from grandparents for fear of being blamed for the child's illness. Moreover, although many drew on a combination of Western medicine, traditional medicine and nutritional cures, they avoided sharing this with health care professionals. Similar findings arose from studies of Taiwanese parents caring for a child with cancer: many parents reported drawing on traditional and Western medicine in trying to restore the child's health, attached particular importance to the support of the extended family and religious beliefs (Taoism, Buddhism and Catholicism), and felt there was stigma associated with a child having cancer and dying (Mu et al., 2001; Mu, Ma Hwang and Chao, 2002).

In some cases working cross-culturally involves engaging with people whose gendered beliefs and practices run counter to our own understanding of the rights and positions of men and women, as for example in working with women who had children far earlier than is usual in the West and who we feel are unable to nurture their children because they are still in need of nurturance themselves; when working with people who regard sexual segregation as more important than we do, where women defer (and are expected to defer) to husbands and other male relatives in relation to their own health and the health of their children, and men answer questions posed to their wives and mothers; and where grandmothers and mothers see it as their responsibility to ensure their daughters are circumcised.

Finding the right balance between respecting and questioning cultural differences can be enormously difficult: while some of the gendered differences mentioned above may appear to be indicators of the submission of women and infringements of human rights from a Western perspective, this may not be the experience of the women themselves. This does not mean adopting a level of cultural relativism whereby one cannot question cultural beliefs and attitudes we see as oppressive and at odds with the values of equality, freedom and personal integrity, including honour killing and female genital mutilation (Rober and De Haene, 2014). Nevertheless, it is important to recognize that prejudice and the desire to defend our own views and experiences can result in ascribing problems to others.

It is also important to take account of beliefs, values and practices that are shared. For example, across all cultures 'parenting' involves some level of nurturance and control: all children need love, even if the child's primary caregiver is not a biological parent. Similarly it is not only 'others' (parents living in mainland China and Taiwan) who are fearful of telling their child they are seriously ill, explore alternative methods of treatment when Western medicine does not appear to be helping, turn to their extended family at times of difficulty and feel responsible when their child is seriously ill.

Communication and language barriers

Language is integral to our ability to structure and provide meaning to experiences, form relationships and express what we need. Consequently, where the providers and recipients of health care cannot communicate in the same language, it is more difficult to take a clear history, assess the severity of the symptoms and understand the needs of the people with whom they are working. It is also more difficult for ill people and their families to make sense of what professionals say, ask questions and reach informed decisions about care. As such, it is hardly surprising that researchers have found a strong link between language proficiency, health status, use of health care services and the outcome of health care (de Graaf and Franke, 2009; Granger and Baker, 2003; Kai, 2013; van den Muisjenburgh et al., 2013). For example, de Graaf and Franke found that a high percentage of GPs and home care nurses working in the Netherlands felt that problems in communication meant that Turkish and Moroccan migrants who died had not received sufficient care or an explanation about their disease that they could understand, informal carers had been unnecessarily overburdened and making appointments had been more difficult. Similar findings emerged from studies of the health care professionals working with non-English-speaking hospice patients and families in English-speaking countries (MacGrath, Vun and McLeod, 2001).

Communication is not confined to the verbal: unless there are significant visual problems, most of us rely on non-verbal cues, including body language and gesture. This is particularly true where words are difficult to understand and hear and when the messages we receive are ambiguous. This can be confusing when people have a different language and cultural background to our own: although the meanings ascribed to some forms of body language and gesture are universal, others are situational, depend on the context and relationship between the people concerned, and vary from one culture to another.

It is beyond the scope of this chapter to offer a comprehensive account of all potential differences but it's worth mentioning, for example, that although in the West moving one's head up and down is a sign of agreement and from side to side disagreement, this is not necessarily applicable elsewhere. Likewise, although a 'thumbs up' gesture conveys approval or appraisal in most Western countries, it is a sign of insult in some other countries. Although eye contact is usually a sign of attentiveness, honesty and respect in Western societies, in many Middle Eastern, Asian, Hispanic and Native American countries eye contact is regarded as disrespectful, particularly when a woman makes eye contact with a man as this is understood to indicate sexual interest. There are also cultural differences in the amount of personal space we need and see as appropriate (Juckett, 2005). Similarly, while some form of physical contact (for example, the shaking of hands) and exchanging information about oneself and family is a way of greeting and recognizing the personhood of another in many societies, this is not the case for certain cultural groups. For example, the religious beliefs of orthodox Jews and Muslims mean it is forbidden to shake hands with, let alone hug, someone of a different gender.

In addition, there may also be differences in the value ascribed to how much one says. In Western societies (particularly the US) saying more tends to be a way of demonstrating power and knowledge. However, in many other societies, people believe it is better to speak more selectively, to listen, gather one's thoughts and compose oneself before responding to what has been said or asked (Greenfield, Quiroz and Raeff, 2000; Wang and Li, 2007). Likewise, people from individualistic societies tend to be more open in showing how they feel, while those from collective societies are more likely to suppress facial expressions, a pattern that is understood to relate to the desire to avoid drawing attention to the uniqueness of the individual and disrupting the harmony of the community (Wong, Bond and Mosquera, 2008).

In drawing attention to these differences it is not my intention to suggest that one needs to be tentative in engaging with people from a different cultural background: instead it has been to illustrate how unwittingly interactions intended to be respectful can come across as inappropriate or even dismissive. For example, a Columbian woman interviewed about her experience of health care said that despite living in the UK for 19 years, she returned home every year for medical check-ups because 'doctors here don't look you in the eye and they don't even touch you' (Gideon, 2013, pp. 173–174). Similarly, working in Kosovo, where social interactions are far more tactile than the UK, opened my eyes to how strange it might seem for distressed and traumatized people to be seen for therapy in the UK where, other than in exceptional circumstances, physical touch between a therapist and client is discouraged.

Interpreting

As discussed in greater detail in Chapter 7, where the recipients of health care are not fluent in the main language of the country, it is preferable to be seen by a bilingual professional who is fluent in their first language. For example, in trying to comfort patient anxiety during the treatment process, it is so much better if one is able to speak the same language. Most of us are more comfortable and less embarrassed about discussing personal and family problems without a third party present. At a more practical level, bilingual or multilingual staff play an important role in pointing out directions that could help the patient recover more efficiently and safely: as aftercare is one of the most critical processes in recovery, a timely recovery may depend on how thoroughly the at-home instructions are understood and followed.

Being seen by a professional who speaks one's language has the additional benefit of allowing for language switching, as required when a child is fluent in English but has limited understanding of their parents' first language. For example, language switching can be used to clarify points of language and inhibit or amplify expressions and connections with feelings. However, when working in a shared 'other' language the boundaries between the personal and professional can become more difficult to maintain: both parties can find themselves pulled into a pattern of over-identification and apparent shared sense of otherness in a foreign world, and colluding in the idealizing of a lost culture and the life that might have been (Akhtar, 2006; Antinucci, 2004; Costa, 2014).

Where, as is often the case, this is not feasible, the NHS provides access to the services of a trained interpreter. Using a professionally trained interpreter reduces the chances of misunderstandings and offers the possibility of discussing issues one is unwilling to share with family or friends (Flores, 2005). However, concerns about confidentiality mean some people are reluctant to use interpreters, and prefer asking someone from their family or a friend to interpret for them (Davies and Bath, 2001). This is particularly likely where past experiences or current living conditions are seen as shameful, where people have migrated from a situation of political conflict and/or there is a desire to hide certain aspects of their lives from the immigration authorities.

Whilst drawing on the services of family and friends runs counter to NHS policy, in general family and friends are trusted and share a similar world-view, and particularly where people feel disempowered, it shifts the balance of power more in the patient's favour (Greenhalgh, Robb and Scambler, 2006). Where parents are unable to speak or read the majority language of the community in which they live, children may take responsibility for interpreting and mediating social transactions involving speech, writing or signing. Unless children are very young, where their contribution is recognized the experience can be empowering, leading to an increase in intimacy and trust with their parent (Cline, Crafter and Prokopiou, 2014). However, as discussed in Chapter 5, language brokering can have more problematic consequences for intergenerational relationships, particularly where children are expected to translate disturbing information.

Interpreting requires enormous skill: depending on the nature of the consultation, interpreters are required to shift between the multiple and potentially conflicting roles of translator, interpersonal mediator, system mediator, educator, advocate and link worker. Because conversations are mediated through a third person, it is often more difficult to establish the person's concerns, check their understanding and know how they are feeling (Flores, 2005; Kai, 2013; Kai, Beavan and Faull, 2011). Similarly, in interpreted conversations patients do not say as much, ask fewer questions, there is less humour, discussion of patients' own feelings and ideas about their social context. Consequently, despite attempts to establish a collaborative relationship, communication can become overly strategic rather than a sincere effort to achieve understanding and reach consensus (Greenhalgh, Robb and Scambler, 2006; Seale, Rivas and Kelly, 2013).

There is also a potential for the power dynamics that dominate the outside world to invade the consulting room: institutional dynamics may mean interpreters find themselves in a subjugated or even disempowered position in relation to the health care professional and the setting in which they are working (Maitra and Krause, 2015). Moreover, although interpreters often act as a bridge between the minority community and mainstream society, this is not always the case. In some situations the interpreter is a bilingual person who is not from the same minority ethnic group, and in others, despite coming from the same country, differences in accent that reflect membership of another socio-economic and/or political grouping can interfere with the possibilities of feeling respected and understood.

In the context of a busy clinic or hospital, it may not be feasible to set aside additional time to debrief. However, where possible, meeting with the interpreter after the consultation provides a space to reflect on potential misunderstandings and questions that might seem culturally inappropriate. It also means there is a space for interpreters to reflect on resonances with their own experiences, including experiences of not understanding, discrimination and dislocation.

> For example, Dalilleh, a Farsi interpreter who left Iran with her parents as a very young child found discussions about a couple's difficulties in learning English and accommodating to life in the UK extremely painful: they reminded her of her own experience of growing up in a home with immigrant parents who struggled to readjust to living in the UK and her embarrassment about their inability to learn English.

Recommendations for practice

To engage sensitively with people who have a different cultural background to ourselves, it is important to have sufficient knowledge and understanding of their cultural beliefs and practices, the contextual challenges they face (including racism, other forms of discrimination and the socio-economic and acculturation stresses associated with migration), and our own cultural experiences, gaps in understanding and prejudices. To achieve this, all health care trainings need to include modules that focus on cultural constructions of health and illness, 'cultural competence' (Cross, 1988) and self-reflexive exercises aimed at increasing one's 'cultural attunement' (Falicov, 2013) with those deemed as 'other'.

It is also important to examine existing clinical and preventative practices, engage with grass-roots methods and resources within the extended family, community and spiritual tradition to ensure that the services provided are accessible, flexible, compatible with people's culture and life experience and address the needs of their community. This includes discussing the cultural ramifications of illness, disability, death and health care with colleagues, community leaders and others from diverse backgrounds, attending relevant trainings and drawing on the research and clinical literature (Falicov, 2013; Guregard and Seikkula, 2014; Maitra and Krause, 2015; Papadopoulos, 2007). Nonetheless, it is also important to bear in mind that the views of any one person, whether an academic, health care professional or religious leader, will never be able to capture the full complexity of the beliefs, practices and experiences of an entire cultural (and racialized) group.

Matching cultural and language background

As cultural and language barriers have the potential to challenge the delivery of patient-focused care, it can be enormously helpful to be seen by a professional with insider experience of the same cultural background who is fluent in the same language. This limits the possibility of misunderstandings arise and exacerbating the sense of 'being out of place' (Probyn, 2004) that so often accompany experiences of illness, migration and cultural diversity.

There is considerable evidence that when people feel some sense of commonality with the health care professionals they see, they tend to require fewer additional diagnostic tests and referrals, recovery is less complicated and there is greater satisfaction (Zoppi and Epstein, 2002). As such, it could be extremely helpful to increase the numbers of trained health care professionals who are bilingual. Indeed, one study found that training GP receptionists to contact patients led to a modest increase in uptake in screening: however, where the receptionists were from the same cultural grouping and shared the same language, the increase in the rates of uptake was far greater (Atri, Falshaw, Gregg et al., 1997).

However, this is not always possible or ideal. For example, where one is from a highly politicized country or feels ashamed of one's life following migration, it may feel preferable to see someone who has no connection with one's past. Moreover, although many health care professionals feel a particular commitment to working with people from their country of origin and/or with a similar background, some do not, as confining one's work to this population has the potential to frame oneself as 'other'.

Furthermore, as mentioned earlier, where there are considerable overlaps in experience, personal–professional boundaries can become more difficult to maintain, pulling both parties into a pattern of over-identification (Akhtar, 2006; Antinucci, 2004). Indeed, speaking the language in which one was brought up rather than trained can trigger visceral memories and cause one to lose one's professional grip in remembering pleasurably other experiences of an earlier time in life (Costa, 2014).

Engaging with cultural differences

In cross-cultural work, clinical interactions are often 'a matter of different persons carrying the baggage of different culture and [bringing] different experiences of power and discrimination into the meeting' (Maitra and Krause, 2015, p. 237). Even if we feel able to empathize with the position of the other, we need to extend our understanding in order to engage imaginatively with their dilemmas, suffering and experience of life: what seems wrong at first may become more meaningful and/or appropriate if we use our imagination and skill and begin with what makes sense to the other. This means viewing the person who is suffering (and/or their family) as the expert of their experience in knowing what hurts, what makes a difference and what risks are and are not worth taking.

Establishing common ground with peoples whose experiences are different to our own involves listening to get a better understanding of what they are going through, encouraging them to bring their ideas about illness and health care to the encounter, and working towards integrating what we are told with what we know about Western medicine. This is important because, with the exception of situations where traditional healers caution people against life-saving medication (for example, telling people who are HIV positive that they should not take ARVs), non-Western methods may prove helpful: even if these other methods do not prove helpful, they need not cause harm. Moreover, validating rather than discrediting people's views reduces the likelihood of a delay in relying more wholeheartedly on Western methods of treatment should other methods fail (Flores, 2000). However, to be able to hold both frameworks in mind and move towards some form of integration, we need to value the cultural context, beliefs, wisdom and practices of the people with whom we work.

This does not mean discounting our clinical experience, training and understanding, but working towards establishing some sense of shared understanding even if moments of understanding are only fleeting. It also means being ready to acknowledge our inability to do so in ways that enhance rather than damage relationships with the people with whom we are working, for example by asking such questions as:

- Can you explain what problems the illness is causing for you?

- What do you think caused the problem?

- Why do you think it started and when?

- How severe do you think your condition is?

- What kind of treatment do you think you need?

- What results are you hoping to receive from treatment?

- What aspects of illness do you fear most?

- How would this condition be treated in the country where you grew up?[21]

Questions like these can help to ensure we are more aware of issues that people see as important. For example, questions about the treatment people would have been able to access in their country of origin can open up discussions about ideas of causality that are influencing their experiences of illness, or lead on to learning what other methods they are using to alleviate their symptoms. However, it is unfair to burden people who have serious health concerns with the additional burden of acting as our 'cultural interpreters'. Moreover they are unlikely to know where our gaps in understanding lie. Furthermore, although many people value the opportunity of discussing their cultural values and practices, we need to tread carefully to avoid positioning the people we are working with as 'other'. It is also important to be mindful of the way in which we ask questions and speak, and remain alert to the possibilities of misunderstandings. In some situations, it is helpful to address tensions arising from experiences of difference within the consultation, for example by asking such questions as:

- It seems like we are of a different age, gender and have different cultural backgrounds: should we think about this now or come back to this later if it seems relevant?

- Is there anything you would like to discuss that we have not considered yet?

- I am interested in how different aspects of our lives influence wellbeing and experiences of support at times of illness, including cultural and spiritual beliefs: can you say how this relates to you?[22]

- I have a feeling that what I have just said/asked seems inappropriate: is that the case?

I asked a Kurdish couple, Zohar and Ahmed, who had serious concerns about their adolescent daughter, whether they ever took a break from worrying about her, for example by going out for a walk or coffee together. Zohar smiled and seemed to view this idea positively. However, her husband responded by saying 'being romantic is not in our culture'. In asking this question, it was not my intention to focus on their relationship but to encourage them to engage with life outside of their home and worries. Paradoxically, acknowledging and laughing about this misunderstanding helped to shift the tone, creating a more collaborative relationship: following this exchange they begin to speak more openly about the difficulties of bringing up children in a context in which they found it difficult learning English, and where the rules of bringing up children and the lifestyles they were exposed to were very different to what they had known.

To discuss such differences openly, people like Zohar and Ahmed need to trust that they are respected, that their beliefs and practices will not be trivialized and that discussions about ethnicity, racialization, gender and age will not have a damaging effect on the care they receive. People also need to feel we can hear, are moved by their experience but are not over-whelmed by what we are told (Rathbone, 2009). This means being clear about our own boundaries, including what we are and are not ready to disclose to others (Maitra and Krause, 2015).

However, it is important to avoid reducing culture to an alternate, enclosed space, underplaying and guarding against discussions about culture, positioning this aspect of identity as more significant than others, and fram-ing people deemed to be 'other' responsible for practices that occur more widely (Daniels, 2012; Rober and de Haene, 2014): it is not only amongst migrants, ethnic and racialized 'others' that women are at risk of being sub-ordinated and oppressed, and that the rights of children are not respected. Likewise, Western notions of individuation are not only less applicable to people from cultures that prioritize greater interdependency but to the posi-tion of most Western women as well (Gilligan and Brown, 1993).

Indeed, cross-cultural work is likely to involve moving beyond our comfort zones and venturing into unexplored areas, including questions about our own existential dilemmas, cultural values and prejudices, and confronting feelings that are uncomfortable to acknowledge, including the shame, anxiety, powerlessness and irritation that stem from privilege and oppression. However, because many aspects of culture and privilege are implicit, we may not realize when our own beliefs, values and styles of communicating limit our ability to hear and engage with someone else. For example, fears of replicating the mistakes of colonialism and of being seen as racist can lead to a level of cultural relativism that makes it dif-ficult to question cultural beliefs and attitudes which we see as oppressive and at odds with the values of equality, freedom and personal integrity (Rober and De Haene, 2014).

There are no predictable routes to follow: often the best we can do is approach one another with some kind of understanding and recognize that there may be misunderstandings we are unaware of. However, unless we attempt to inhabit the unfamiliar, there is a risk of becoming over-whelmed and disempowered, seeing others as less human and progressive and discounting their experience (Maitra and Krause, 2015). Indeed, as in all work with illness, intercultural work involves dealing with the constant tension between sameness and difference and the need to be mindful of the particular while remaining sensitive to the universal, being able to listen, make informed guesses, lay aside our assumptions, take risks and draw on our shared experience of humanity.

5
INDIVIDUAL AND FAMILY EXPERIENCES OF MIGRATION

Most of the earlier attempts to understand the causes, processes and consequences of migration were aimed at establishing a model that would be applicable to all forms of migration. That was at a time when travel and communication were less available and most migrants were expected to settle in the country to which they moved. Since then, the rates of migration have intensified, with greater numbers of migrants and refugees drawing from and moving to an ever-widening number of countries. At the same time, the globalization of production, distribution, exchange and evolution in technology and social networking have opened up societies in ways that were unimaginable before (Braziel and Mannur, 2003). As such, most people's lives are bound up with the entanglements and consequences of dispersion at some level (Brah, 1996).

Diasporic studies have had a considerable impact on understandings of migration. The concept of diaspora refers to the longing and mental fragmentation experiences of dispersion tend to evoke. It is concerned with belonging, with the ways in which people make sense of 'borderland identities' (Rosaldo, 1989), where instead of living according to one cultural or meaning system, people are faced with negotiating the similarities and differences between two or more systems. Although diaspora was originally confined to forced migrations, its use has been extended to any grouping that retains a sense of national, racial and/or ethnic identity when dispersed across national, geographic and social divisions (Brah, 1996; Papastergiades, 2000).

Migration is, and has always been, a family affair. In the past, where the prospects of employment were limited, young men moved to seek work to earn enough money to send back and build a home, or to bring wives and children to join them. However, the demographics of international migration have shifted: at present half the world's migrants are women who leave as the primary migrant, rather than to join family members as in the past. Although women work in all sectors of the labour market, a high proportion work in areas associated with traditional gendered roles such as teaching, health care and domestic work, including caring for children and the elderly (Ehrenreich and Hochschild, 2003; Lutz, 2008).

While many mothers and fathers leave their children in the care of other family members (usually women), some are able to bring their children with them or send for them at a later stage. Others move after having children or to join their migrant adult children in later life. Indeed, in some contexts migrating for work is an almost expected aspect of life, as in the Caribbean (Chamberlain, 2006) and Philippines (Parrenas, 2014). However, regardless of whether one chooses or is forced to leave, and whether the move is permanent or temporary, family ties, obligations, hopes and memories are integral to experiences of migration (Falicov, 2013).

Until recently, relatively little attention was paid to the experiences of non-migrant kin. This may reflect uncertainty about whether a family continues to be a unit when some members move and start their 'own' family. Because most of the earlier scholars of migration were migrants themselves, this omission suggests a reluctance to engage with experiences that could challenge their views of self, family and migration, for example guilt about parents, sisters and brothers who remained in situations of political conflict, and the contrast between their own opportunities and obligations and those of their non-migrant kin. However, even though non-migrants do not move from one geographic territory to another, the migration of a parent, child, sister or brother means that the 'emotional territory' in which they live is different to what it might have been: while migrants face disruptions to anticipated experiences of family that are a consequence of their own decision to leave, non-migrants are faced with re-establishing agency and adjusting to disruptions that relate to someone else's decisions rather than their own (Falicov, 2013).

Over the last 20 years there has been a shift to exploring how geographically dispersed families 'forge and sustain the multi-stranded social, economic and political relations that link together societies of origin and settlement, creating transnational social fields that cross national borders' (Basch, Glick Schiller and Blanc-Szanton, 1994, p. 6). This includes looking at the ways in which remittances, economic ties, rituals, stories and memories shape relationships between those who leave, those who stay, those who come and go, and subsequent generations of children and grandchildren. Transnational studies have shown how the stories and memories families share (including stories of home, the arrival, alienation and connections with the host nation) transmit values, beliefs and expectations across generations (Chamberlain, 2006; Chamberlain and Leydesdorff, 2004; Haagsman and Mazzucato, 2014; Parrenas, 2014). They have also shown that looking to family memories can be more complicated when experiences of family are troubled, when one's cultural traditions are seen to be inferior to those of the country in which one lives and when it is difficult to disentangle family memories from memories of living in an oppressive society (Al-Ali, 2002; Altschuler, 2008a). Indeed, studies of Italian migrants living in the UK (Fortier, 2000) and Chinese migrants in the USA (Wang, 2004) illustrate how it is not only the stories one chooses to tell but those one omits to tell that recruit children and grandchildren into idealized or denigrated constructions of their parents' past and country of origin.

Separation and loss

Experiences of migration are far from uniform: they vary depending on such factors as whether migration was voluntary or coerced, whether the family unit moved together or sequentially, the proximity between one's country of origin and current place of residence, age, gender, health status, financial opportunities, socio-political factors, prior experiences of support, loss and trauma, and whether or not people moved within their own country before migrating, for example, from impoverished rural circumstances to urban areas (Bornstein, 2013; Falicov, 2013; Fortier, 2000).

For many, migration offers access to far greater physical, economic and political security, fluidity in gendered roles, better professional and educational opportunities and more independence than seemed possible at home. Indeed, situations of uncertainty and disorganization offer the possibility of a 'third individuation' (Akhtar, 1995), of developing a different and more comfortable understanding and experience of oneself and others. For many people this is impossible: the practical and emotional challenges associated with dislocations in social, financial and geographic experience mean life is dominated by loss, loneliness, economic uncertainty and exposure to prejudice.

Moreover, even if migration offers access to better opportunities, all migrations are accompanied by some sense of loss and disarray (Falicov, 2013). Geographic journeys tend to be accompanied by unconscious inner journeys, anxieties and fears about losing loved ones, aspects of self and a sense of being held (Grinberg and Grinberg, 1984; Neyzi, 2004). Experience that sustained and anchored one's identity before, including interactions with family, friends and colleagues, are absent, even if only temporarily. Some families spend long periods apart before being reunited. Many are confronted with very different lifestyles and forced to make adjustments that challenge core ideas of what family, couple, intergenerational and sibling relationships entail.

Refugees and asylum seekers face an additional set of challenges: many will have endured traumatic experiences in their home country, on their journey to another country and/or in detention centres, to be faced with the practical and emotional stresses of trying to secure a residence permit, living in poverty and adjusting to life in a markedly different society in which their qualifications are not recognized (Heeren et al., 2012; Kirmayer et al., 2011). Drawing on his own experience, Said argued that exile creates an 'unhealable rift [...] between the self and its true home' whereby 'the achievements of exile are permanently undermined by the loss of something left behind for ever' (Said, 2002, p. 173).

As such, it is unsurprising that studies of clinical populations found a strong link between migration and increased rates of depression, marital conflict and identity crises (Golding and Burnham, 1990; Hyman, Guruge and Mason, 2008), particularly amongst people who are poorer and less educated. However, the link appears to be weaker amongst non-clinical populations: many first-generation migrants experience far better physical and mental health than second-generation migrants or native-born peers (Suarez-Orozco, Rhodes and Milburn, 2009). As mentioned previously, this pattern has been attributed to 'selective migration' (the notion that people who migrate tend to be physically as well as psychologically more robust), the hope and strength new beginnings can inspire, and fact that first generations are usually able to draw on at least two frames of reference: those related to their country of origin and the country to which they move (Bhugra, 2004; McDonald and Kennedy, 2004).

One of the more complex challenges migrants and their non-migrant kin face is how much to hold onto or let go of the past. Holding onto 'uchronic imaginings' (Portelli, 2000), to how life might have been if history had taken a different course, can be enormously sustaining: it allows those who live elsewhere to remain an ongoing 'emotional presence' (Boss, 2006) and constructs traditional values and lifestyles as enduring despite experiences that challenge this. However, prioritizing these imaginings can mean the differences between anticipated and lived experience remain at the forefront of one's mind, 'freezing' understandings of self, family and community. The gap between physical absence and psychological presence tends to be particularly intense for people who hold onto the dream of a return when this is impossible (for example, when contact with their country of origin is cut off), with unrealistic reunion fantasies limiting the possibilities of engaging with new ideas, relational networks and the language of the country in which they are living (Falicov, 2013).

In contrast, although letting go of the past can speed up the process of acculturation, it limits the possibilities of reworking the past in the context of the present and drawing on memories and familiar social values that can be sustaining in situations of flux. For example, on migrating to Israel in the 1950s and 1960s, Moroccan Jews faced considerable external pressure to adjust their lives to fit in as well as internalized pressure to avoid being seen as outsiders. These pressures led to an erosion of the positions of their religion, community and patriarchy, without anything else being put in its place. What made this more difficult was that, as in many other countries, the policy of dispersal limited the possibility of rebuilding ethnic community links (Shavit, 2013).

As discussed previously, current experiences of loss have the potential to trigger unconscious as well as conscious thoughts and feelings that relate to past loss. The likelihood of the past influencing responses to the present is particularly important to bear in mind in working with refugees who have experienced rape, torture and other forms of brutality (McColl, McKenzie and Bhui, 2008; Roizblatt, Biederman and Brown, 2014; Sluzki, 1993).

Even where experiences are less traumatic, the combination of 'culture shock' (Handlin, 1973) and reduced access to the relationships and concrete objects that were intrinsic to experiences of self tend to challenge the newcomer's psychic organization, creating a sense of flux reminiscent of earlier separations and evoking feelings that relate to conscious and unconscious memories of the past (Akhtar, 1995). This may account for the frequency with which people who moved when younger express a desire to retire 'back home' and re-establish links with the people and places that were central to their previous lives as they get older (Hernandez and McGoldrick, 1999; Rutter and Andrews, 2009; Walters, 2002).

For example, Hammerton (2004) found that people who moved from Britain to Canada in the 1950s tended to emphasize triumph over material and cultural obstacles in the early post-migratory years, and only expressed concern about broken family ties when they approached retirement, their children were older and access to social networks in their country of settlement had reduced. This suggests that earlier accounts of success were a defence against facing the losses and uncertainties posed by migrating.

Indeed, it can be difficult to mourn as even though migration may have resulted in the loss of face-to-face contact with family and friends, familiar customs, language, foods, music, rituals, geography and climate, unlike death these losses are not absolute or irretrievable: in many cases, everyone is still alive and it is possible to imagine a return or reunion. It is also possible to miss home, not know what and where home is anymore, and refuse to go home, all at once (Wood, 2013). Moreover, the place to which one returns is usually very different to the place one left, partly because one has changed, and partly because of circumstances 'back home'. When people who fled Kosovo during the war of 1999 returned, places that had represented the embodiment of safety and special memories were infused with memories of destruction, death and betrayal: their houses, places of communal gathering and cinemas had been destroyed and people they had known before were missing or dead.[23]

Understanding responses to migration

Based on extensive work with immigrants and his own migration from Argentina to the US, Sluzki (1979) proposed that most immigrants go through a series of phases in coming to terms with migration, which include a preparatory stage, during which periods of elation may be followed by multiple anxieties and dismay. This is followed by the actual act of migration, a transition with few rituals that may take a few hours as with an aeroplane journey, or far longer as tends to be the case for refugees and asylum seekers. There is often a period of overcompensation after this when loss and dissonance are underplayed in the interests of survival and adaptation. This is usually followed by a period of de-compensation, during which people are faced with coming to terms with altered life circumstances and the dissonance between the beliefs and customs of their country of migration and the country in which they live. Sluzki draws attention to the potentially long-lasting consequences of migration in discussing ways in which experiences of loss and intercultural conflicts transmit loss from one generation to the next.

However, responses to migration are far more varied. As Falicov (2013) suggests, to make sense of individual and family responses to migration it is important to take account of the factors related to migration/acculturation, ecological context, family organization and family life cycle:

Migration and acculturation:

- Type of migration (for example, whether they are legally entitled to remain or undocumented)

- Composition of separations (for example, whether children moved with a father, mother or as an unaccompanied asylum seeker)

- Trauma experienced before, during and/or after migration

- Balance between the losses and gains

- Uprooting of meaning – physical, social, cultural and political

- Transnationalism – relationships between migrants and non-migrants

- Changes over time

- Process of acculturation

- Spontaneous rituals
- Second-generation transnational exposure
- Adolescent–parent bi- or multiculturalism.

Ecological context:

- Poverty
- Work, school
- Neighbourhood
- Isolation
- Ethnic community
- Virtual community
- Spiritual resources
- Cultural understandings of illness and health care (including interactions with health and care professionals)
- Racism, other forms of discrimination and anti-immigration reception
- Contextual stressors – language, social network.

Family organization:

- Separations and reunifications
- Long-distance connections
- Other people in household
- Kin care and transnational triangles
- Remittances
- Gendered transformations
- Polarizations about migration
- Boundary ambiguity.

Family life cycle:

- Cultural ideals and meanings
- Timings

- Transitions

- Rituals

- Socio-centric versus individualist constructions of family

- Patterns of child-rearing

- Intercultural developmental dilemmas (for example, autonomy versus family loyalty, parent–adolescent conflicts)

- Pile-up of transitions

- Absence of crucial life cycle markers.[24]

It is important to distinguish between stressors that are endemic to immigrant experiences and stressors that relate to pre-migration trauma, experiences that took place during transit (witnessing the drowning of loved ones, being adrift at sea for long periods before being rescued), experiences of asylum, temporary settlement, violence when staying in a refugee camp, as well as longer term settlement in the host country (Perez Foster, 2001). My own experiences suggests it is also important to take account of stresses less obviously related to migration, including stresses related to intergenerational and sibling tensions and other forms of loss.

Intergenerational transformations

A wide range of factors affect the impact of migration on parent–child relationships including the actual circumstances of migration (whether children are born before or after migration, parents move leaving their children in the care of other relatives, or as below when adult children move leaving their parents behind), differences between the cultural beliefs and family values of the country of settlement and country in which parents grew up, the socio-political context positions in the life cycle and stresses that are unrelated or predate migration.

When adult children leave parents behind

In many cases, an adult child moves in order to seek better employment and/or further their education. Where, as is often the case, parents support their child's decision and the move signifies the realization of their own dreams, many are ready to accept the problematic consequences this has for them in the interests of their offspring, and hide what they find troubling, as reflected in studies of parents 'left behind' in Albania (Vullnetari and King, 2008), Kyrgyzstan (Abelzova, Nasritdinov and Rahimov, 2009), India (Miltiades, 2002), China (Giles and Mu, 2005), Thailand (Knodel and Saengtienchai, 2007) and South Africa (Altschuler, 2008a; Marchetti-Mercer, 2012). However, as discussed in relation to illness, although hiding one's own difficulties might be aimed at protecting children, maintaining emotional connection and avoiding being seen as too needy, it can introduce a level of artificiality which interferes with the possibility of the authentic connection parents and children aspire to, and migrant children's understanding what is wanted or needed (Alvarez, 1999).

Depending on finances and other practicalities, migrants and parents are often able to keep in contact by intermittent visits, phone calls, sharing photographs and where necessary providing financial assistance. However, other than occasionally or at times of emergency they are rarely able to offer one another the practical and emotional support that is needed during difficult periods. While local paid carers, neighbours and professionals can and do play a significant role in supporting older non-migrant parents and other relatives, this cannot make up for moments of loneliness, of being able to interact in a more ordinary way, for example by meeting for a drink, walk or to watch television together. Similarly, as helpful as the advances in communication technology can be, emails and Skype calls cannot replace the 'emotional refuelling' (Akhtar, 1995) face-to-face interactions offer (Antman, 2012; Mulder and Cooke, 2009). This means that parents and their migrant children may be faced with coming to terms with the disparities between their expectations of family relationships, filial responsibility and lived experience.

In other situations, parents migrate to join their children in later life. Moving at this stage of life can be enormously challenging: in addition to leaving the familiar and adjusting to life in a new context, older adults are likely to be facing retirement, their own increased physical and mental decline and that of their peers. It is also more difficult to learn a new language and adjust to a different cultural context when one is older. Increased frailty and difficulties in establishing a new social network mean that illness and/or the death of one's partner can result in shifts in patterns of power and dependency that are uncomfortable for both parties. Where several children have settled in the same place, siblings will be faced with renegotiating their relationships in the context of parents' increased frailty.

A further potential complication is that grandparents' difficulties in adjusting can reactivate and intensify intercultural conflicts between their children and grandchildren. This is not necessarily the case: the arrival of one's parents at this stage of life offers migrant adults opportunities to reflect on, remember and reclaim aspects of the past that have lain dormant because they seemed irrelevant to the people they see on a daily basis. As importantly, grandparents can act as a bridge enabling younger generations to connect with their parents' original culture, customs and homeland (Falicov, 2013; Hernandez and McGoldrick, 1999).

When parents leave young children behind

In many situations, financial and other pressures mean parents are forced to leave their children behind on a temporary or permanent basis. As mentioned earlier, although men were more likely to leave to seek work elsewhere before, increased numbers of women are now moving to support their families, leaving their children in the care of others. However, this is not really a change: throughout the world women have been moving from rural to urban areas or from Third to First World countries to support their family by caring for the children of other parents (Ehrenreich and Hochschild, 2003; Hondagneu-Sotello, 2007; Lutz, 2008).

To date, relatively few studies have focused on the effects of parental migration on non-migrant children. Nonetheless, those that have been conducted suggest that parental migration can have positive as well as negative consequences. For example, remittances from abroad can alleviate the budget constraints non-migrant families face, resulting in a decrease in child labour and improved schooling and child health (Alcaraz, Chiquiar and Salcedo, 2012; Antman, 2011, 2012). In her study of children whose mothers left the Philippines to work elsewhere, Parrenas (2005) found that many were well adjusted.

However, the consequences for other children are more problematic. Indeed, despite being well adjusted, many of the children Parrenas interviewed felt the absence of parental support, guidance and shared experiences of everyday life (including eating together and bedtime rituals) outweighed the financial benefits, expressing regret about the loss of family intimacy, having to accept commodities rather than affection as reassurance of their parents' love and missing out on the pleasure and comfort of daily interaction.

Most studies suggest that children suffer more when a mother is absent but others suggest the opposite (Gao et al., 2010). However, it is difficult to disentangle children's experience of their parent's absence from the effect on the rest of the family. For example, where gendered roles are highly stratified and a father is absent for long periods of time, mothers tend to assume responsibility for tasks that had lain in the father's domain before, more commonly assuming responsibility for financial income and disciplining children. However, it can be difficult to assume responsibility for areas of family life one has little experience of (for example, disciplining boys). Moreover, in many situations, older children need to assume greater responsibility for such tasks as domestic chores and caring for younger siblings to free their mother to focus on other tasks. Consequently, even though children continue to receive maternal care, the increased burden their mother is carrying affects the quality of that care (Graham, Jordan and Yeoh, 2014).

In contrast, when a mother moves to work elsewhere, grandmothers and other women tend to step in to offer 'other mothering' (Parrenas, 2005). Where this is not the case, fathers who act as the primary caretaker may be forced to work long hours outside the home so that, as when a mother is absent, children may miss out on the quality of parental care they need. Moreover, in most societies, caring for children is accorded less status than paid employment and challenges deeply held beliefs about gendered roles. As such, even if the father supported and/or was the driving force behind the mother's decision to work elsewhere and is committed to caring for their children, giving up on one's own chances of paid employment can be extremely challenging.

Nonetheless, these changes in roles and responsibilities can have positive implications for the ways men and women see themselves and one another and relate to their children. Moreover, provided children receive sufficient support, having to assume greater responsibility for their own lives can be empowering: it offers children space to grow independently and develop skills that will help them when they become adults (Asis, 2006).

To make sense of the relationships between migrant parents and their 'left behind' children, it is also important to take account of the ways in which transnational ties are maintained, evolve and weaken. This includes whether or not children are raised by loving and responsible grandparents (or other relatives), whether non-migrant relatives support the parent's decision to work elsewhere, the relationships between the adults concerned, their readiness to allow the child to embrace both carers, and whether migration is embedded in the cultural memory of the family and society (Chamberlain, 2003, 2006; Falicov, 2007). For example, it is easier to maintain emotional contact where the times apart are as short as possible and where it is possible to connect with one another by phone, email, letters, by sending one another photographs, special foods, clothes and, where necessary, schoolbooks. Nevertheless, it is important to remember that non-migrant relatives may need to work long hours outside the home, and that in common with many other families, transnational families do not always function smoothly.

Many parents find living apart from their children extremely painful (Ehrenreich and Hoschild, 2003; Hondagneu-Sotello, 2007). However, factors such as shame and reticence about drawing attention to their own distress mean they tend to avoid seeking help until confronted with psychosomatic symptoms, depression or when, subsequent to being reunited with their children, children become rebellious or depressed (Smith, Lalonde and Johnson, 2004):

> Adel left her baby Lisa in the care of her own mother in the Caribbean in order to earn sufficient money in the UK to support her family. When Lisa was 12, her mother brought Lisa to live with her in the UK. However, despite attempts to remain in contact, when they met they felt like strangers to one another. Having never lived together before, Adel's attempts to make up for lost time and fears about the more liberal life style of adolescents in the UK meant she was far more restrictive of Lisa than her grandmother had been, resulting in blow-ups she and her daughter found enormously upsetting.

> The possibility of rebuilding their relationship was complicated by the fact that in coming to live with her mother, Lisa was forced to say goodbye to the people who had been her primary source of support before; her grandmother, other relatives, friends and teachers. A further complication was that Adel had a new partner with whom she had a baby. In working with this family, it was important for Adel to hear what her daughter found difficult and for Lisa to hear her mother. Exploring the impact of migration on their lives helped to normalize some of the changes they were facing, and to begin to relate differently to one another. It was also helpful sharing stories about experiences that took place while apart as a way of catching up on one another's lives.

When children are born subsequent to migration

Many families thrive when children migrate with their parents or are born subsequent to migration, but the consequences are more complicated for others. Unless families move 'en masse', parents are unable to draw on the wisdom of other relatives when faced with difficulties they cannot resolve and turn to children for support instead. While acting as parents' main source of emotional support can be empowering for children and create a special sort of intimacy, it can interfere with intergenerational boundaries, limiting parents' ability to set realistic boundaries and children's engagement in age-appropriate activities (Grinberg and Grinberg, 1989; Mendoza, Javier and Burgos, 2007; Sluzki, 1979).

It is often assumed that migration is easier for children as, unlike their parents, they tend to be more connected to their immediate family than the wider community of their country of origin. However, as with adults, children's experiences vary considerably, informed by such factors as their age at the time of moving, the nature and duration of separations from, and reunifications with, parents, siblings, grandparents, extended family and other people central to their previous lives, exposure to racism, prejudice and other hardships.

Moreover, children are rarely consulted about the decision to move, or leave friends, school and non-migrant family. Unaccompanied asylum seekers and undocumented children are particularly vulnerable, as they are subject to apprehension and the deportation of family members at any point. For example, although 19-year-old Marianne had been living in the UK since the age of 6 it was only when she started applying for a university place that she realized she had none of the legal documents she required: on attempting to rectify this her application to remain was turned down by the Home Office and she was told she would be deported 'home' to Nigeria, despite the fact that she has had no contact with her family since they arranged for her to be sent to the UK and does not know if they are alive (Tickle, 2015).

One of the other challenges parents and children face is that the desire to succeed and assimilate in a new country can mean aspects of loss and cultural dissonance are underplayed by the first generation and re-emerge as a clash between first and second generations, or in the form of disdain for those 'left behind'. In many cases, parents' own struggles in dealing with traumatic experiences, concerns about protecting their children and fears about being reported to the authorities mean children are not given an opportunity to understand and make sense of their parents' experience or their own (Falicov, 2013; Tongomoo, 2015). This means they are left to make sense of 'postmemories' (Hirsch, 1999), of the losses associated with their parents' past that they have not been told about and cannot understand:

> Gail's experience of growing up in a home with a mother who spent the Second World War in hiding and a father who had been sent to a concentration camp meant that her childhood was haunted by 'unspecified fears', powerlessness and feelings of shame she could not understand. Despite attempts to ensure her children's lives were very different to her own, looking back she feels the haunting presence of the past meant she was unable to provide her children with the sense of security they needed.

As with Gail, where childhood is dominated by unstated and unknowable fears about one's parents' past, the symbolic importance of parent–child bonds to both parties can make it difficult for parents and children to disentangle their own struggles and achievements from those of the other. Indeed, migrants who struggle to separate from their family and country of birth often work through these separation issues in relationships with their children (Falicov, 2013; Suarez-Orozco, Todorovo and Louie, 2002). Where parents are traumatized, extremely isolated, worried about finances and family back home, and/or struggling with depression and psychosomatic symptoms they may be 'emotionally absent' (Boss, 2006) despite their physical presence (Phinney and Ong, 2007).

However, as reflected in my study of the impact of migration from apartheid-based South Africa to the UK and the experience of working in Kosovo, encounters with the next generation can lead to reassessing the past. Where parents have moved from an oppressive or war-torn country, the desire to avoid being seen as shameful in the eyes of their children, the 'tokens' of their new life, can lead to rethinking their earlier stance. Likewise, encounters with the next generation can lead to rethinking the importance attached to living apart from one's non-migrant family (Altschuler, 2008a):

> 45-year-old Mary framed her decision to leave apartheid-based South Africa as a way of escaping an oppressive political system, and even more importantly, of distancing herself from parents she saw as needy and controlling. However, as her UK-born son became older, his longing for more contact with his grand-parents, aunts, uncles and cousins, and interest in what she saw as 'relics' of the past (pictures and objects from her parents' home) confronted Mary with how much she, her son and the rest of the family had lost.[25]

Access to two or more cultural frameworks

Growing up in a different time context means that parents and children often see the world differently (Bourdieu, 1991). However, this is more pronounced when migration has taken place, particularly where the beliefs and child-rearing practices of the country in which families live are very different to the context in which parents grew up. In these situations, parents are faced with bringing up children in relation to dual cultures, balancing the need to adapt to the customs and laws of their new country (acculturation) with maintaining some sense of continuity and identification with their country of origin (enculturation). The struggles to negotiate these differences, find a compromise and meet in between can intensify the more usual tensions associated with adolescence and other life-cycle transitions, impacting on parents' sense of competence and ability to 'be there' for their children:

> Rezan and Mehmet, a Kurdish couple who left Turkey about 25 years previously, talked about the difficulties of parenting in a context in which 'we haven't known the rules and regulations of bringing up a child here'. Their 19-year-old son was becoming increasingly aggressive and his 16-year-old sister, who had seemed to enjoy school before, had become increasingly withdrawn and was

thinking of leaving school. Their difficulties in learning English, and Mehmet's experience of long-term unemployment, meant that both parents felt like failures and were unable to recognize what they had and could still offer their children.

With this in mind, much of the work focused on parenting, on creating a space in which it was possible for Rezan and Mehmet to reflect on their experience, including aspects of experiences they found shameful. However, the work also involved bringing experiences of competence and control to the fore, including exploring what Rezan and Mehmet felt they had been able to offer their children, what aspects of parenting they had enjoyed, and how their children knew they were cherished. This led to sharing stories of providing their children with love, ensuring they had food, clothing and attended school. It also led to reflecting on what their children had gained from being connected with more than one country, sharing memories of visits to Turkey and the importance of their children's relationship with their now deceased grandparents. However, it was also important to look beyond the past and focus on the future (Penn, 1985), to imagine what their family might look like in years to come.

Parents from cultures where the norm is to tell a child what to do and expect obedience are likely to find this difficult to maintain with children socialized in a society in which children have more of a voice and are allowed greater individuality. What makes these situations particularly uncomfortable is that where parents have moved to secure a better life for their children, intergenerational conflicts related to adaptation can feel like an affront to the sacrifices one has made. Intergenerational conflicts often centre on socializing with opposite gender friends, developing friends from other cultures, rights, freedoms and expectations of academic performance. Conflicts with daughters tend to relate to cultural imperatives about dress, deportment, socializing with the opposite sex and the risks of pregnancy. Some teenage girls respond by leading a double life, keeping relationships secret and dressing differently when at school or in the community. Others subordinate their feelings and actions to the will of their parents, which can result in becoming depressed, anxious and preoccupied with difficulties in cultural and family adaptation.

Because boys are not at risk of becoming pregnant, they tend to be allowed greater freedom and experience less parental scrutiny. However, they are often subject to higher expectations for academic achievement. Boys who are unwilling or unable to meet these expectations may end up rejecting their parents' culture and gravitating to counter-culture groups, confronting parents with the knowledge that the next generation is unlikely to succeed in the way in which they had hoped. As with the family discussed above, when parents (particularly fathers) are unemployed, reduced status and limited control in the outside world can result in becoming more controlling within the home (Falicov, 2013).

Where disciplinary strategies accepted and valued in one's country of origin are not only discouraged but illegal, parents have to guard against drawing on familiar models of discipline and learn new ways of relating to avoid falling foul of the law and appearing shameful in the eyes of their children. Some studies indicate that where there are considerable cultural differences, parents tend to exert stricter controls than would have been the case in their country of origin, suggesting strictness is an attempt to protect oneself and one's family from risks associated with exposure to a different socio-cultural system (Portes and Rumbault, 2001; Renzaho, Green, Mellor and Swinburn, 2010). However, instead of being protective, this approach can have damaging consequences. Several studies have found a link between disciplinary crises and adolescent suicide: Lau, Jernewall, Zane and Myers (2002) found that Asian children of immigrants who were less acculturated were at greater risk of attempting suicide in situations of high parent–child conflict than their more acculturated counterparts.

This suggests parents should relax their controls and assimilate more. However, maintaining some traditional rituals with the first generation can go a long way towards restoring and maintaining family and relational resilience in stressful circumstances (Falicov, 2013). Where families retain aspects of their traditional culture, family relationships are warm and supportive and boundaries are flexible but clear, children do better in terms of their general health, mental health and education. In addition, parents are more likely to remain more influential in their children's lives and children are more likely to retain a strong and positive sense of belonging to the same ethnic group as their parents (Berry et al., 2006; Phinney and Ong, 2007). As this work suggests where children are able to maintain ties to competence-producing aspects of their parents' cultural values and traditions, there is less risk of family relationships deteriorating and children are more protected against cultural conflicts and negative influences outside home. Families appear to be more resilient where parents are able to maintain or restore a sense of continuity and coherence by selectively maintaining some aspects of their previous life's and discarding or underplaying others. In contrast, abandoning these traditions too readily is likely to have problematic consequences for intergenerational relationships.

This is more difficult where parents and children do not share any language, as the gap in experience can become so large that families do not have the resources to resolve cultural conflicts. Moreover, although there is often a shift towards embracing the culture of the dominant group after migrating, this is less likely or feasible in situations of racial and ethnic discrimination. For example, Dustman, Frattini and Theodoropoulos

(2010) found that, despite the fact that the second-generation ethnic minority immigrants they studied were better educated than their parents' generation and their white British-born peers, they were less likely to have jobs and earned lower wages, even when they had the same qualifications as white British-born peers.

However, in most situations continuity and change happen side by side. Reflecting on her position as the first generation born to parents who moved from Pakistan to the UK, Syal (2015) said that much of her adolescence was spent trying to fit in: being seen as too Western for the parents who brought her and her siblings up communally, and too foreign for the 'cool kids' at school. However, rather than turning her and her peers into a confused 'mongrel' generation, the experience of questioning their belonging, and of seeing society from two different viewpoints enhanced her generation's capacity for creativity and entrepreneurship in carving out careers in business and the arts.

Language brokering

Many immigrant parents are unable to speak or read the majority language of the country in which they live. Because children tend to learn a new language more quickly than their parents, many children contribute to family life by acting as 'language brokers' (or interpreters). In these situations, children can find themselves in a position of mediating social transactions involving speech, writing, signing forms and communicating. This may mean assuming major responsibilities for the social, administrative and economic lives of their families and for interactions with health care professionals and schools.

Debates about the consequences of language brokering for children have been dominated by Western cultural assumptions about the nature of childhood, including the assumption that children need to be protected from most adult concerns and tasks and only gradually start to engage in more adult-style responsibilities (Crafter, O'Dell, de Abreu and Cline, 2009). For example, concerns have been raised that expecting children to engage with 'adult' affairs, such as their parents' health and financial problems, will undermine the innocence and freedom from anxiety that are conducive to strong emotional growth (Cohen, Moran-Ellis and Smaje, 1999). Another concern is that language brokering might affect intergenerational power, destabilizing a family structure that has already been challenged by the experience of migration (Suárez-Orozco and Suárez-Orozco, 2001).

Although these concerns are valid, they fail to take account of cultural differences in expectations of parent–child relationships, that interpreting may be seen as 'one of those things that you do to help the family'. For example, in a study of immigrant adolescents who moved from the former Soviet Union to Israel, language brokering took place within family settings where interdependence, rather than separation and autonomy, was integral to adolescent development (Dorner, Orellana and Jiminez, 2008). Assuming language brokering will have an inevitably problematic effect on families underestimates the many nuanced ways in which migrant children and parents negotiate their different and often contradictory positions of power. Similarly, these concerns fail to take account of the empowering consequences of knowing one is trusted to tell the 'right' story, strengthening the bond between the child and their parents (Dorner, Orellana and Jiménez, 2008; Song, 1997). Moreover, there is considerable evidence that language brokers often outperform their non-brokering peers academically, and that their social interactions with teachers and peers tend to be more sophisticated (Cline, Crafter and Prokopiou, 2014; Dorner, Orellana and Jiminez, 2008; Morales and Hanson, 2005).

However, the consequences are more likely to be positive where parent–child relationships are not fraught, where children are not caught up in battles between their parents and when language proficiency is not used to make claims that relate to other aspects of their relationship. Interpreting is less problematic when it takes place in a relatively private setting which reduces the chance of causing embarrassment to the interpreter and their parents, and when children are not expected to forgo schooling and other age-appropriate activities. It is also less problematic when children are not expected to share information that is inappropriate, harmful or distressing to their parents or potentially shaming information about themselves, for example a teacher's concerns about their schooling or concerns about their compliance with medical treatment (Morales and Hanson, 2005; Shen, Kim and Chao, 2014; Wu and Kim, 2009). Indeed, in these situations it is not unusual for children to censor or embellish what is said. Moreover, where children are expected to interpret for parents in negotiations with the authorities (for example, in arguing their need to be re-housed) and the request is not granted it can be difficult to know whether the decision would have been different if parents had been able to speak on their own behalf.

Where interpreting appears to be causing tension between parents and adolescents, working with families to increase adolescents' understanding of their parents' positions (including the sacrifices they have made in order to ensure their children had better opportunities) and parents' understanding of the adolescents' position (including the pressures they experience when expectations feel too much) can help in reducing the likelihood of adolescents responding by acting out in risky ways (Shen, Kim and Chao, 2014).

Schooling

One of the greatest challenges facing migrant, but more particularly refugee, children on arrival in a new country is adapting to a new environment. However, for this to be possible, schools, teachers and their peers need to adapt as well. Although additional research is needed to understand how education services need to adapt to help children progress at school, this is likely to require changes in national policy that celebrate diversity, including changes to the national curriculum, and additional training on working with cultural diversity, addressing language barriers, racism and bullying. Children's adaptation is also likely to benefit from initiatives focused on the interface between school, the family and community, including offering parents language and adult education classes and arranging social events to help parents network with others. Other initiatives that have proved helpful include changes to the classroom environment, offering additional language classes where needed, establishing peer/buddy schemes and collaborative exercises so that children can learn about one another, and employing bilingual teaching assistants (DfES, 2004; Doyle and McCorriston, 2008; Hamilton and Moore, 2006). As working with children who have been traumatized can be enormously draining it is also important to set up a support structure that includes mentoring and opportunities for teachers to reflect on personal–professional connections (Fox, 1995).

In areas where a high percentage of children are immigrants and refugees, few schools have access to bilingual teachers, support staff and interpreters that cover the full spectrum of all language groups. With this in mind, some schools have begun to offer young interpreter schemes in order to assist children in this process. As discussed above, provided children are not expected to assume a level of responsibility that places them in a difficult position and does not compromise their own opportunities for learning, helping newly arrived peers understand what is happening, adapt to a new school environment and feel less isolated can be enormously empowering, and has the advantage of celebrating their language skills (Cline, Crafter and Prokopiou, 2014).

Schools can play a significant role in helping families negotiate intercultural conflicts, by providing children with opportunities for academic learning, learning about the society in which they live and engaging with peers. Likewise, schools offer parents opportunities to engage with teachers and with other parents. When children find academic work particularly difficult, it is obviously important to assess the nature of their difficulties and where relevant refer them on for remedial help.

However, academic difficulties (including language difficulties) may be bound up with difficulties related to migration. In these situations, information about the family's experience of migration can offer useful insights into the challenges children face, including who came first, where they came from, which language dominates in the home, the status of that language in the wider society, and settled-ness of others from the same region or country. For example, children who move to join or grow up in more closed communities may have less need to speak English. Indeed, some families subscribe to the television networks and newspapers of their home country and do not engage with events dominating the country in which they live. Although this enables parents to maintain some sense of continuity between their present and past lives, it can mean that their children grow up dislocated from the local culture. Moreover, unless children attend one of the more fundamental faith-based schools, they have to find ways of negotiating their connection with the culture of home with the culture they encounter outside of home without undermining relationships with their parents.

Another issue to bear in mind is that where a father comes first and learns to speak English before being joined by the rest of the family, children are likely to be exposed to differently accented English at home and school, and their parents' 'mother tongue' at home. Gendered roles and expectations are also important: for example, where culture dictates that women do not leave the home alone and children attend English language school, mothers may rely on their children to translate on their behalf.

Refugee children are likely to face additional challenges: political conflict in their country of origin and the journey to safety may mean their schooling will have been disrupted. Trauma can impede the ability to learn and cause fear about people in authority. Hostile discrimination and the rejection of their peers make this even more difficult. When parents' support is lacking, academic achievement tends to decrease: depending on where they are from, refugee parents may not be able to speak English, do not understand the concept of parent–teacher meetings and do not expect to be engaged with their children's schooling. Moreover children's attempts to assimilate as rapidly as possible in order to distance themselves from horrific experiences can create tensions between parents and children that are difficult to acknowledge or address (Kia Keating and Ellis, 2007; McBrien, 2011; Rousseau and Guzder, 2008).

Nonetheless, it is important to avoid assuming that all forms of migration, including experiences as a refugee, have a damaging impact on intergenerational relationships. For example, although migrant and refugee children living in economically stressed situations are likely to be required to carry out essential tasks (such as cleaning, tidying and babysitting) more frequently than those from families with greater financial resources, providing these tasks are manageable and children are still able to engage in age-appropriate activities, acting as 'family helper' can be extremely empowering and is very different to becoming a 'parentified child' and being robbed of one's childhood (Falicov, 2013).

Likewise, as discussed in relation to language brokering, many children find nuanced ways of dealing with the advantages they have had as a result of being exposed to a different cultural and educational system by alternating cultural codes according to the context in which they find themselves, and avoid using their experiences in ways that threaten relationships with parents, including differences in education.

Couple relationships

Many couples thrive on moving to a new country, strengthened by a spirit of adventure, the hope of new personal and professional opportunities, freedom from the constraints of the society in which they had lived, and distance from family and other social networks. The absence of family and familiar networks may mean partners look more to one another in trying to resolve dilemmas, developing a greater sense of closeness and mutuality.

However, this is not always possible: following migration, social networks tend to be smaller and less reciprocal than before, leading to individual and interpersonal stresses that interfere with the possibility of maintaining a relationship both partners find satisfactory. Where one or both partners are extremely isolated, the pressure to make up for the support of family living elsewhere can create a level of dependency that feels intolerable. Many couples struggle financially because their qualifications and previous work experience are not recognized, and lack of fluency in English means they are unable to re-qualify or demonstrate their true capacities. Indeed, research and clinical reports of increased rates of depression, anxiety, family conflict and violence amongst migrants (particularly illegal migrants) attest to the potentially negative consequences role strains, threats to identity, loss of cultural referents and the isolation of living in different socio-cultural and geographical settings can present (Falicov, 2013; Hyman, Guruge and Mason, 2008; Shirpak, Maticka-Tyndale and Chinichian, 2011).

There is considerable evidence that a long-term satisfactory relationship offers a buffer against some of the more complex stresses associated with migration (Cheung, 2008). However, most studies of the impact of migration on couples focus on married heterosexual people who are young and in their middle years: far less attention has been paid to the positions of people who are not formally married, older couples and those in a same-sex relationship. Although many of the opportunities and challenges they face will be similar, unlike younger couples, older couples are likely to be facing retirement, increased frailty and the illness or death of their peers. These losses have the potential to re-evoke and exacerbate feelings that relate to earlier experiences of loss, including the losses associated with migration. As such, they may which can require a level of support from one another (or from adult children) that feels intolerable.

Much of what was said in relation to heterosexual couples applies to those people who are in a same-sex relationship as well. What is different is that where the family is unsupportive of their sexuality and homosexuality is illegal or frowned upon in the wider society, migration can free people to celebrate their relationship with one another and own their sexuality in a way that was not possible back home (Mallon, 2013; Walker, 1991): in Daniel's case, leaving Uganda, a country where homosexuality is illegal, was a bid to escape from hiding who he was from his family as well as the authorities.

The immigration policy of the country to which one moves has a significant impact on the challenges couples face. In 1997, The United Kingdom began providing limited immigration rights to bi-national lesbian and gay couples who could prove they had been living together for four years. This inequality ended with the Civil Partnership Act of 2005, which provides bi-national same-sex couples with immigration rights equal to those enjoyed by opposite-sex couples. This is not the case in many other countries: even where one is entitled to apply for partner to enter and remain in the country, very often there are no clear guidelines and criteria for processing of these types of applications, leading to delays, inconsistencies and allowing prejudice to inform decisions which compound the stresses of migrating (Rickard, 2011).

New immigration rules were introduced in the UK in 2012 restricting the rights of citizens wanting to bring their foreign spouses to live with them. The change in law has a greater effect on low-to-middle income families: currently, where a British citizen has a disposable annual income below £18,600 (with an increase for each dependent child), one is unable to bring one's spouse into the country (other than in exceptional circumstances, for example in some cases of illness). This means that the so-called 'sponsor' (in real terms a husband or wife) has to choose between home and family, between whether to leave the UK to be with one's spouse, or stay and spend significant periods apart.

Negotiating and resolving differences

Just because people migrate does not mean that the more ordinary couple differences disappear or are easy to resolve. For example, regardless of whether one has or has not moved country, it is not unusual to have differences in approaches to parenting, in how much time to spend with one's family of origin, investment in activities outside of home, the extent to which one adopts a more optimistic or pessimistic attitude to challenges and the tendencies to hold back or be more open in sharing how one feels and thinks.

However, couples whose lives are located and dislocated through migration are likely to be faced with other differences as well. For example, it is not unusual for polarizations to develop which arise from ambiguities about leaving and staying. This could involve one partner holding on to sadness while the other is more preoccupied with the benefits of migration, or one partner trying to replicate a sense of family life that is similar to what it was back home while the other is keener to integrate and dis-identify with the past.

Hardly surprisingly, the divorce rate is higher amongst certain migrant groups (Carballo and Mboup, 2005): even after accounting for the fact that birthplace groups have different age structures and marriage patterns, Khoo and Zhao (2001) found that divorce for migrants to Australia was twice as high as the host population. Where couples separate or divorce, the absence of family support and culturally sensitive support can compound the loneliness and low self-esteem that so often sets in at such times, with significant consequences for physical as well as mental wellbeing. Although divorce has a significant impact on both partners, where job opportunities are limited and social status is bound up with being married, the consequences for women tend to be more problematic. However, this is not the whole picture: the UK policy of prioritizing housing for women (mothers) can mean men are left homeless. Where separation or marital problems result in one parent returning to their country of origin, there is a risk of losing touch with one's children, impacting on children's wellbeing. This is not necessarily the case: where returning is a way of escaping a violent relation, the consequences for parents and children are likely to be far more positive.

In all walks of life, it is easier to accommodate to change when the decision is shared. However, this is less possible when a 'tired stayer' forgoes this opportunity despite wanting to move, or one partner is a 'reluctant' or coaxed leaver and the other a reluctant stayer (Abraham, Ausperg and Hinz, 2010; Bonney, McCleery and Forster, 2002; Boyle et al., 2008; Challiol and Mignonac, 2005):

> David was offered the chance of promotion provided he moved from the USA to Britain. His partner Jessica agreed to forgo her own career prospects in the interests of David's career and the family's financial prospects. However, when they moved she resented the loss of parity, economic and other more personal losses this entailed, leading to tensions they found difficult to address. Their

children's experiences seemed to mirror these differences: while their older daughter found it difficult to adjust, her younger sister seemed to thrive and adjust with little difficulty. Consequently, in working with David and Jessica, it was important to disentangle their experiences from those of their children, and from the pulls of their respective families of origin. However, it was also important to disentangle other long-standing differences from differences related to the decision to migrate. This led to drawing up some form of 'contract' about what needed to be different to enable them to move forward.

When couples move from a society in which gendered roles and family patterns are highly stratified to one where they are more fluid, couples are likely to be confronted with examples of families and lifestyles that challenge previous ideas of right and wrong: familiar ways of being a man, woman, husband, wife or parent may not be feasible or even desirable, resulting in adjustments that would have seemed unacceptable at home.

In some situations, both partners value the transformations that enable women to secure economic security and experience greater autonomy and respect (Palriwala and Oberoi, 2008). However, adapting to these transformations in roles and expectations can be enormously difficult. For example, although labour force difficulties (particularly the un- or under-employment of male immigrants) and changes in family structure are two of the most difficult challenges migrant couples face, strains in gendered roles are quoted as the major cause of marital conflict, separation and divorce, particularly where women's economic role increases with little change in her husband's gendered attitudes (Guruge et al., 2010).

Where women are able to learn a new language and engage in the labour market, their increased economic position and social responsibilities can change the distribution of power, enabling them to assume more responsibility for household decisions and control over family resources. Increased economic power also means they need not remain in an unsatisfactory and/or abusive marital relationship (Hyman, Guruge and Mason, 2008). However, in many situations, invisible male power influences the extent to which traditional gendered roles can change: for example, where men find it difficult to accept their wives' greater freedom to dress, socialize and make decisions for themselves, some react by exerting old patterns of control, such as controlling their finances and insisting on having many children (Maciel, van Putten and Knudson-Martin, 2009). Although women face similar difficulties in entering the labour market as well, many men experience unemployment as a threat to their identity as 'good husbands', and in some cases attempt to reassert power and control through physical and emotional abuse (Hondagneu-Sotelo and Messner, 1994; Pratt Ewing, 2008; Shirpak, Maticka-Tyndale and Chinichian, 2011). Moreover, as reflected in my work with Bihar, a Kurdish woman whose

unemployed husband was violent to her, shame about being found wanting, and/or desire to protect elderly parents, mean many abused women
avoid telling anyone in Britain or their family back home.

Freedom from the constraints of the culture in which people were
brought up and/or loneliness can result in developing an intimate relationship with someone who might have seemed unacceptable or unavailable before. Indeed, intermarriage between people from different ethnic
groups is often seen as an acid test of integration: although all marriages
require some level of compromise and negotiation, marriage across
ethnic or religious boundaries points to a time when questions about
ethnicity, religion and 'race' might be seen as heritages to be drawn on,
rather than incommensurable identities that can never be compromised
(Woods, 2015).

Using this criterion, much of post-war migration to Britain has been a
success. West Indian, Chinese and Irish migrants have widely intermarried
with their neighbours, their schoolmates and work colleagues, an increase
reflected in the growing number of people who identified themselves as
'mixed' in the 2011 census compiled by the Office for National Statistics
(ESCR, 2012; Jivraj and Simpson, 2015). Intermarriage is less prevalent
amongst other ethnic groupings. Although cultural stereotyping, other
forms of stress and family permission inform the likelihood of intermarriage, religion appears to be an important factor: migrants whose faith has
no tradition in their country of settlement tend to intermarry less often
than those whose religious backgrounds are more common. For example,
the rate of ethnic endogamous marriages[26] in Western Europe is highest in
Hindu and Muslim communities (Lucassen and Laarman, 2009).

Engaging with other practices and beliefs offers access to the wider
society, enabling one to feel less out of place. However, rejecting practices
and beliefs that have been integral to who one is can exacerbate feelings
of estrangement. Where couples in this position are struggling, it can
be helpful to work towards replacing the devaluation and shame with
respect, pride and enjoyment of one's heritage (Falicov, 2013). Moreover,
even if couples are attracted by their difference and desire to establish a
relationship that is different to the expectations of the society in which
they grew up, subsequent experiences (particularly illness and other forms
of loss) can re-awaken the desire for the familiar.

Transnational marriage

The rapidly growing phenomenon of commercially or kin-arranged international marriage is having a transformative effect on gendered power in
'sending' as well as 'receiving' countries (Belanger and Linh, 2011). For

example, in her study of migration, marriage and employment amongst Indian, Pakistani and Bangladeshi residents in the UK, Dale (2008) found that about a third of UK-born men and women from the Indian subcontinent marry a partner from 'back home', more so amongst those from Pakistan and Bangladesh than India. This figure is slightly higher for women which suggests that marriage migration is not being used as a back-door route for the economic migration of men to the UK. The finding that women with degree-level qualifications were less likely to marry a man from 'back home' is consistent with suggestions that these women have greater power to negotiate their own marriage partner and/or have parents who are more willing for them to do so.

People living in diasporic communities often seek brides from the home country, assuming they will be docile and transmit traditional values to their children. The reality may be very different: where migrant brides are able to learn the language, are not isolated and work outside the home, exposure to different social values and lifestyles can result in developing different aspirations for themselves and their family. In contrast, more highly educated women who resist traditional patriarchal arrangement by marrying someone from the same culture who lives abroad can find their dreams of establishing a more egalitarian relationship are dashed by the aspirations of a less educated and more traditional husband, in some cases leading to domestic abuse or divorce. Living abroad also means that when difficulties arise, she and her partner cannot draw on the wisdom and buffering of family. However, abuse and divorce are less likely where women have considered this possibility and maintain contact with transnational networks that look out for them (Bloch, 2011; Maciel, van Putten and Knudson-Marin, 2009). They are also less likely where women find nuanced ways of bargaining with men. For example, Hirsch (2003) found that Mexican immigrant women learned to bargain with men in 'modern' ways, but did so in a less confrontational way than usual in the USA: in keeping with their original culture, they framed their bargains as in the best interests of the family rather than themselves.

The tradition of arranged marriage has operated successfully within many communities and countries over a long period of time. However, this tradition has come under greater challenge more recently, with questions focused on whether arranged marriages inherently violate human rights, particularly women's rights, whether they are being used to abuse international immigration systems ('sham marriages'), whether arranged marriages offer greater stability for raising children, and whether these couples have a more or less loving, respectful relationship (Grillo, 2011; Pande, 2014). There is an important, albeit sometimes fine, distinction between forced and arranged marriage. Arranged marriages take place with full agreement and consent from both parties, whereas in forced marriage one or both parties do not consent to the marriage, and an element of duress, physical, emotional or both, is involved. As reflected in Sanghere's (2009) account of his mother's marriage to a man with a history of schizophrenia, some women are coerced or agree to marry men who would otherwise not have been acceptable. However, marriage is not only an individual bond but a family project: by living abroad emigrant daughters are accorded greater status as a result of their ability to send financial remittances back home, altering the living standards and status of their family (Beck and Beck-Gurnstein, 2014; Belanger and Giang Linh, 2011).

Internationally arranged marriage confronts men with somewhat different challenges. Although men who migrate as a groom (for example, by marrying an immigrant's daughter) may be able to gain entry to a country seen as more favourable, this may mean accepting a style of living that would be derided back home, as when men find themselves living with and financially dependent on their wives' family. Back home, in some areas the higher value of bride prices resulting from arranged international marriage means it is more difficult for single men to marry someone locally.

Sibling relationships

Relatively little attention has been paid to the impact of migration on sibling relationships. This is an unfortunate omission because, as discussed in relation to illness, adult negotiations of similarities and differences are informed by childhood experiences of relating to someone who is, at one level, very similar but at another level 'stands in one's place' (Mitchell, 2003, p. 10). Consequently, the meanings associated with a brother or sister's decision to migrate are likely to be imbued with feelings related to far earlier negotiations of similarity and difference. Moreover, staying or leaving is likely to mean siblings' responsibilities and opportunities are different (Carling, 2008).

Where siblings have a supportive relationship with one another, differences tend to be underplayed. However, where relationships are more fraught, differences in experiences may be attributed to migration even if they are unrelated. In addition, although growing up in the same country does not determine how one views particular events, the social and cultural context in which sibling relationships were conducted will have been similar (Edwards, Hadfield, Lucey and Mauthner, 2006). As such, where some siblings have stayed and others have chosen or felt forced to leave a highly politicized country, the political is likely to inform the 'identity claims' siblings draw on in making sense of their shared and different experiences (Al-Ali, 2002; Altschuler, 2008b).

Reflecting on his older brother Peter's migration from apartheid-based South Africa, Alex began by speaking about the 'huge' sense of loss he felt when his brother, the person who had been his primary support after the breakdown of their parents' relationship, moved to the UK. However, greater emphasis was placed on the 'resentment that he hasn't been here to help' with their elderly mother: although Peter and his wife help 'a little' on their return visits to the country, Alex said 'it's not enough as they should be compensating more – for their huge absences'. What Alex found particularly difficult was that, despite his assuming primary responsibility in caring for their mother, in her eyes Peter would always be 'the much preferred son'. These feelings were tempered by the fact that having previously seen Peter's migration as heroic and his own decision to stay as cowardly, his current view was that his brother had run away from his responsibility to his country and family.

Alex's emphasis on the 'huge' loss he felt when his older brother left reflects Marchetti-Mercer's (2012) finding that many non-migrants experience their siblings' emigration as a vast loss, which some describe as akin to death, bringing about significant changes in social networks and relationships. His emphasis on the value of being able to turn to his brother for support when their parents divorced attests to the comfort, camaradie and companionship of being closely connected with someone in a similar position (Mauthner, 2003). This is reflected in accounts of the advantages of migrating with, or to the same place as, a sibling and one's children being able to draw on the support, friendship and guidance of aunts, uncles and cousins living locally:

> For Rachael, whose childhood memories of growing up in apartheid-based South Africa were dominated by having to hide that her mother was mentally ill and that her parents were born Indian but 'declared white by application', migrating with her older sister was particularly important because 'there wasn't anyone who, who, you know, had our lives', who knew that it 'wasn't sort of making oneself different, it was just a fact that we were'. In their case, the estrangement of being out of place that accompanied migration echoed far earlier experiences of the shame bound up with an embodied and racialized sense of 'being out of place' (Probyn, 2004).

Where siblings move with their parents as children, it can be enormously helpful to look to one another for support when the stresses of migration mean parents are less available. Differences in positions within the family (including birth order), interests and abilities mean each child's experience of family and acculturation is not necessarily the same (Song, 1997). Nonetheless, brothers and sisters are likely to have a similar understanding of the challenges of negotiating life in a different context (for example, knowing how to behave when the patterns of friendship, environment, subjects and level of teaching in school are very different) and balancing parents' expectations and maintaining connection with cultural traditions while making space for the new.

In some situations, the desire to emulate and follow an older sibling means younger siblings pay more attention to their schooling to equip themselves to be able to leave (Chamberlain, 2006). In a study of the effects of migration on children in rural Pakistan, the overseas and internal migration of brothers increased the pace of learning but sisters' migration had no effect, attesting to the importance of understanding the multiple factors that contribute to educational achievement, including gendered expectations and access to schooling (Kuhn, 2006).

Reunions

Reunions offer transnational families a chance to affirm that they remain important to one another and engaged with one another's lives. However, coming together for a limited period is never able to capture the full complexity and intensity of experiences that were lost, missed and unwitnessed. As such, reunions may be times when the difference between 'real' and imagined experiences of family, and the opportunities and responsibilities of migrants and non-migrants, come to the fore (Gardner and Grillo, 2002; Olwig, 2002).

For example, the desire to make up for gaps in time and face-to-face contact can mean it is difficult to raise issues that might not be resolved before parting. Likewise, it can feel difficult speaking too positively about one's life in a new country for fear of causing resentment or envy. Although 'editing out' potentially problematic issues might be aimed at rebuilding or maintaining relational connection, paradoxically it limits the possibilities of establishing the authentic connection both parties aspire to, leading to blow-ups and disappointments that are confusing to all (Alvarez, 1999). Living some distance apart also means that despite attempts to remain in touch, migrants and non-migrants are likely to be out of synch with one another's lives. As reflected in the account of Ruth, who remained in South Africa when her children moved to the UK, USA and Australia, this can be particularly challenging for grandparents and their grandchildren:

Ruth: 'I kind of feel that they – they forget us between visits. That means a re-establishment each beginning – and it's a beginning again – and they've changed so much in the last year since you've seen them. You know – what

Annie's favourite colour was last time you saw her she hates this year and so gifts are impossible – and – um, it's just almost an artificial situation – everybody's on their best behaviour which isn't exactly normal.'

In other situations, where migration was partly based on a desire for more distance from family, even if one is more aware of the costs of migration when together, disagreements that erupt during these times can become a validation of the decision to live apart. However, this is not always the case: heightened awareness of how little time there is to be together can increase both parties' willingness to put their differences aside.

In some cases, the possibilities of seeing one another are constrained by finances and difficulties in securing a visa: it is more difficult to travel and stay in touch in a situation of political conflict where the 'global power geometry' (Massey, 1991) means there are particular concerns about the influx of migrants from one's country of origin.

The growth in technology has opened up new ways for transnational families to maintain a sense of being connected in contexts of dispersal, for example by emails and watching the same soap opera. Likewise Skype calls offer the possibility of seeing as well as talking with one another in 'real time'. However, differences in time zones mean connecting in real time is difficult: for example, although Skype could have allowed Ruth[27] and her children to light candles ushering in the Jewish Sabbath (a ritual that embodied their shared sense of family and Jewish identity) 'together', differences in time zones meant this was impossible.

The complexities of negotiating what it means to be a family when parents, children and siblings live apart are particularly relevant to understanding reunions to mark significant transitions in the life cycle (Olwig, 2002). For example, when a close member of the family dies, provided finances and other practicalities allow, many migrants join their non-migrant family in the country in which they grew up to fulfil the traditional rituals associated with death, and/or in keeping with the deceased's preference and religious beliefs fly the body back 'home'. As with all gatherings to mark a death, coming together is an opportunity to affirm the importance of the deceased and the survivors to one another. However, in situations of migration, these reunions tend to be brief and take place in the context of a more final parting. Consequently, coming together can highlight how much has changed. In some cases, mourning is complicated by sadness and guilt about not having been able (or not having made the effort) to see the deceased, the person who had been a source of emotional nourishment whose presence evoked special memories of the past. Where the deceased held the family together and represented migrants' identification with their country of origin (as is often the case with parents), their death can confront migrants and their non-migrant siblings with questions about future relationships with one another (Altschuler, 2008b; Gunaratnam, 2013).

> When asked about his experience of migration, Charlie (who had left South Africa about 20 years before) framed his response in terms of loss, illustrating this with the events surrounding the recent death of his mother-in-law. Practicalities like school and financial difficulties meant that he and their children were not able to go to South Africa with his wife to attend the funeral. As a result his experience was that 'the funeral was not one of those family – family things'. They compensated by holding a gathering to mark her death in London. However, neither of his children had shed a tear about their grandmother or talked much about her since. This has left Charlie wondering what she meant to them and whether they had really known her, suggesting that her death confronted Charlie with the extent to which his children's and his own experience of family had been transformed by migration.

Real and imagined encounters with death can lead to re-remembering and re-envisaging the past, altering understandings of oneself and others (Umberson, 2003). It is obviously impossible to undo the past and make up for what was lost. However, where relationships are strained, exchanging memories and mental images of events that took place prior and subsequent to migration (including details that renew and increase knowledge of one another) can go a long way towards generating empathy for one another and restoring a sense of family coherence (Falicov, 2013).

Recommendations for practice

In addressing the challenges faced by people whose lives are located and dislocated through migration, five domains of experience are important to bear in mind: migration–acculturation, the ecological context, family structure and positions in the family life cycle (Falicov, 2013) and experiences that predate the decision to migrate. These issues are central to initiatives aimed at helping people rebuild a sense of community, more intensive psychotherapeutic work, and as health care professionals, making sense of the resonances with our own experiences, thoughts and feelings.

Rebuilding a sense of community

Most situations of migration involve a loss of 'social capital' (Bourdeau, 1991), of the shared norms, values, understandings and networks that facilitate cooperation within or among groups. Some people deal with these losses and changes in identity by becoming diasporic members of virtual communities. This includes maintaining a strong connection with family and/or investing energy in communities back home, including donating their skills or offering financial support to religious, medical and schooling projects (Ormond, 2013).

Others focus more on rebuilding a sense of community in the place in which they are living. This can happen in an organic way: for example, many people, including my grandparents who moved from Lithuania to South Africa, migrate to a place where there is a friend, relative or acquaintance who can offer support in finding work, accommodation and advice on negotiating life in a new country. In some cases, rebuilding a sense of belonging centres around places of worship and religious gatherings. Particularly in the larger cities, there are often distinct ethnic neighbourhoods in which sights, flavours and smells of one's country of origin are reproduced and where cultural memories and traditions are kept alive and recreated. However, confining oneself to these circles can be restrictive, increasing the likelihood of children who are keen to integrate distancing themselves. Moreover, distinct areas of ethnic settlement tend to evoke mixed feelings amongst the rest of the population: although they carry the allure of the exotic and offer an opportunity to 'taste' another culture, they can become symbols of difference and the presence of new identities, lifestyles, social divisions and inequality, exacerbating anxieties around integration, citizenship and nation building (Phillips, 2015).

Rebuilding a sense of community with people from the same country is more complicated when migration relates to civil conflict because it is impossible to know what role one's compatriots played in the conflict. Where post-migration life has been more difficult than anticipated, many people are reluctant for news about their circumstances to reach family and friends who decided or felt forced to stay. Rebuilding some sense of community is particularly complicated where one is isolated, cannot speak the dominant language, where health is compromised and one does not understand how the local services work. In these situations, migrants are likely to benefit from information and advocacy in relation to schools, health and social benefit schemes, and opportunities to learn English and engage with other people.

Across the UK, a wide range of innovative programmes have been established aimed at helping people construct a greater sense of belonging, including befriending and horticultural projects (which combine gardening with therapy), photography, walking groups, and opportunities to prepare foods and share stories that generate memories and familiar experiences with other immigrants. Some projects use writing as a medium for processing, sharing and disseminating ideas and experiences.[28] Others use mindfulness exercises (exercises which focus one's awareness on the present moment, while calmly acknowledging and accepting one's feelings, thoughts, and bodily sensations), sport (particularly football), drama, dance and traditional craftwork in tandem with psychotherapeutic approaches to enhance the wellbeing of all migrants including refugees, asylum seekers and internally displaced people. These projects offer a space in which people are able to express themselves freely around issues of immigration, flight, gender, sexuality, religion and politics: where people have been traumatized, non-verbal creative activities like dance and painting can provide a vehicle for expressing the uncontainable and speechless horror that continues to haunt people's lives (Harris, 2009; Koch and Weidinger-von der Recke, 2009). Initiatives like these are equally applicable to working in refugee camps: for example in our recent work in a camp in Northern Greece, Idomeni, a group session for Farsi speakers offered three 14 year old unaccompanied asylum seekers from Afghanistan a chance to tell their stories, and in the absence of their own parents, draw on the wisdom lthe older members of the group.

Where adults and children seem unable to recognize the strength their cultural heritage could offer, drawing a 'tree of life' that traces all aspects of their heritage offers a way of connecting with cultural roots, skills and the special people who live elsewhere. The Tree of Life Technique has been used with people in many different contexts: it was first used with children affected by HIV/AIDS in sub-Saharan Africa (Ncube, 2006), but has subsequently been applied to working with people who have experienced other forms of hardship in Australia, Brazil, Canada, Russia, Nepal, the UK, the USA (Denborough, 2008; Hughes, 2014) and refugees in the camps of Calais and elsewhere. It involves groups of people drawing their own 'tree of life' and talking about their 'roots' (their family origin and where they come from), the 'ground' (their current lives, who they live with and what they do), 'trunk' (their knowledge, talents and special skills, for example sensitivity to others), 'branches' (hopes, dreams and the history of these hopes and dreams) and 'fruits' (the gifts they have been given). The participants are then encouraged to join their trees into a 'forest of life' and discuss the 'storms' that affect their lives, how they respond to these storms and protect themselves and each other.

Group experiences can be particularly helpful for refugees and asylum seekers, as they help in rebuidling some sense of connection in a context in which people feel isolated and disconnected. With this in mind, a wide range of community and non-statutory organizations have set up projects offering after-school recreational activities and homework clubs for children, parenting groups, language courses, advocacy and legal advice. In some areas, concerns about the disenfranchisement of young refugees between the ages of 16 and 21 have led to the development of mentoring schemes and language classes aimed at encouraging people between the ages of 16 and 18 to continue their education and avoid being drawn into drug taking and other forms of risky behaviour. For those who are more cautious about face-to-face interactions, social media sites offer an opportunity to connect with others with similar experiences.

Whilst projects like these offer a forum for discussing difficulties, as importantly they offer a non-pathologizing and empowering context for developing a new social network, providing a buffer against loneliness, alienation and discriminatory experiences: even if the people one meets are from different countries, engaging with more experienced immigrants can help those with less experience bridge the gaps between their past lives and the present. Where projects are seen to promote wellbeing and avoid using the labels of mental illness, they are more likely to be experienced as non-stigmatizing by the communities they serve. These projects tend to be most successful and self-sustaining when they are not only initiated by health care professionals but in liaison with potential service users and community leaders.

Psychotherapeutic work

The economic and socio-political stresses associated with migration and confusion, alienation, shame and/or guilt associated with leaving or being left means that some people are in need of professional support. Symptoms precipitated or aggravated by migration (such as depression, psychosomatic conditions, addiction and family conflict) can arise at the time of departure, and when reunions and any significant changes in the life cycle occur.

In all work with people who are struggling, it is important to create an atmosphere in which migrants feel free to explore and reflect on their experience, including experiences they find troubling or even shameful. Although migration may not be the main or only reason for their difficulties, it can have a profound effect on experiences of self and others. Consequently, reflecting on the ways in which life has been affected by migration opens up the possibility of a less pathologizing understanding of self, family and responses to the emotional, economic and socio-political stresses associated with migration. As discussed in relation to situations of illness, where one aspect of experience (in this case migration) has become the primary frame for viewing experience it is important to raise comments and questions that bring other aspects of experience to the fore, including particular family dynamics.

For example, exploring the connection between intergenerational and intercultural conflicts can lead to a wider understanding of the challenges parents and children face in negotiating their connections with two or more socio-cultural and language systems. Likewise, encouraging couples to reflect on their shared and individual views about the differences between their current situation and the way their couple and family relationships would have evolved if they had stayed back home can lead to a different understanding of the past, as well as what they want and need from one another in the present.

Where families have spent long periods apart, exchanging memories and mental images of events that took place before and during their separation (including small details) can help in making meaning of these separations, renewing and increasing their knowledge of each other and re-establishing some sense of continuity and coherence (Falicov, 2013). Likewise, where migration has led to being cut off from the rest of the family, it can be helpful to explore what would need to change before it is possible to re-engage with one another. In many cases, living apart means it is not feasible to meet together. In these situations it can be helpful to encourage the person to imagine how they might feel if they were in the other person's position and how that person's views of the past might have changed over time. Where the idea of reconnecting feels too risky, often the best we can do is work towards minimizing the impact of these cut-offs and ensuring these splits are not replicated by the next generation.

However, although it is important to bear witness to stories of loss, trauma, hopelessness and failure, it is also important to explore stories of strength and resilience. This includes asking what has helped people through difficult situations before, about the personal qualities and strengths that helped them survive and whether it would be possible to draw on what they have learned in overcoming current difficulties. Indeed, the very fact that refugees and other migrants were able to move and restart their lives in a new country is, in itself, an indication of resourcefulness.

Where parents seem paralysed by guilt, exploring what they feel they have been able to offer their children, how their children know they are treasured and what children have gained from being connected with more than one country can help parents recognize their strengths and resourcefulness and the benefits of their decision to move. Likewise, where immigrant children are struggling at school, asking whether there is anyone in their class who knows what it means to have lived in more than one country and can speak more than one language can go a long way towards celebrating their achievement and dispelling the notion that they are stupid.

Recovering stories of agency and resilience is particularly important where people have been persecuted, violated and stripped of their voice, as is often true of refugees and asylum seekers. In many cases, powerful feelings are only able to come to the surface when one is silent (Rober and de Haene, 2014). Nonetheless, although the establishment of trust and ability to identify and empathize are critical to engaging with people in distress, the capacity for inner dialogue and reflection are reduced when traumatized, limiting the possibilities of external dialogue and interpersonal interactions (Guregard and Sekkula, 2014). It can be extremely difficult to make sense of traumatic experiences when there is no sense of stability in one's life (Agger, 1992). As such, it is often more helpful to begin by focusing on practical and social issues, including daily and occupational activities, concerns about being unable to work and what sort of coping skills people draw on in managing anxiety and flashbacks from the past.

It is always important to take account of the potential inequalities in power between our positions as health care professionals and the people with whom we work. However, this is particularly important when experiences of authority have been abusive (Bryant, Sutherland and Guthrie, 2007). For example, questions aimed at encouraging people to reflect on their experience may recall experiences of being interrogated by immigration authorities and the fear that signs of mental distress might have a negative impact on applications to the Home Office. In other cases, as discussed by Rachel Hopkins in Chapter 7, the work needs to extend beyond the clinical context: one may need to intervene more directly, for example by acting as an advocate or as an intermediary between the family, community and institutions like school.

Personal–professional resonances

Work with migrants from a different cultural background to one's own offers an opportunity to extend understanding of difference and resilience under challenging circumstances. However, this requires a commitment to honour diversity, question 'normative' theories and find culturally sensitive solutions to the problems people face (Maitra and Krause, 2015). This includes familiarizing oneself with their cultural beliefs and traditions associated with intergenerational and couple relationships in order to develop an understanding of the nuanced forms of continuity and value changes at play and the socio-political context of their lives, including economic stresses and exposure to prejudice (Falicov, 2007; Maciel, van Putten and Knudson-Marin, 2009).

However, listening to and identifying with people who have been through horrific experiences can be overwhelming, giving rise to secondary traumatization and a sense of 'survivor guilt', giving rise to irritation, exhaustion, disbelief and scapegoating the complexity of needs, legal status, challenges of working via an interpreter and the often horrific nature of the refugees' accounts can engender feelings of helplessness, sympathy, rage, and the need to rescue and disregard one's usual professional boundaries, invoking dependency and disempowerment that are difficult to acknowledge, let alone address (Daniels, 2012). Consequently, it is important to reflect on our own responses in order to empathize with unfamiliar people and places, recognize how others see one's culture, and identify voices of pain and disquiet as well as hope and initiative.

6

INTERSECTION BETWEEN MIGRATION AND ILLNESS

This chapter focuses on the intersection between experiences of illness and migration. The case examples discussed here illustrate that when difficulties arise, placing migration and its consequences central to discussions about illness and mortality can help to construct a less pathologizing understanding of self, family and others. They draw attention to the importance of listening, bearing witness to pain and exploring the impact of the past on the present. However, they also illustrate the need to highlight stories of strengths and resilience and attend to transference and counter-transference phenomena: to personal resonances with the experiences of the people with whom we are working.

The philosopher Derrida (2000) proposes that the foreigner is a figure that questions our own existence and belonging: he speaks of an otherness that is not a spatial problem but relates to the cultural and experiential distance between you and me. Likewise, in discussing the journey from the world of the healthy to the world of the ill, Sontag (1991) and Probyn (2004) speak of the otherness-within, of the shame of 'a being out of place' that disturbs our sense of feeling at home with ourselves and in the world. In both situations, conscious and unconscious traces of otherness, of other times, places and experiences of self intermingle with day-to-day personal and family life, informing the kind of care required from professionals, family and friends.

As outlined in Chapter 5, experiences of and responses to migration vary considerably, informed by factors related to the process of migration, experiences of cultural diversity, acculturation, racism, other forms of discrimination, family structure, positions in the life cycle and realities of daily post-migration life. In many situations, migration has a moderating or even positive effect on experiences of illness: moving to a country where the health care is more advanced can provide access to better treatment and pain relief, in some situations at no extra cost. Many people show great courage and determination in the face of serious illness and/or migration-related challenges: many migrants and refugees are able to draw on the strategies they developed in adapting to previous situations of difficulty when faced with the diagnosis of a life-limiting condition (Hubard, Kidd and Kearney, 2010; Mizrahi et al., 2008). Where people have found it difficult to integrate and engage with the wider community, illness can become a 'third space' (Bhabha, 1994): a catalyst for developing a deeper connection with people of the country in which one is currently living than seemed possible before. Moreover, the intersection between migration and illness can allow for positive transformations in experiences of family, including transformations in gendered roles and patterns of power.

However, this is not always the case: in other situations, illness, disability and the threat of death exacerbate the stresses people are already facing in adjusting to life in a different socio-cultural, geographic and political place. This is particularly hard when one is unable to access support from family and friends previously central to one's life. What makes it even more difficult is that experiences of not being how 'One Should, Ought and Wants to Be' (Yngvesson and Mahoney, 2000, p. 17) can stir up earlier feelings of loss, fragmentation and trauma, including the otherness of not belonging.

Where migration involves moving to a country where the culture is markedly different, it can be hard to disentangle illness-related feelings of estrangement from the estrangement of engaging with a health care system in which perceptions of causality, methods of treatment, and interactions between the ill person, family and health care professionals are very different. This is even more complicated where language barriers and racialization mean one's behaviour is more likely to be scrutinized and found wanting. For people who have been tortured, incarcerated and/or physically and sexually abused, even the most routine technical procedures such as having a needle inserted into one's arm in order to draw off fluid or introduce medication, or metal barriers being placed at the sides of the bed to prevent falling (as is often the case before being given an anaesthetic) can evoke terrifying flashbacks of the past, including events that lie beyond consciousness.

In contrast, when non-migrant relatives are ill, disabled or face the possibility of death, the health care one is able to access is familiar and many of the structures on which one's life is grounded remain the same. However, even though non-migrants have not moved from one geographic location to another, the 'place' they inhabit at times of illness is likely to be different to what it would have been had their adult children, parents or siblings not chosen or felt forced to leave. Financial and other practicalities mean that in most cases, family living elsewhere are unable to offer the practical hands-on support that is needed, other than for brief periods of time. Even if migrant family members are able to care for non-migrant relatives for a more protracted period of time, this is likely to require considerable financial investment and putting aside the rest of one's life. Although some transnational families are able to negotiate these challenges with relatively little difficulty, where relationships have been fraught experiences of caring and being cared for may be imbued with feelings of indebtedness, re-evoking past resentments about decisions to migrate.

Although this is starting to change, relatively little attention has been paid to the challenges health care professionals face in working with migrants, refugees and asylum seekers. However, as reflected in a study of the experience of doctors, many remain haunted by memories of situations in which they were 'reduced to nods and smiles' (Richardson, Thomas and Richardson, 2006, p. 93), where the care they were able to provide fell short of what was needed and wanted, and anxiety about working across differences was compounded by lack of knowledge about cultural and religious values, and the tensions between cultural sensitivity and anti-oppressive practice. Similarly, staff working in accident and emergency departments have expressed concerns about the frequency with which language barriers mean ambulances are called out for situations that were not urgent (Betancourt, Green and Carillo, 2000; Clarke, Finley and Campbell, 1991; Hultsjo and Hielm, 2005; Richardson, Thomas and Richardson, 2006).

As reflected in the following two diagrams, illustrating the intersection between illness and migration it is important to hold at least four dimensions of experience in mind: illness, migration, family factors and the socio-economic and economic context in which people live:

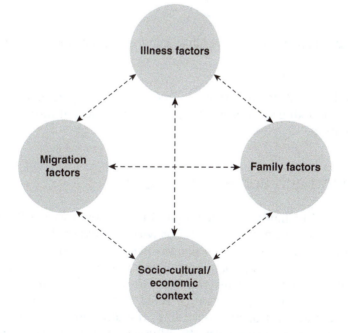

Figure 6.1 Mapping the intersection between illness and migration

Illness factors	Migration factors
Onset	Journey and type of migration (forced or chosen)
Course	Trauma pre-, during and following migration
Prognosis	Uprooting of meanings (physical, social and cultural)
Incapacitation	Natural of losses and separations (migrates alone, with a parent/partner)
Degree of uncertainty	
Treatment	Balance between stresses and benefits, possibilities and restraints
Expectations of health care system	
Prior and current experiences of medical care and healing	Reunions and spontaneous rituals
	Acculturation and exposure to other socio-cultural and language system
	Residency status

Family factors	Socio-cultural/economic context
Family structure	Cultural and language barriers
Family life cycle	Dominant discourses re: illness, migration, outsiders, gender, sexuality, age and 'race'
Particular family dynamics	
Polarizations, gendered and age related shifts arising from illness and migration	Educational and employment opportunities
	Position of the ethnic community
Prior experience of loss and trauma	Contextual risks (war, political, racism, drugs, violence, gangs)
Resiliency, resources and access to social support	
Relationship between migrant and non-migrant kin	Contextual protectors (access to material, professional and other resources, including social network, language, religion and other forms of spirituality)

Figure 6.2 Migration, illness, the family and the socio-cultural/economic context

In addition, it is important to reflect on the personal resonances aroused by working with people whose lives have been informed by illness and migration.

Childhood and adolescent illness

As discussed in Chapter 3, when a child is diagnosed with a life-limiting condition, parents must come to terms with the loss of the dream of having a 'normal' child. Very often parents need to ask more of one another (including emotional support and changes in childcare arrangements) to ensure that their ill child receives the care that is needed and the lives of the rest of the family are as unaffected as possible. Similarly, depending on age and level of understanding, the affected child has to find a way of coming to terms with the physical symptoms associated with their condition and treatment, fears for the future and the differences between their own lives and that of their siblings and peers in a context in which their parents and other close relatives may be struggling to contain their own feelings of loss, anxiety, and in many cases shame and guilt. As reflected below, although migration is not necessarily the main or only determinant of how parents and children respond, it can have a profound effect on the challenges one faces and support one is able to receive and provide.

On living apart at times of childhood illness

When a child is seriously ill, providing relationships are supportive, the compassion and practical assistance of trusted family and friends can be enormously sustaining. However, unless other family members and close friends have moved as well, this is rarely feasible for migrants, particularly in the early post-migration years. The practical and emotional demands of caring for a seriously ill young child without being able to turn to one's extended family and close friends can stretch relationships to a point that feels intolerable. Consequently, at what is likely to be the most disruptive and demanding time of their lives, parents are less able to draw on the relationships and structures on which their earlier lives were grounded, limiting their ability to contain their child's worries as well as their own, and children's readiness to turn to them for support. Although friends, neighbours and colleagues are sometimes willing to step in to help, it takes time to build relationships with people who have the strength and willingness to accompany one through what may be a harrowing journey.

In some cases, distance from close family and traditional social structures can be liberating: it frees parents to respond to their ill child, adjust to the intergenerational and gendered shifts caring for a seriously ill child often require, and engage with health care professionals as they see fit rather than having to take account of the anxieties and views of other family members. However, where migration and other family dynamics have resulted in a cut-off in relationships, illness can result in rethinking and reworking relationships with one another:

> I was asked to see American-born Dana, a single mother, and her 13-year-old daughter, Sophie, who had been diagnosed with Crohn's disease a year before. The family were referred because the medical team felt the tensions between mother and daughter were having a negative impact on Sophie's health and compliance with the treatment. Over the course of this work, it became apparent that Dana left the United States in her early twenties in order to establish more distance from her family of origin. However, the combination of the

breakdown in her relationship with Sophie's father about two years previously, and the worry and tensions associated with trying to ensure Sophie ate properly and did not over exert herself, confronted Dana with what had been lost: neither of them was able to draw on the wisdom of grandparents, aunts and uncles when their relationship became more strained and when Dana's anxieties about Sophie's health meant she was unable to engage with Sophie's own distress and fear. Moreover, whilst Dana was in occasional telephone and email contact with her parents, she dismissed their advice, including the suggestion to allow Sophie more freedom, as she felt they would have thought differently if they were present and able to see how pale and exhausted Sophie became at times. Furthermore, although Dana resented the fact that her parents were not more supportive, a mixture of shame and pride meant she underplayed the difficulties they were facing in speaking with them.

Consequently, much of the work focused on separating these different layers of experience. This involved exploring alternate ways of addressing the impact of illness upon their relationship, including what they wanted and needed from one another in the present, how migration might be affecting the challenges they were facing, the possibilities of healing the rifts between Dana and her parents, and disentangling Sophie's experience of her parents' divorce and her father's disappearance from her life from that of her mother.

Families face somewhat different challenges when children develop a disabling condition as a result of travelling to a country where there is a greater chance of contracting an infectious disease. Most parents find it enormously difficult coming to terms with the fact that their child is disabled. However, this is likely to be even more difficult when the disability is a result of having contracted an infectious disease during a visit to one or both parents' country of origin to mark a significant family event, such as a wedding or christening. This is even more challenging when one parent had felt it was too dangerous to travel but had been overruled.

In other cases, experiences of illness and death offer families the chance to show that they remain in touch with the realities of one another's lives:

Gillian, the oldest of four children, was the only one in her family to have left South Africa. Rather than framing migration as disruptive, she draws upon her family's history of moving from Eastern Europe in framing migration as integral to her understanding of what it means to be a family. She illustrates this by saying that when her daughter died shortly after the diagnosis of a rare malignant tumour 'there wasn't even a question about it – they [her sisters and brother] all came the next day – they came'. Her emphatic statement 'there wasn't even a question' frames sibling relationships as enduring, despite living apart.

Gillian's account of her daughter's death also shows how experiences of illness and death can become a vehicle for developing a greater sense of connection with people in the country to which one moves: the support she, her partner and children received from local friends, neighbours and parents of her daughter's classmates increased her sense of being part of a community, a 'circle of care', shifting her relationship with the people she had previously thought of as other: 'the English'.

Hierarchical skews

Where people are unable to speak English, the NHS offers access to a trained interpreter. However, as explored in Chapters 4 and 5, because children tend to learn a new language more easily than adults, they are often expected to act as language brokers during medical consultations. Although this may fit with the family's understanding of filial support and desire for privacy, it can mean children are party to information parents would otherwise have wanted to shield them from. Whilst there is always a possibility of misunderstandings and mistakes arising when translating from one language to another, the chances are greater when one cannot understand the information one is expected to translate, placing children in a difficult position when problems arise. An additional complication is that acting as parents' bridge with health care professionals can lead to hierarchical skews that interfere with the quality of care children receive (Cohen, Moran-Ellis and Smaje, 1999: Suárez-Orozoco and Suárez-Orozoco, 2001). Moreover, where parent–child and couple relationships are fraught, interpreting can be used to play one parent off against the other (Shen, Kim and Chao, 2014; Wu and Kim, 2009).

Although Aysen and Bayram had moved from Turkey to the UK about 20 years before, neither of them spoke English. Rather than drawing on a professional interpreter, they preferred to rely on their 12-year-old son Ahmet to translate on their behalf in meetings with the medical staff. This made it difficult for his mother Aysen, the person who took primary responsibility for his care, to confront him when he failed to adhere to his diabetic regime. Her sense of not belonging and reluctance to portray her family as shameful or problematic meant she delayed raising her concerns with the medical team. An additional complication was that, like many parents of children with a chronic condition, Aysen and Bayram disagreed about how strict they should be with their son and whether to be more open with the professionals responsible for his medical care.

In working with this family, it was important to focus on questions of adherence and the way in which the parents negotiated their differences. It was also important to focus on the intergenerational consequences of migration and language barriers. However, it was similarly important for the medical team to take account of the family's experience of difference and work towards helping the parents, particularly the mother, feel more ready to trust them with their concerns.

Medical migrations

Where there are significant concerns about the medical care that is available and families are able to access sufficient funding (through private or EU health insurance funds), children with a life-limiting condition may be sent abroad for a second opinion and/or treatment (Bookman and Bookman, 2007; Ormond, 2013). This can have an enormously positive effect on their physical health, offering access to cutting-edge methods of assessment and treatment.

However, depending on where they move to and from, children and parents may be faced a health care system where the paradigms of illness are very different, where perceptions of causality, attitudes towards disclosure, the communication of suffering, spirituality, understanding of childhood, children's right to information and interactions with health care professionals are at odds with 'back home' (Kleinman, 2006; Papadopoulos and Lay, 2007).

In some cases, being treated elsewhere means families spend time in a society where expectations of the roles of men and women are very different. As in situations where children living in rural areas are treated in a supra-regional centre in one of the larger towns, very often one parent accompanies their child while the other stays behind. This may be manageable for a short period of time. However, difficulties tend to arise when this is for longer, particularly where parents need to assume responsibility for tasks that clash with traditional gendered roles.

When 6-year-old Mahmud was diagnosed with a rare form of cancer, concerns about the quality of care he could access locally resulted in his family deciding his mother should take him to the UK for treatment, leaving his two younger siblings in the care of their father. However, as helpful as this was to Mahmoud's physical health, it was difficult to separate experiences of illness from the experience of moving to an unfamiliar environment in which Mahmoud and his mother could not draw on their usual support system and were unable to speak with the health care professionals without the help of an interpreter. Although an interpreter was booked to attend pre-set appointments, it was difficult to communicate with the staff and other parents and children on a more 'ad hoc' basis, or eavesdrop on other conversations on the ward.

Furthermore, being treated in the UK challenged cultural norms of what it means to be a family: in the society in which Mahmoud and his mother had been living, it was unusual for a woman to take responsibility for interacting with people in positions of authority (like health care professionals). Likewise, although Mahmoud's siblings were well cared for by their father and other close relatives, it was unusual for a father to assume this role and they missed the person who had been their main source of support until then: their mother.

In some cases, concerns to ensure their child gets the best possible treatment mean that both parents accompany their son or daughter. Providing their relationship is supportive, this can be enormously helpful, particularly since they cannot draw on the structures and other relationships upon which their lives have been grounded. This is more difficult when parents have other children and dependent relatives as someone else from their family or wider community has to step in to care for them, compounding the disruptive consequences for the children, their parents and the rest of their family. It is also more difficult when the parents' relationship is fraught and/or they have separated or divorced but financial constraints force them to live together for what is often a protracted period of time. The emotional intensity of situations where a child is seriously ill can rekindle more positive feelings for one another, increasing the parents' capacity to negotiate and reach shared decisions. However, the reverse is also true: the desire to avoid being drawn back into a relationship that felt unacceptable can result in blow-ups that impact on decisions about their child. In these situations, one or both parents might value the opportunity of reflecting on how they manage this situation and claim the emotional as well as physical space each of them needs.

When it becomes apparent that a child will not survive, the complicated process of being connected with two or more worlds is made even more complex by having to decide where one's child should die and their remains should rest. Just because one's child is dying does not mean parents will agree upon the best course of action. For example, one parent may be keen to return, fulfil traditional rituals and mourn with the rest of their family and community, while the other might be reluctant to do so, particularly when the pain control their child could access would not be as good as in the UK. Likewise, one parent may be more willing to accept the reality of impending death, while the other agitates to continue active treatment. Similarly, although one parent may believe it is better for the child to die in their home country, their partner may disagree as going home means giving up the dream of a cure and the supportive structure of the health care team, people with an in-depth understanding of their child's last days. Returning is also likely to be more difficult where children have been treated in a country where there is greater fluidity of gendered roles, where mothers were able to experience greater autonomy than in their home country.

The possibility of providing appropriate care is greater when we understand the cultural and religious practices of the people with whom we work, including beliefs about anticipations of death (Becker, 2002; Maitra and Krause, 2015). Nonetheless, actions ascribed to culture may have less to do with culture than an outsider's uncertainty about what is acceptable and feeling unable to ask:

> The staff working in a neonatal unit assumed that a mother's decision to sit a little way from her newborn baby (a child born with a genetic defect) reflected cultural taboos against becoming too engaged with a baby who is likely to die. However, when encouraged to sit closer, this mother accepted gratefully, suggesting she had not realized she could move the chair from where it had been placed when she entered the room.

Adult illness

As discussed earlier, many people are able to transcend the challenges illness presents with relatively little difficulty and/or see this as an opportunity for introducing constructive change. Nonetheless, being diagnosed with a life-limiting medical condition and having to accommodate one's lifestyle, personal and professional aspirations to maximize the chances of healing and surviving can be enormously difficult, with profound consequences for experiences of self and others.

Whilst some people prefer to deal with this situation on their own, for others being able to turn to people one knows and trusts is not only extremely supportive but helps in rebuilding a sense of continuity between the past, present and anticipated future (Little et al., 2002). However, unless one moves with a partner or other family members, this is rarely possible for migrants, particularly people who are isolated and moved fairly recently: even relatively minor conditions like a cold or backache become reminders of how alone one is when no one else notices how unwell they are, suggests seeing a doctor, brings food into the home or can be asked to collect medication from the pharmacy.

Where the condition is more severe, even if others are willing to help, exhaustion, worry and the 'diminishment' of self (Roose and Neimeyer, 2007; Weingarten, 2013) that accompanies many situations of illness tends to reduce the desire to be with others and feelings of entitlement to support, limiting the likelihood of turning to recent acquaintances for help. What makes this even more difficult is that experiences of bodily estrangement can re-evoke feelings and memories that relate to prior trauma and other forms of estrangement, including the estrangement associated with trying to fit in while knowing one does not, even if migration took place some time before.

Parental illness

When a migrant with dependent children is seriously ill and undergoes debilitating treatment, non-migrant parents, sisters and brothers may be able to take time out of their ordinary lives in order to support them and help care for their children. However, as mentioned earlier, it is rarely possible to do so on an ongoing basis. Although providing and receiving the practical and emotional support on a short-term basis is likely to be enormously helpful and enables families to affirm they can be relied upon and remain central to one another's lives, being together at such times in the knowledge of having to part once again can increase awareness of the possibility of more permanent parting, bringing the differences between 'real' and imagined experiences of family to the fore (Gardner and Grillo, 2002; Olwig, 2002). Moreover, having spent large periods of one's life living apart, it can be difficult living together in close quarters, particularly at a time of heightened emotionality. Where relationships have been fraught, even where past differences have been resolved, the emotional intensity and experience of living together for a protracted period of time can trigger conscious and unconscious feelings related to old disagreements and misunderstandings. Even though some of these difficulties may be a consequence of having lived apart for so long, talking about family dynamics can seem trivial or even selfish, particularly where the person one is frustrated with is in pain, undergoing debilitating treatment and facing the possibility of death.

Living together and being cared for by one's family is particularly complicated when the condition is stigmatized, as is the case for women in sub-Saharan Africa who, like Nonkosi, return home having contracted the HIV virus from becoming a sex worker in order to support their children and other relatives. However, even when the condition is not stigmatized, blow-ups and misunderstandings can arise that draw families back into past splits and polarizations.

Where parents have lived and worked abroad, the diagnosis of a life-threatening illness can result in returning to one's home country, particularly when the condition is terminal and non-migrant family are willing and able to offer the sort of support one cannot access elsewhere. This can be enormously helpful, particularly where family relationships are not fraught, as it ensures that one's children will be cared for by people one trusts. However, taking this step means children are faced with saying goodbye to friends and the life they have known at a time when so much else in their lives is uncertain, compounding the challenges of coming to terms with their parent's impending death:

> For example, Tessa and Joanna moved to Australia with their parents at the ages of 2 and 4, and returned to the UK with their mother after she was diagnosed with a terminal form of cancer. As their father had been killed in a road accident several years before, their maternal aunt became their primary carer after their mother's death. Although Tessa and Joanna had spent time with her on holidays to the UK, they did not know her well and resented her trying to 'step into the shoes' of their mother: as such they veered between turning to her and pushing her away.

In other cases, the difficulties of living apart and trying to bridge gaps in contact relate to interactions with the ill or dying person's partner as well as their children:

> Susanne came from New Zealand in her early twenties to study in the UK where she later settled with Genya, a Russian-born man she met at university. She sought help after being treated for an aggressive form of breast cancer. Although Susanne chose to be seen on her own, her more personal concerns were bound up with concerns about relationships with her mother and partner and worries about her children. On meeting Susanne, she said that her mother Barbara had come from New Zealand to look after her grandchildren, William (5) and Natasha (3), while she was in hospital and recovering from surgery. In common with many young children, William and Natasha found it extremely difficult being cared for by someone other than their mother, particularly since whispered conversations and her mother's absence from the home meant they suspected something worrying was happening. In this case, the added complication was that because they were very young and had not seen their grandmother for a year, she felt more like a stranger and was unfamiliar with the patterns of their daily lives, their likes, dislikes and which toy they took to bed with them at night.

> Moreover, having spent little time together before, her mother and partner were forced to live together at a time of heightened anxiety. Whilst Genya recognized his wife's need for additional support, he found his mother-in-law's presence intrusive and continued to work full time, despite being offered compassionate leave. Likewise, whilst Susanne valued her mother's support, she was wary of becoming too reliant on her, and resented the fact that her presence

meant her husband was less of a support to their children as well as herself. Consequently, although the work involved exploring Susanne's more personal existential concerns, it also involved reflecting on the more relational concerns she was facing, for example through 'imagining the other', by imagining how she might feel if she was in her mother's place.

As with Susanne and Genya, loneliness and/or freedom from the constraints of the structures and beliefs of the culture in which one was brought up can allow one to develop an intimate relationship with someone who seemed unavailable or even unacceptable before. Many of these relationships are stable and fulfilling. However, even if this decision was based on a desire to distance oneself from the sort of society in which one grew up, illness, disability and confrontation with mortality can re-evoke a desire for the familiar:

Both Anna and Carlos were born in Chile and moved to the UK in their early twenties. Their different backgrounds meant it was unlikely they would have met if they had not left: Anna was from a wealthy, educated but largely apolitical family and came to the UK to study, while Carlos was from a poor farming community and left after being released from prison for activities seen to be anti-government. Although they were drawn together by a shared cultural heritage and sense of dislocation, they were also attracted by their difference, underpinned by the desire for a 'corrective family script' (Byng-Hall, 1995): the desire to establish a couple relationship and experience for their children that was very different to that of their family of origin.

When Anna was diagnosed with oesophageal cancer, they were faced with differences they found difficult to acknowledge and resolve. Having grown up in a family in which she was protected and seen as vulnerable, Anna cherished the fact that Carlos saw her as strong and independent and was reluctant to ask for help. However, becoming ill increased Anna's longing to be cared for: she was reluctant to ask for help, feeling that Carlos could not provide her with the support she needed. Moreover, having distanced herself from her parents and siblings, although she now wished she could turn to them she felt unable to do so.

In contrast, Carlos's fear of losing Anna triggered feelings related to earlier loss and trauma, including flashbacks of his experience of imprisonment and torture, limiting his ability to engage with Anna's fear and distress. Although Anna had respected that Carlos found it difficult to talk about distressing issues before, she now needed him to hear and understand how she felt. When this seemed impossible, Anna turned to friends for support, leading to complications that exacerbated the difficulties both partners were experiencing in coming to terms with the fact she was terminally ill.

Consequently, much of the work focused upon illness-related challenges, including what they could and could not ask of one another, concerns about their children, shared and individual experiences of loss and fears for the future. However, as with Susanna, it also involved exploring the links between their experiences of migration and responses to illness. Although a number of other factors were also important, placing migration and its consequences central to discussions provided Anna and Carlos an alternate frame for reflecting on their relationship and the care of their children, opening up the possibility of reviewing their differences in a way that did not automatically position one person as right and the other as wrong. Discussions about migration also led to exploring the connections with their families of origin and what needed to change before Anna felt able to be more open with and reach out to her family.

Exposure to increased scrutiny

People whose responses are different to what is regarded as usual in the country they move to have an increased risk of their behaviour and symptoms being treated with suspicion:

> The questions American-born Daniel asked the medical team were based on a legitimate right to information about his condition (a malignant melanoma) and his desire to explore alternative methods of treatment. However, because his style was more forthright than was usual in Britain he was seen as rude and aggressive. Moreover, although Daniel appreciated the fact that, as a British citizen, he was able to access to free health care, he resented the lack of choice this entailed. In addition, because he thought the chances of survival would have been higher had he been treated in the United States, he felt needed to be vigilant ('demanding') to ensure he received the best possible care.

As mentioned in Chapter 3, it can be difficult to know whether to view 'medically unexplained symptoms' (Swoboda, 2007) as 'real' (as indicative of organic disease or malfunction that is not yet evident) or expressions of an underlying depressive or anxiety disorder (Burton et al., 2011; van der Feltz-Cornelis et al., 2012). However, where the person reporting these symptoms has moved from a country where constructions of illness and treatment are markedly different, it is also difficult to know whether these symptoms reflect a different appreciation of illness and how the body operates, or a cry for help from an isolated and depressed person. Indeed, although the exact nature of the links between the physical and psychological have yet to be deciphered, there appears to be some link between social marginalization, exposure to racism, other forms of violation and experiences of somatic pain (Carter, 2007).

For example, Faduma, a 40-year-old Turkish mother of three children, visited her GP clinic frequently complaining of a range of symptoms, including stomach-, back- and headaches. Although Faduma thought these symptoms meant she was seriously ill, her GP saw them as an expression of the social and emotional challenges she was facing, including guilt about leaving her non-migrant parents, difficulties in adapting to life in a new context and learning English, worries about her children's schooling and living with an unemployed and alcoholic husband.

Consequently, in working with Faduma, it was important to respect her symptoms at a physical level, including the stress of contending with symptoms no one understood, and explore what sort of help she might have sought in her country of origin before attempting to address the links between physical and emotional distress. As in work with other migrants, particularly refugees, the work extended beyond these clinical sessions: this included acting as an intermediary and advocate by attending a meeting at her children's school with her and exploring the possibility of accessing additional community support.

Nonetheless, in some cases it is more difficult to avoid questioning what one is told and sees: as when there are suspicions that symptoms are being used to increase migrants' access to disability and housing benefits, and when faced with symptoms arising from family and marriage practices less acceptable or illegal in the UK (such as female genital mutilation or marriage between cousins).

Illness and the position of non-migrants

Even though non-migrants do not move from one geographic context to another, the fact that their children, siblings and/or parents migrated means their experience of illness, disability and threat of death is likely to be very different to what they would have been if their loved one had not left.

For example, where young people leave in search of better prospects of employment elsewhere in later life parents are faced with managing situations of illness and increased frailty without them. In other cases parents move to join their children at this stage of their lives. This enables them to receive the hands-on practical and emotional support they need and allows their children to fulfil their and their parents' expectations of filial care. However, moving at this stage of life means spending one's last days in a country where the culture and climate may be very different, without the structures upon which one's life has been grounded: isolated from friends and colleagues and where, other than one's children, no one knows who one is and what one's life has been like. It is also more difficult to establish a new social network at this stage of life, particularly when unable to speak the main language. Consequently, parents who move at this stage are inclined to be more reliant on their children than would otherwise have been the case, which can give rise to tensions, expectations and disappointments that are difficult for all concerned.

The situation tends to be different for 'left behind' parents: for example, although Beryl supported her children's decisions to leave apartheid-based South Africa, she had not anticipated that her husband would have a stroke at 65, and how difficult it would be caring for him without the hands-on support of her children. However, she underplayed her difficulties when speaking with them.

As reflected in the small but growing body of research focused on the experience of non-migrant parents in countries like China (Giles and Mu, 2005), India (Militiades, 2002), South Africa (Altschuler, 2008a; Marchetti-Mercer, 2012) and Turkey (Coles, 2001), like Beryl many non-migrant parents and other non-migrant relatives find it extremely difficult deciding when and whether to alert family living elsewhere that they are seriously ill, have had a fall or, as is often the case in late life, when memory deteriorates to a point where living alone is starting to be risky. A number of factors could account for Beryl's tendency to underplay difficulties including the fear of pushing her children away by appearing too needy and the desire to protect them from anxiety and/or herself from the sadness and disappointment of knowing they could not (or are unwilling to) drop the rest of their lives to help her. Holding back may have been an attempt to retain her identity as a strong and competent person and avoid facing her own mortality in a context in which the person she had spent so much of her life with was deteriorating before her eyes. Regardless of the motivation, the tendency to underplay difficulties means it is more difficult for migrant children to know what is needed, wanted and when to put their lives on hold to return and to offer hands-on support.

Where migrant adult children are kept informed about parents' health concerns or discern that things are difficult by reading between the lines, they may be able to play a significant role in supporting their parents and non-migrant siblings from a distance through regular emails, phone and Skype calls, providing financial assistance and assuming more caretaking responsibility on visits back home. Where parents do not understand what they have been told or they or their children feel the quality of the medical care they are receiving is inadequate it may be possible to phone or meet the medical team when they do visit to help parents make sense of what is happening, contribute to decisions about care and, if need be, set up a better care package. However, because it is rarely possible to offer this sort of support on a more ongoing basis, as reflected below, experiences of illness and the threat of death can confront parents and children with the gaps between their lived and anticipated experiences of what it means to be family:

> Jack, a 70-year-old cardiologist who left South Africa in his early twenties, remained haunted by the memory of his elderly mother saying she hoped he would come back, and not seeing her again until she was dying.

With some exceptions (Altschuler, 2008b; Marchetti-Mercer, 2012), relatively little attention has been paid to the ways migrant and non-migrant siblings negotiate their differences when their parents' health begins to deteriorate. Living closer tends to mean non-migrants assume greater responsibility for parental care than their migrant siblings. This may not be problematic. However, even if the relationship has always been supportive long-term caregiving can be extremely burdensome. This is particularly challenging when parents are severely incapacitated, the financial costs are considerable, and when non-migrant siblings have little respite and continue to be responsible for their own dependent children.

One of the other complexities migrant and non-migrant families face is that non-migrant parents tend to be confronted with many other losses at this time of life including retirement, the illness and death of friends and close relatives, and are therefore more isolated than before, stretching parent–child (more usually the non-migrant child) relationships to a point that feels intolerable (Surbone et al., 2006). Even if siblings live in the same town, it is not unusual for relationships to become strained and for family members to disagree about such issues as the need for additional care, treatment options and a move to residential care (Davies and Nolan, 2003; Kramer, Boelk and Auer, 2006). However, differences in caring responsibilities that arise from migration can re-evoke feelings that relate to earlier negotiations of differences, limiting siblings' ability to hear one another. Some of these differences may relate to the fact that siblings who see their parents more often are likely to be more aware of the extent to which parents' health has deteriorated:

> Sheila's brother Brian moved from the UK to work in Hong Kong. As a result she assumed primary responsibility for looking after their parents as they became increasingly frail. When their mother, and later their father, showed symptoms of dementia, Sheila became increasingly worried about the risks of accidents in the home, felt unable to cope, tried persuading them to move into residential care and looked to her brother for support. However, because Brian's visits to the UK were for limited periods of time, he was less aware of their confusion and gaps in memory and opposed this, compounding Sheila's own guilt about taking such a step. What made this particularly difficult was that,

regardless of how much she had done for her parents, she felt they respected and valued Brian more than herself.

Despite the desire to work collaboratively, the emotional intensity of coming together for a limited period of time and facing one's parents' (and probably one's own) mortality can result in blow-ups that are difficult to understand. As such, it may be impossible to reach decisions about a parent's care without disentangling the past from the present, ideally by discussing this together and – if this is not feasible – separately. Where migration is from a highly politicized country, this may include trying to disentangle the political from the more personal.

As discussed in Chapter 5, reflecting on the migration of his older brother Peter from apartheid-based South Africa, Alex, who continued to live in the country, said that having previously seen Peter's stance as heroic and political, his view had shifted to seeing his migration as a way of escaping responsibility for the political as well as the family.

However, it is important to avoid generalizing: in some cases migrant siblings play a more central role in the care of non-migrant parents. Moreover, although living apart can mean it is more difficult healing the rifts that arise, this is not necessarily true: where relationships have become strained, concerns about parents' health can become a 'third space' (Bhabha, 1994), opening up the possibility of a better understanding of one another.

Later life and confrontation with death

Despite considerable advances in the management of chronic conditions, relatively little is known about the ways in which older people from ethnic minorities, including migrants, view chronic illness or manage this in their everyday lives, even though there is a greater prevalence of chronic illness amongst certain ethnic minorities. In view of the fact that many migrants are extremely isolated and growing evidence of a strong link between loneliness and health (Jaremka, Fagundes, Bennett et al., 2013; Jaremka, Fagundes, Glaser et al., 2013; Jaremka et al., 2014; particularly in later life (Victor et al., 2012), this omission is extremely unfortunate. For example, insufficient attention has been paid to the fact that people from ethnic minorities do not necessarily subscribe to mainstream Western medical tenets, such as the belief that individuals can control their environment and the value of taking responsibility for one's health. Although people living in Western societies tend to view death as the ultimate disruption, for people of other cultural and religious backgrounds death represents a form of continuity: it is part of the ongoing wheel of life.

As discussed in Chapter 4, experiences of culture and ethnicity are not static but continually redefined and renegotiated. For many people ethnicity is the embodiment of their most central values; this tends to become increasingly important as they get older and are faced with deteriorating health and the threat of death, as was true of my father (Becker, 2002). As migrants get older, very often the meanings attached to life and death become more closely connected with their homeland (Hammerton, 2004). Consequently, where finances allow, some people move between their country of settlement and origin when they retire: this enables them to maintain links with their non-migrant family and country of origin and, where migration involved a significant climate change, avoid weather they find particularly challenging.

However, going 'home' is less feasible when older adults and/or their partners are frail and ill. Having lived elsewhere for a long time, they are unlikely to be able to draw on a supportive network in their country of origin: family and friends of their age may be frail or ill too or have died (van der Geest et al., 2004). Moreover, where they have established a family in the country of settlement, returning would mean living apart from their children at a time when they are likely to need increased support. In contrast, for those who are less settled and have family remaining in their country of origin, their gaze is more likely to turn back to the homeland where most of their family live. In some cases the desire to return is thwarted by financial constraints. For others, returning home or moving to join migrant children when ill would mean spending one's last days in a place with less developed medical treatment and pain relief, hastening the likelihood of death. Where, as is often the case, elderly parents move to join their children when they become more ill and frail, they are likely to be able to draw on the support of their children and grandchildren. However, it is impossible then to turn to friends one has known throughout one's life when faced with illness, the death of a much-loved partner, or when parents and adult children disagree on aspects of medical care.

Anticipations of death have the potential to re-evoke feelings related to past loss. Consequently, sitting together in a hospital or hospice with the said and unsaid can trigger memories of previous partings, of sitting together at airports and train stations, in the knowledge of a more permanent journey into the unknown (Clifford, 1997; Gunaratnam, 2013). The dying person may be admitted to a hospice or another form of residential care where the staff members have little knowledge of their cultural and religious practices. In these cases, people who have been particular about following religious dietary restrictions may be unable to say what they want and need, or indeed to know what they are being fed. Although relatives and neighbours may be able to speak on behalf of that person, they may not attach similar importance to their religious and cultural beliefs and practices.

Relatively little is known about the ways in which migrants view their homeland and the possibility of dying elsewhere in later life. Regardless of whether or not migration has taken place, fears about severing links with one another and the past mean that, provided the dying person's mental capacity is not compromised, the last few weeks, days and hours include sharing much-loved recipes and life stories, adding names to photographs, re-discussing inheritance and talking about family secrets. Where migration has taken place these discussions are likely to be infused with unexpressed questions about whether or not cultural and religious traditions will be maintained after the death and what the next generation's connection with what had previously been one's home might be. Where memory fades and confusion sets in, visions of earlier times and places blend with the present, making it impossible for loved ones to ask the questions they never knew they had, or did not have the courage to ask before, including questions about life 'over there' and family who stayed behind (Gunuratnam, 2013).

Questions of connections to more than one country are rendered even more complicated by having to decide where to die. In some cases, religious and cultural traditions result in a very particular form of homecoming as dead bodies and sealed caskets are taken back to their country of origin, adding to the emotional, practical and financial challenges survivors face (Gunaratnam, 2013). For many people, the homeland represents a source of stability, the repository of memories of youth, family and friends who died some time before. However, for those who were forced to leave in traumatic circumstances, one's homeland is likely to be a source of painful or even shameful memories, of chaos and disorientation:

> For Rachael, whose experience of growing up in apartheid-based South Africa was dominated by having to hide that her mother was mentally ill and that she was born Indian but 'declared white by application', the death of her brother-in-law, the husband of the older sister whose support had sustained her through difficult times, re-evoked shameful memories of the past.

Nonetheless, real and imagined encounters with death can become another sort of 'third space' (Bhabha, 1994), allowing for the possibility of re-remembering and re-imagining the past, altering understanding of oneself and the other (Umberson, 2003). Consequently, anticipations of death can provoke the pull of a distant homeland and the desire to bring together the various strands of one's life, showing how experiences of identity may be place-based even though they are not place-bound, as with Joe, a man who moved from to South Africa in 1938:

> Joe's decision to leave Germany was primarily motivated by a desire to escape a country in which being a Jew meant his life was at risk. However, his other motivation was to escape a father whom he saw as cold and cruel. Joe went on to develop a strong identification with his country of settlement, South Africa, devoting much of his life to fighting apartheid. Nonetheless, when faced with death, he told his children he wanted to be buried in Germany, the country associated with troubled memories of his positioning as a Jew as well as memories of his father, whom he never saw again as he died in a concentration camp. This suggests that, faced with death, Joe reached some form of reconciliation in relation to his father and 'fatherland', even if this anticipated reconciliation or return would only take place after his death.

> It is difficult to refuse the wishes of someone who is dying (Pipher, 1999): Joe's wish meant that his children had to transport his body to be buried and return to Germany when they wanted to visit his grave, suggesting desire to ensure that they remain connected with and develop a better understanding of what had previously been his home.

When, as is often the case with parents, the deceased held the family together and represented migrants' attachment with their country of origin, migrant and non-migrant siblings are likely to be faced with questions about their future relationship. Gatherings to mark the death of a loved one are an opportunity to affirm some sense of continuity, signalling the importance of the deceased and others to one another (Gardner and Grillo, 2002; Olwig, 2002). However, the powerful emotions surrounding situations of death and the intensity of being together in the knowledge of separating once more mean that it is not unusual for blowups to occur, reminding the survivors of the value of living apart.

Mourning tends to be more complicated when living apart interferes with the possibility of healing the rifts that can develop:

> About a year after Tanya had come to study in the UK, her mother called to say that her father, a man in his mid-fifties, had died following a sudden heart attack. Difficulties in coming to terms with the sudden and unexpected death of her much loved father were compounded by the fact that, although Tanya was able to attend his funeral in the US, on returning to the UK she was surrounded by people who had not known her father. What made this even more difficult was the fact that her father had been her main source of support when she was diagnosed with Crohn's disease as an adolescent. However, their relationship

had been more troubled following her decision to study abroad. Moreover, although she had agreed to go home for the December break, she decided to delay her return until the summer, which meant she did not see him again.

There is considerable debate about whether Jewish identity (or identities) is based on religious affiliation, culture, ethnicity, biology or a combination of all of these factors. Nonetheless, much of the literature prioritizes legacies of exile and oppression: this is reflected in the idea that, for Jews, instead of cultural identification being located in place, it is more rooted in genealogy and traditional customs (Boyarin and Boyarin, 1993). Indeed, the Jewish tradition of placing a stone on someone's grave before leaving the cemetery as a sign to others that someone has paid their respects to the deceased alludes to experiences of dispersal and a sense of belonging that is not only rooted in place. Consequently, traditional customs and cultural sites, including places of worship, offer migrants an opportunity to feel part of an 'imagined community' (Anderson, 1983): even if people have not met before, aspects of experience are assumed to be shared.

However, Tanya's sense of isolation, guilt and despair about losing her father meant she was reluctant to attend synagogue services to say the traditional memorial prayers as there would be no one there who knew her father or what she and he had meant to one another. It is obviously impossible to undo the past. However, in working with Tanya it was important to revisit aspects of the past, reflect upon and reimagine what her leaving might have meant both for herself and her father and what he would have wanted for her now.

In other situations, political factors interfere with the possibility of mourning and making sense of one's connection to the deceased and one's homeland:

Ali felt he made the right decision in leaving Iran to avoid another term of imprisonment. However, he was haunted by the fact that his parents died a year after he left but he was not able to support them or attend their funerals. What made this even more painful was that he was unable to share memories with anyone who knew his parents and knew him when they were alive: although other people from his village had also come to the UK, they lived a long distance away.

In some situations, young children are left holding on to grief their migrant parents cannot contain:

Greta and Hans, who had moved from Holland to the UK about 10 years previously, sought help as they were worried about the way in which their 6-year-old son Jan had changed following the death of his maternal grandmother: he had become increasingly withdrawn, found it difficult to sleep and was afraid of separating from his mother. In an initial meeting, Greta and Hans revealed that on hearing her mother had been in a traffic accident and was in a critical state, they had gone to Holland, leaving their son in the care of a close friend. Although they suspected Greta's mother would not survive, they decided to wait until their return before telling Jan about his grandmother.

When asked about Jan's previous experience of separation, it became apparent that although Hans worked abroad fairly often, this was the first time Jan had spent a night without his mother. It was therefore possible that he had come to equate death with separation. As with Tanya, feelings of guilt and regret seemed to increase Greta's struggle in mourning her mother. They had considered returning to Holland but decided to stay because of Hans' work: although Greta had agreed with this decision she was tortured by the thought that if they returned she would have had more time with her mother and might have been able to prevent her death.

Greta's distress meant that there were times when she found it impossible to avoid crying in Jan's presence. As mentioned in discussing responses to illness, when children are not told what is happening, they draw on what they see in order to make sense of what is happening: although Jan knew his grandmother had died, his mother's distress meant he was worried something was wrong with her as well. Consequently clinical work focused on helping Jan come to terms with and understand his grandmother's death, and individual sessions with Greta. Greta and Jan were also offered an opportunity to reflect upon their experience as a couple. This included exploring the way migration had compounded their difficulties in coming to terms with this sudden unanticipated death. Discussions about migration led to the realization that the death of Greta's mother had increased their sense of belonging in the UK: the support they had received from their son's school, parents of other children in his class, friends and colleagues gave them a greater sense of belonging to a community, which resulted in a decision to hold a ceremony to mark the death of Greta's mother with the people with whom they shared many aspects of their lives in the UK.

Refugees and asylum seekers

Most research and clinical literature fails to take account of the opinions refugees and asylum seekers have about experiences of illness and health care. However, the few studies that do exist indicate that although many refugees and asylum seekers were generally pleased with the NHS care they received, there were areas where they experienced difficulties, including access to hospital-based specialists and medication as well as access to and the confidentiality of interpreters. In addition, most people stated their preference for GPs who offered advice rather than prescriptions. These concerns illustrate the need to be aware of and acknowledge the impact different systems of care can have on individuals' expectations of health care. They also illustrate the need to ensure all sectors have access to equitable care (Bhatia and Wallace, 2007; O'Donnell et al., 2008).

Most of the challenges discussed in relation to all forms of migration are applicable to refugees and asylum seekers. However, others emerge from their particular positions as refugees. For example, people who have been caught up in political conflict are likely to have faced unspeakable horrors, including situations in which they or their family were at risk of being killed and/or where fear, anxiety and the desire to protect themselves and/or loved ones meant they acted in ways that ran counter to their deepest values. Having invested all their energies into survival and making a dangerous journey to safety, it is not unusual for the rates of suicidal ideation, suicide attempts and 'successful' suicide to increase on reaching safety (Aspinal, 2009, 2010; Perez Foster, 2001; Ratkowska and De Leo, 2013).

In addition, the struggle to survive means that health care is unlikely to have been a priority; consequently, people may have delayed seeking care until their symptoms became pronounced, impacting on the chances of treatment and survival. Moreover, even when asylum has been granted, it can be difficult to prioritize one's own health when worried about family or friends who were too young, frail or ill to escape:

> Soon after arriving in the UK, Fefo, a woman who fled Uganda after refusing to engage in actions she found inhumane, began experiencing a range of debilitating symptoms, including breathlessness, tightness in the chest and pain in one arm (symptoms which could be indicative of angina). However, worry and guilt about the elderly mother she had left behind meant she found it difficult to think about her own health needs and seek professional care.

The urgency to leave means many refugees do not have intact or retrievable medical records, impacting upon the possibilities of appropriate assessment and treatment (Aspinall and Watters, 2010; Fisher, 2004). For example, when people whose family have died or are dispersed present with symptoms suggestive of a genetically transmitted condition, such as Huntington's chorea, it is more difficult to construct a clear and accurate account of the illness history of the family. This is particularly problematic when working with unaccompanied minors as they are unlikely to have much understanding about their own health history, that of their parents and many other aspects of their history (Chase, 2013).

In other situations, distance from other adults one knows and trusts mean parents act in ways that run counter to their deepest held beliefs, for example by sharing far more with their children than they would otherwise have done or leaving them in the care of strangers to attend to their own health needs. Other challenges relate to access to care: for example, although asylum seekers who are in end stage renal failure are able to receive certain forms of treatment free of charge, they are unlikely to be placed on the transplant list even if they have been told this is needed.

For refugees who bear the physical and psychological scars of imprisonment, torture, rape, deprivation and other traumatic experiences, the trauma, bodily fragmentation and invasions associated with illness, treatment and assessment (for example, a vaginal examination) can re-evoke conscious and unconscious memories, flashbacks and physical sensations that make it difficult to trust people in positions of authority, including health care professionals. An additional complication is that flashbacks from the past can interfere with the possibility of providing a coherent claim to the Home Office, affecting the chances of securing asylum and full entitlement to health care: attempts to deal with trauma by distancing oneself from the emotion associated with these experiences may mean that one's account is unconvincing as it comes across as too dispassionate (Bogner, Herlihy and Brewin, 2010).

Rape has long been recognized as a weapon of war: physical and psychological acts of violence against targeted individuals are carried out in order to break individuals and fragment families and communities, invoking such fear and shame that victims and their families remain silent. One of the more common responses to rape is to 'dissociate', to try to separate self from body in order to manage the overwhelming feelings of shame, humiliation and pain. Drawing on their work with men and women who have survived rape and other forms of torture, Avigad and Rahimi (2010) discuss the importance of working towards enabling the person to bring soul and body together again through confronting 'damaged' aspects of oneself and gradually allowing this to become part of one's personal narrative, and where possible, narrative of the family.

However, many people are torn between wanting and not wanting to find words for the unspeakable trauma they have faced. There are also likely to be times when as health care professionals we are ambivalent about encouraging people to reflect on traumatic events for fear of what might be unleashed, for example:

> I was asked to see Liu, a woman who had been repeatedly raped in her country of origin. Liu began by saying she had been raped but then shifted to her worries about the four children she had left behind before becoming tearful and saying she was too exhausted to go on. Rather than encouraging her to

continue I decided to sit with her in silence. The decision was informed by clinical experience, my reluctance to push her to say more than she was ready to and the understanding that in some cases, powerful feelings are only able to come to the surface when one is silent (Rober and de Haene, 2014). However, it was also informed by my own anxieties about the risks of compounding her distress and the more personal fears her story evoked for me.

In some situations language barriers mean asylum seekers rely on the documents they possess that are written in English to explain their concerns, which contain information they may not have wished to divulge:

> While waiting for a Tamil speaking interpreter to arrive, Daman introduced himself by showing me the papers he was using to support his claim for asylum, which included graphic details and pictures showing how his genitals and fingers had been mutilated as a result of being tortured. Although Daman may actually have wanted to share some of these details he was not in control of how much information was disclosed.

Unlike Daman, most people die during torture. Moreover, many are too disabled and destitute to make their way to safety. A certain element of chance and, to some extent, resources and resilience enable a minority to arrive in the country they are aiming for. However many go on to present with a wide range of health problems, particularly chronic pain, post-traumatic stress disorder (PTSD), anxiety, depression and other forms of distress without the traumatic experience ever having been disclosed or identified (Amris and Williams, 2015).

Survivors of political torture often contend with a sense of invisibility arising from feelings of shame, guilt and anguish that are so deep and beyond ordinary human existence they are impossible to express in words: shame emerges from an experience of intense powerlessness and unwilling passivity, guilt from wondering whether one could have done something to avoid arrest, detention and torture, and anguish about the possibility of having advertently betrayed loved ones or colleagues. During torture, pain is used to destroy and deny the very idea of relationships. If torturers succeed, they turn victims into informers, unwilling allies of the very people who are harming them. Even if they say nothing, people on the outside can never be sure whether the survivors 'turned' – whether they provided information that puts others at risk. What makes this even more difficult is that those who are tortured are usually made to believe they are alone and can expect no help, comfort or compassion from the outside. As such, they tend to emerge hyper-vigilant, fearful and mistrustful (Nutkiewicz, 2007).

Experiences of torture mean many survivors have an uneasy relationship with health care providers: people advised to attend torture treatment centres because they are petitioning for political asylum are often unclear about what to expect and whether doctors and therapists work for the government and the court system. Having been abused by people in authority, victims of torture can find it difficult to trust and to know when it is safe to stand one's ground and whether it is possible to fight for what one wants and needs. In addition, torture draws on medical expertise: in some cases doctors and psychologists have been implicated in their experience of torture (Miles, 2006). In common with many other refugees, some torture victims will not have encountered Western styles of healing before, particularly psychotherapy. This means it takes time for clinicians to explain what they can offer and explore the challenges people have faced and are facing.

In working with survivors, it is important to take account of PTSD and other conditions that can be diagnosed. However, this can have the unintended consequence of medicalizing and pathologizing the survivor: as significant as the triggering traumatic event may be, it is also important to focus upon other stressful aspects of life including the loss of family, paid employment, educational opportunities and displacement through expulsions, exile and flight. In many situations the idea of a cure or healing is an unattainable goal. Healing requires the opportunity to achieve justice and bear witness to an uncontainable and uncontrollable past. However, this is generally not open to the survivor. Moreover, all too often the health care workers these survivors meet are not equipped to deal with the complex moral, relational and existential issues arising from torture.

Furthermore, while some people find relief and comfort from trying to put their experiences in to words, for others this is too risky. When traumatic memories have been blocked out and people are too fearful of facing the past, survivors are left with excruciating chronic pain. In these situations, often the best we can offer is to alleviate the anxiety, suggest ways of distraction from pain, and work towards increasing their ability to function in everyday activities (Patel, Kellezi and de Williams, 2014; Montgomery and Patel, 2011).

Recommendations for practice

In working with immigrants, refugees, asylum seekers and non-migrant kin with health problems, the primary concern is to focus upon the issues they find troubling. Depending on the responsibilities and expectations of our professional role, this might include asking about the symptoms they are experiencing, providing some explanation of why these symptoms may have developed, if needed, recommending additional tests and, where possible, intervening to alleviate their symptoms and reduce suffering. For people who are extremely isolated, even if language and cultural barriers mean it is not always possible to understand what is said and needed, consultations with health care professionals may be one of the only opportunities of feeling held, of being with a person who takes one's concerns seriously and can be trusted to maintain confidentiality.

Access and training

A wide range of initiatives have been introduced aimed at ensuring migrants are able to access the medical and psychosocial care that is needed at times of illness and death. However, despite considerable improvements this continues to be problematic.

Greater emphasis needs to be placed on establishing a clearer understanding of the needs of particular migrant and ethnic groups and on increased engagement with stakeholders (including patients, families and representatives of local community organizations) and advocacy groups knowledgeable about migrant and minority ethnic group issues, particularly where there is distrust of the medical system. As health care professionals, it is important to increase our understanding of the challenges arising from experiences of migration, trauma and the cultural and religious traditions of the people with whom we work and find sensitive ways to address these experiences. Since GPs tend to be people's first port of call, it is also important to increase the level of support and training they receive to improve communication, reduce the stigma associated with refugee status and extend their skills in addressing the challenges refugees and other migrants face (Bhatia and Wallace, 2007; O'Donnell et al., 2008). In addition, Primary Care Trusts could supply information to newly arrived refugees on how to access services.

Extending the clinical brief beyond the session

In many situations, work with immigrants, refugees and asylum seekers involves engaging with other agencies and finding out about and linking people with resources within their community. This may include acting as an advocate or intermediary supporting people in realizing their rights in the UK, for example the right to rehabilitation, accessing services and housing benefits. This is particularly important in working with adults and children who have survived torture (Avigad and Rahimi, 2004).

Voluntary sector community organizations can act as a bridge in identifying and addressing the needs of particular migrant groups (Falicov, 2013). Migrants who are extremely isolated are likely to benefit from information in relation to health care, social benefits, and opportunities to learn English and engage with other people to rebuild some sense of community in the place in which they are living now. Faced with loss and fragmentation, some people may need help and encouragement to engage with activities that lead to connecting with others. In view of the strong link between loneliness and ill-health, this is particularly important in later life (Jaremka, Fagundes, Bennett et al., 2013; Jaremka, Fagundes, Glaser et al., 2013; Jaremka et al., 2014; Victor et al., 2012).

As Fortier (2000) found in her study of Italian immigrants living in London, organizations representative of the home culture have the potential to reify and reinforce asymmetries in gendered roles and responsibilities around health care. It can feel uncomfortable or even dangerous to connect with compatriots when little is known about the role they played in situations of political conflict and oppression, and where shame about one's current life means one is reluctant for news about one's situation to reach non-migrant family or friends.

Nonetheless, particularly where people feel uncomfortable with local services, transnational networks play a significant role in health care and emotional survival. In many cities, social networks are used to secure treatment for formal as well as informal health care, including care that incorporates biomedical and traditional practices, challenging assumptions about the uni-directional flow of medical knowledge and treatment from what is regarded as the more developed North to the South. Indeed, studies of Latin Americans in London (Gideon, 2013) and Bolivians in Spain (Escandell and Tapias, 2010) indicate that in some cases, where finances are stretched, compatriots get together to raise funds for people to see Latin American or Spanish-speaking doctors.

Placing migration central to discussions of illness

The complexities of living some distance from one's extended family and country of origin and adjusting to life in a different environment mean that exploring how migration impacts on illness and health care can help in reframing struggles that seem indicative of personal failure as almost inevitable responses to the challenges associated with being ill and facing the threat of death in contexts of migration, bringing experiences of self, family and health care that are underplayed into increased visibility.

Provided sufficient trust has been established and people feel their views will be respected, conversations about migration and cultural adjustments offer insights into the differences between people's current lives and the lives they might have led in their country of origin, including the support structure they might have been able to draw upon previously. It can also be helpful to explore the relational, gendered and intergenerational transformations that so often arise in accommodating illness as well as migration, the challenges of responding to illness when one is less able to access the support of family and friends, and exposure to racism and other forms of prejudice.

Asking about the sort of health care people would have been able to access before can lead to discussing people's understanding of the cause of their symptoms, including their spiritual beliefs: this is particularly important because many people turn to religion and other forms of spirituality when faced with life-limiting illness, anticipations of death and other difficult situations. Similarly, discussions about cultural and language barriers offer an opportunity to think about situations where communication has been particularly difficult, helping to reduce the likelihood of misunderstandings. Where experiences of migration and/or illness have led to feeling demoralized and ashamed, it is also important to bring experiences of strengths and resilience to the fore. This includes considering the relational, spiritual and other resources people have drawn upon in the past, what helps in maintaining their sense of determination and self-esteem at difficult times, and whether any of the previously useful strategies could help in accommodating the challenges presented by illness.

It is impossible to undo the past and make up for what was lost. However, situations of flux and heightened emotionality can become a 'third space' (Bhabha, 2004) that allow for a different understanding of oneself, others and the context in which difficulties evolved. Where relationships have become estranged, and/or migrants and their non-migrant kin have avoided sharing their concerns with those living elsewhere, it can be helpful to encourage people to reflect on the 'internalized other' (Tomm, Hoyt and Madigan, 2001), to imagine how they might feel if they were in the other person's position, and what might need to happen before they feel ready to breach the gap and share their concerns with one another Where it is possible to meet, exchanging memories and mental images of events that took place prior to, or during, their separation (including small details that renew and increase knowledge of one another) can help in regenerating empathy for one another, remaking meaning of these separations and restoring a sense of family coherence (Falicov, 2013).

It is also important to avoid pushing people into discussions they are unwilling to consider and ensure discussions about migration do not increase their sense of being seen as 'other'. Likewise, it is important to remain alert to our own prejudices and the more complicated feelings that can arise from attempting to bridge the gap between our own experience and 'unfamiliar lives' (Levinas, 1994). However, this touches on challenges that are pertinent to all work with illness and death: the capacity to take risks, engage with uncertainty, learn from mistakes, and to be moved by the suffering of another without being overwhelmed by the feelings their situation evokes in ourselves.

7

WORKING WITH MIGRANT PATIENTS IN GENERAL PRACTICE

Rachel Hopkins

As a general practitioner (GP) in inner city London, the majority of my work is with patients who are first- or second-generation migrants to the UK. My interest in this area of work was initially sparked as a new GP, some two decades ago, finding consultations with patients from different cultures fascinating but also frustrating. I would often end a consultation with the feeling that despite my best efforts and the use of an interpreter when required, I had somehow failed to meet my patient's expectations, or to understand something they had been telling me. Sometimes patients were clearly cross and frustrated with me; sometimes I just had a feeling that communication had not gone well, and sometimes patients returned without following my advice. I realized that although my education as a doctor had been comprehensive biomedically, and my training as a GP had covered a more holistic 'bio-psycho-social' approach (Brody, 1999) as well as considering the interrelationship between doctor and patient (Balint, 1957), I had very little education on working across cultures.

About this time, I took a course in systemic approaches to working in general practice and developed an interest in narrative and systemic approaches in the consultation, initially under the tutelage of John Launer, who has written widely in this area (Launer, 1995, 1996, 2002). I used these ideas to develop my cross-cultural work with patients, taking a narrative and systemic approach. Systemic theory is concerned with interrelationships and context at many levels; systemic approaches in general practice can involve appreciating the social, family and cultural context of the patient, and making connections (Asen and Tomson, 1995). Narrative approaches to the consultation value the stories that patients tell about their experiences and see the consultation as an opportunity to co-create a more useful narrative with the patient (Launer, 1996, 2002). This was also the time I first met Jenny Altschuler, who came to our practice to offer a family therapy service to our patients and supervision to the GPs. She helped us to think more widely about the family in our work, and we started to discuss the effects that migration had on the families we saw.

My own cultural background is white and British, and I was born and grew up in North London in an academic family. My parents shared interests in the human condition and understanding human emotions, relationships and behaviours. We spent some time living in Hong Kong and in the USA: my own small experience of economic migration. I remember hearing my parents talk about the experiences they had in working in a very different culture in Hong Kong, and my own first attempts at cross-cultural communication talking to my Chinese nanny. I recall feeling 'different' in school in the USA and my attempts to fit in as quickly as possible. Perhaps this background drew me into general practice and stimulated my interest in cross-cultural work.

I work as a partner and GP trainer in a busy practice. In the course of my work, I meet patients from all over the world and from a wide variety of backgrounds. The area has changed over the years, and while we used to receive many new asylum seekers, they are now mainly resettled outside London due to government dispersal policies. We have well-established Somali, Bengali and Turkish communities and many newly arrived migrants who have arrived by choice to work, study, or to join family. I very much enjoy meeting and getting to know patients from such varied backgrounds. However, it is sometimes a challenge to meet all their needs, with the complications of different cultures, language and expectations. In this chapter I want to discuss some of the practical and clinical issues that can arise in caring for migrant patients, with reference to my own working environment. Many of the same issues may also be relevant in secondary care or other health care environments.

Practicalities of health care for migrant patients

One initial challenge for new immigrants is navigating our health care system. Migrants may be unfamiliar with the GP service and so turn to accident and emergency departments, or expect referral onward to hospital for conditions usually treated in primary care. Some migrants, from resource-poor countries, may not have had previous experience of preventative care and so may be less likely to respond to invitations such as for cervical screening (Abdullahi et al., 2009). Particularly difficult can be controlled access to hospital care for patients who have not had a primary care service in a gatekeeper role before and who are used to accessing specialists directly. These challenges for patients can easily lead to inappropriate use of services or misunderstandings with health professionals.

Patients often base their expectations on their country of origin. For example, a new patient, Helga, a banker from Germany, came to her GP to request a hospital gynaecology referral. She had no symptoms, but wanted a smear test done, a procedure usually done by the practice nurse in the UK. Her GP's initial response was one of irritation that a hospital referral was 'demanded' as she felt her own skills were belittled, whilst Helga was at first bemused and angered by the lack of care offered by the NHS when she was not referred to a gynaecologist. Appreciating that there is a different health care system in Germany, where access to specialists is direct, meant that the GP could explain the UK system to Helga who was then more satisfied with the new arrangement.

Other new migrant patients, in greater need, such as asylum seekers, may come to their GP frequently for support with a range of social issues, such as housing and immigration, as well as health problems, because primary care is potentially one of the few accessible places to meet a professional with interpreters available (Fang et al., 2015).

Valmir, newly arrived from Kosovo as an asylum seeker, shouted furiously when the GP explained she only helped with health care, not housing. On further questioning it emerged that Valmir was quite desperate, living with his sick wife and small children in temporary accommodation, with his own medical problems and insecure immigration status. He couldn't focus on his health care needs until the family's needs for secure living had been sorted out. After understanding the context, the GP helped Valmir to get a solicitor to help with housing and immigration. Only then could Valmir work with his GP on his own and his family's health problems.

Migrants from resource-poor countries, who have previously had limited access to medical care, can also feel put out by the offer of primary care (O'Donnell et al., 2008; Fang et al., 2015). In many countries, hospitals hold the main resources for medical treatment of patients and community clinics are considered very inferior. Procedures such as blood tests, X-rays and injections are seen as important; therefore, patients may feel that their problems are not taken seriously when treated in primary care. For example, Abdirahman, who had recently arrived from Somalia as an asylum seeker and was suffering from chronic pain down the entire right side of his body, demanded to be sent to hospital 'so the computers can diagnose me properly'. I have found it helpful in understanding these issues to ask newly arrived migrant patients about their previous experience of health care, about what they would normally do in their country of origin, and what they are hoping for from the doctor here. It can take some time for new arrivals to get to know their GP and realize the potential benefits of continuity of care from a local service.

Patients from countries with different health care systems in which prescribing medication is very important can feel that the lack of prescription (such as for self-limiting illnesses such as coughs and colds) means lack of suitable care. It can be helpful to prescribe simple home remedies such as paracetamol or linctus, to avoid overuse of antibiotics and maintain the doctor–patient relationship when patients are very concerned not to receive a prescription. However, this may have the disadvantage of perpetuating the custom of visiting the doctor for a prescription for minor illness. There is plenty of business for private doctors in London who are prepared to prescribe antibiotics for colds, if NHS GPs do not oblige, or patients may buy these online or bring supplies from countries where they are freely available. Asking the patient how important a prescription is for them, or what they are used to taking, can help to establish parameters for negotiation.

Other practical difficulties for health professionals and patients may arise when new migrants arrive with complex health problems, but without comprehensive documentation. For example, an elderly parent may come to live with family due to frailty, or a serious illness. Difficulties for the UK health professional may include reports written in other languages, medication without international labelling or lack of information on medical history other than through the patient, who may have very little understanding. This confusion can potentially be dangerous to patients, who may then not receive all the care they need.

An example of this confusion occurred when an elderly woman, Maria, arrived from Bolivia to join her daughter Patricia, who had lived in the UK for many years. Maria had run out of her medication some days before she came to visit the GP. She had boxes with labels in Spanish which appeared to include steroids and warfarin; both potentially dangerous to stop. A third medication was a painkiller not licensed in the UK. There was no clear medical history other than 'stroke' and no dosage information on the medications, or information on the indications for them. With Patricia's help, some information was faxed from the Bolivian hospital, in Spanish, so that the GP was able to continue the medication more safely and substitute a UK alternative for the medication not used here. Maria's health was very poor and Patricia needed a lot of ongoing support from the primary care team to care for Maria at home.

In another example, a middle-aged woman arrived from Iraq to join her husband, speaking no English. Through an interpreter she was able to say only that she had 'stomach problems' and had had 'an operation'; however, no written reports were available. This lack of information meant that her GP had to start from the basics to establish the diagnosis through examination and arranging tests in the UK. It can take many visits to the GP or hospital before such complex issues are resolved, especially where no previous information can be obtained and translated. This process is time-consuming for doctors and potentially risky for patients.

Difficulties around migration and medical care can also occur when patients move between countries, accessing health care in more than one location. Many UK-based immigrants choose, or need, to have some health care undertaken 'back home' where they are familiar with the language and setting, perhaps while they are there on holiday visiting family. This can mean coming back to the UK with reports in other languages, or no written information, but having had surgery or investigations or having started new medication. This can be very difficult to integrate smoothly into NHS health care. For example, Iwona had her smear test while home in Poland, and reported to her practice nurse, Sally, that it was normal. However, without a copy of the result Sally could not enter it into the practice system. And even when Iwona brought a copy of the result, she continued to receive invitation letters from the NHS national cervical screening service, as they do not change recall dates based on smears outside the NHS system. Similarly, Hassan chose to have his hernia operated on in Turkey, but complications set in after his return home to the UK, which were more difficult to treat without documentation of his procedure.

Other patients save up their health care issues to be dealt with in the UK, for example their annual diabetic check or other chronic disease checks, although living for much of the year in other countries. This is particularly popular with patients who have grown up in the UK but now live partly abroad, as they are used to the NHS and prefer to consult in English. It is also often done by people who live for part of the year in countries with limited access to health care.

Many people, such as elderly people sharing time between migrant and non-migrant kin, or wives visiting husbands working in a different country, now live between countries, for example by spending summer in the UK and winter in Ghana, Bangladesh or Spain. International students also move back and forth for terms and holidays. This international lifestyle may cause little trouble for health care for healthy young people, but can be complicated for those with chronic medical issues which may be diagnosed, understood or treated differently in other countries. 17-year-old Tamara, an international student from the Middle East, gave a history of weight loss surgery three years ago that had resulted in complications. She was on unusual medication given to her in Germany, and the indications for it were not clear. The medical documentation she brought with her was in Arabic and German. Her British GP was not familiar with the use of bariatric surgery in children or the treatment Tamara was taking, could not read the documents and took some time to understand the issues and to arrange suitable follow-up; by this time Tamara had finished her course of studies and returned home.

The international mobility of patients can cause difficulties for recall systems when patients may not always be in the UK for follow-up. NHS systems are not designed with these mobile patients in mind. For example, our practice was recently inspected for adherence to performance-related pay criteria and were informed we were in breach of regulations, as we should be sure to remove from our practice list everyone who is abroad for more than three months at a time. However, there is no obvious way to know where a patient is when they do not respond to an invitation, or to monitor movements into and out of the country. Also, as discussed in Chapter 2, NHS staff should not be put in the position of acting as 'border officials'.

More importantly, international mobility can cause difficulties in child safeguarding. For example, little Nikolas came to live with his grandmother in London. He had kidney problems, but his grandmother didn't seem to be giving him his medication reliably, and it was unclear if she held parental responsibility so that she could consent for the treatment he needed. Social services started an investigation, but by then grandmother and Nikolas had left the country.

Other practical problems can include medications licensed in some countries and not others: for example, buproprion is used as an antidepressant in the USA but is only licensed for smoking cessation in the UK. There are also conditions diagnosed in some countries but not in others: for example, 'constitutional' low blood pressure is diagnosed and treated in Germany but not in the UK while 'neurasthenia' is diagnosed in China for many cases that would be labelled 'depression' in the UK (Kleinman, 1980). Conditions may be treated differently in different places, such as ear infections treated with steroids in Italy, but not in the UK. Patients may also enter the UK on medication not recommended in the NHS, due to it being less cost-effective or not recommended in guidelines. This can lead to extra expense for the NHS or protracted negotiations by the GP to change the medication. These international differences lead to extra complications for health care professionals and confusion for patients accessing health care in different countries.

Cultural differences in illness experience

Challenges in communication between doctor and patient can arise due to different cultural norms in expression of, and understanding of, illness and disease. As discussed in Chapter 4, anthropologists distinguish between illness and disease as separate concepts: illness as the patient's lived experience and disease as diagnosed by doctors based on the medical model (Fitzpatrick et al., 1984; Kleinman, 1978, 1980, 1988). However, it is important to consider that illness experience is socially constructed by all cultures, not just 'exotic' or unusual cultures, and that doctors, applying a medical model of *disease*, often fail to understand their patients' *illnesses* and so fail to hear or understand their stories (Kleinman, 1988; Helman, 1981, 1985).

The way that patients experience illness and express their concerns is determined by multiple factors, relating to the individual, their family, their culture and their previous experience and expectations of health care systems. However, health care professionals, particularly doctors, are trained in a medical model which assumes that physiochemical and biological changes in the body from disease are the principal factors underlying patients' symptoms and their expression. There have been many criticisms of this narrowness of the medical model, such as by Illich and Habermas (Illich, 1991; Habermas, 1989). These authors criticize the medical model as rigidly overemphasizing the biochemical aspects of illness while denying the importance of patients' personal experiences and social situation. Doctors' duty to look for and treat disease can undermine their ability to understand and care for patients' illnesses. Kleinman attributes much of the misunderstanding to doctors' and patients' very different beliefs about illness/disease and introduces the idea of 'explanatory models' (Kleinman, 1988). Explanatory models are those beliefs that explain why an illness/disease started, what causes exacerbations and what might heal it. The concept of explanatory models can be very helpful in thinking about the different ideas that patients and their doctors may have and why there may be problems with mutual understanding.

There have been many ethnological studies of folk illness beliefs in non-Western cultures. For example, Good's study of an Iranian folk illness known as 'heart distress', Krause's study of 'sinking heart' in Pakistanis in Britain and Pachter's of 'empacho' in Latino children in the USA (Good, 1977; Krause, 1989; Pachter, 1992). These anthropologists all describe illnesses that cannot be directly correlated with any biomedical 'disease', but exist for the cultures that suffer them. Patients' experience of illness therefore may not fit in with their doctor's ideas about disease. This may lead doctors to dismiss, or fail to hear, patients' stories, while patients may not appreciate their doctor's advice when it does not fit with their illness experience.

As an example, an elderly Bengali lady, Mrs Begum, consulted about her painful leg; her GP diagnosed osteoarthritis in her knee and advised physiotherapy and pain relief. However, the patient kept returning dissatisfied, until the GP was able to hear her concern that her leg was shrinking away and would eventually disappear. The doctor had great difficulty hearing this concern, as it was very distant from the medical model of her training, or her own cultural heritage. However, hearing it eventually enabled her to make a stronger connection with her patient, and appreciate why her advice so far had been unhelpful. Another patient, from Vietnam, confided in her doctor how her dead relatives appeared to her at night and helped her and other friends with their problems and pains. Her doctor's first thought was to interpret this via the medical model and consider hallucinations or delusions; however, on reflection, this was best framed as part of the illness narrative, to be heard respectfully and seen as a source of support and comfort, rather than considered as a symptom of biomedical disease.

Some illness beliefs that seem strange to biomedical doctors are more common in non-Western cultures; for example, illness being caused by djinns, black magic or spirits. However, people educated and brought up in a Western medical tradition also hold a mixture of biomedical and folk health beliefs. Such folk beliefs include the widely held idea that getting cold causes colds and folk cures like 'starve a fever, feed a cold' (Helman, 1981). Blumhagen's paper 'Hypertension: a folk illness with a medical name' looked at folk beliefs about hypertension, a medical disease, in urban mainstream USA (Blumhagen, 1980) and illustrated the wide gulf in explanatory models between patients experiencing (folk) illness and doctors treating disease in a mainstream Western setting. These studies illustrate how non-biomedical 'folk' beliefs about illness are not limited to 'exotic' or non-Western cultures, but can be present in a wide variety of consultations. For example, Tony, from the USA, complained to his doctor of multiple symptoms such as fatigue, bloating and general malaise. He was sure his problems were due to 'total body Candida' or 'leaky gut syndrome', a Western folk illness not correlated with any medical disease, although it uses a medical term 'Candida' (Anderson et al., 1986). This created considerable tension in the consultation, as the patient expected his doctor to treat his condition and his doctor was wary of alienating him by denying its existence. This illustrates how there can be cultural tensions between medical culture and lay culture in any consultation, even when both patient and doctor are 'Western' in outlook.

Challenges in communication tend to be more noticeable the greater the difference in culture between doctor and patient. In her book *The Spirit Catches You and You Fall Down*, Anne Fadiman (1997) describes in delicate and compassionate detail the tragedies that followed the misunderstandings between US paediatricians and a Hmong family from Vietnam whose daughter developed epilepsy. The Hmong conceptualize epilepsy as related to the spirit world and those with epilepsy as having special gifts. The family also had no experience of long-term medication (such as anti-epileptics), only of short courses. Even with the use of interpreters, there are no correlates in Hmong language for most Western medical concepts. These factors led to the parents not following medical advice. The paediatricians had no understanding of Hmong concepts, just as the family had no understanding of medical thinking.

However, the doctors had the greater legal power and eventually had the child removed into foster care, leading to great family distress. Tragic misunderstandings such as these would be less likely if doctors were educated to ask about patients' explanatory models in an open-minded way (Kleinman, 2006), rather than focusing all their attention on bio-medical factors.

Cultural differences between doctor and patient are common, if not always so stark as in the case of the Hmong. However, particularly when patients have migrated from countries with very different culture and education, they may hold lay health beliefs that can be very different to medical models. For example, many people from cultures in Latin America, India and China classify illnesses and foods into 'Hot' and 'Cold'. With foods, this doesn't depend on their temperature or spiciness, but on a perceived inner quality (Helman, 1981, 1985). This can be mystifying to health care professionals who haven't been brought up in these cultures, and their doctor's lack of understanding is equally mystifying to patients who assume these beliefs are universally understood. Amharat, a middle-aged woman from Afghanistan, asked her GP if she could eat Hot food, given her menstrual problems – this meant nothing to her doctor and at first was not even heard. This could potentially lead to health problems, as Hot food could include red meat and other iron-rich foods useful for maintaining iron status in menstruating women. An elderly Bengali couple laughed out loud with shock when their well-meaning GP advised drinking more water to help with constipation. Fortunately, their interpreter was able to explain that constipation was a Cold condition that needed Hot treatment and that water was considered Cold, and so the GP was able to advise tea instead, which was more culturally acceptable. Another elderly Bengali patient was noticed to have poor adherence to one of his tablets. He explained eventually that this was because it was yellow. This seemed mystifying, until he identified this colour as Hot and he felt, therefore, that it would make him worse.

Patients' illness experiences that fall outside the medical model of disease may often now be labelled as 'medically unexplained symptoms' (MUS). Such symptoms are often vague or variable, and may include fatigue, nausea, abdominal discomfort and chronic musculoskeletal pain. Some of these symptom patterns are classified by doctors into syndromes like irritable bowel syndrome, fibromyalgia or chronic fatigue syndrome. However, patients may have their own preferred 'folk illness' explanations, such as 'total body Candida' or 'sinking heart'. Labelling these symptoms as MUS can be unhelpful, for example implying that there is no available treatment and implying that the symptoms are 'all in the mind' (Creed, Henningsen and Funk, 2011). It may be more useful to work with patients using labels that the patient finds helpful, whether this is a currently popular medical term such as 'fibromyalgia' or a term preferred by the patient (Kleinman, 2006).

Illness symptoms that do not fit with biomedical diseases are common in patients of all backgrounds (Budtz-Lilly et al., 2015), but may be experienced or expressed differently in different cultural groups. This may be linked with particular cultural experiences of 'folk' illnesses, patterns of acceptable expression of distress, or to the experience of migration or trauma. Doctors are often mystified by patients with 'total body pain' or non-neurological weakness down one side of the body.

Sometimes such symptoms seem to link to life experiences. For example, Afia, born in Pakistan, was a mother of five. Her husband had died soon after they moved to the UK, leaving her to bring up the children alone as all the extended family had stayed in Pakistan. She suffered from pain over her entire body and walked slowly and bent over. Her pain worsened considerably when her daughters went out without her permission or wore non-traditional clothes. Having spent some time trying to 'diagnose' the biomedical cause of the pain and failing, and trying to take a psychological approach which Afia did not accept, her GP instead spent time listening to how Afia's life progressed and her worries over her daughters' marriages and advised on simple pain relief, exercise and support from a local women's group.

Patients may often keep strong ties with their home culture, both within their UK community and with family back at home. This may include use of traditional remedies (Ceuterick, Vandebroek and Pieroni, 2011) and consulting traditional health practitioners, either in the UK or on trips 'back home' (Rochelle and Marks, 2010). This can be a great source of help and support to families, but can also sometimes lead to problems. Some traditional remedies can be dangerous, for example the treatment of 'tooth worms' by the removal of deciduous tooth buds (Longhurst, 2010). Others may delay the use of potentially more effective treatments. For example, a very frail, elderly Chinese lady was brought by her family to the GP. She had been unwell and losing weight for several months, and had consulted Chinese traditional practitioners. On examination, the GP was mystified by round bruises over her abdomen and worried about some form of elder abuse. Fortunately, the daughter was able to explain that these were the result of 'cupping', an alternative medical practice that involves creating suction in cups placed on the skin. However, examination also revealed signs of advanced cancer. It is possible that the use of traditional treatments had delayed access to more effective cancer treatment.

In another case, a 7-year-old child from an Ethiopian family had a serious skin condition that required a very long course of medication. His family were clearly frustrated with the slow progress of his medical treatment and distressed by his appearance. However, his mother had a good relationship with her GP and was able to confide in him that they planned to stop the child's medication and travel back to Ethiopia to visit a holy shrine for a cure. This allowed the GP to negotiate with the mother to continue the medication during the trip. The child returned cured, and although the GP and the family held different explanations for this, it was a satisfactory result for all.

Traditional remedies can also cause misunderstandings. A health visitor was horrified on visiting a new mother, originally from Thailand, to find her giving her new baby a brown-coloured liquid in his bottle. This was a herbal tea which the grandmother had sent at some expense to help with the baby's colic. The health visitor needed great sensitivity to explain her advice that the baby should only be fed on breast milk or infant formula, and to suggest other things to help with colic. These cases illustrate the importance of asking patients from different backgrounds about traditional treatments they are using, in order to facilitate understanding and dialogue.

Female genital mutilation

A problematic and sensitive area of traditional practice is female genital mutilation (FGM). This is the traditional practice of cutting and/or repositioning the female genitals; for example, by removing the clitoris, or cutting and sewing together the labia to reduce the vaginal opening. It is traditionally carried out by older women, without the use of any anaesthetic or antiseptic practices, in parts of Africa, the Middle East and Asia. FGM is potentially dangerous to health, as it is associated with infection and bleeding at the time of cutting, and later urinary infections, sexual difficulties and psychological damage (Simpson et al., 2012). FGM, unlike many traditional practices, is illegal in the UK, as is taking children to another country to have the procedure.

When FGM is undertaken for girls in UK immigrant families, it is usually in the school holidays on trips 'back home', and is hidden from health care professionals and teachers. There are now leaflets available for families in various languages to explain that this is illegal, and help them to stand up to family pressure for cutting 'back home'. These leaflets may also help health professionals discuss this issue with parents, for example at travel clinics (UK Government, 2015).

In clinical practice in the UK, FGM is mainly seen in adult women who had the procedure in childhood in their home country (Simpson et al., 2012). Sometimes women are suffering from the complications of FGM but can be too embarrassed to come forward for help or may not be aware of services available in the UK. The current focus on education on the harms of this procedure, in order to prevent the practice being perpetuated, may have an inadvertent effect of making women who have already undergone this feel ashamed or 'mutilated'. There is also a growing tendency to treat women as potential perpetrators against their own daughters, rather than as survivors of a harmful traditional practice. This can potentially make patients wary of seeking health care.

For example, Fatima had been unable to have intercourse without severe pain since marriage two years ago. She was eventually brought to her GP by her sister-in-law, who spoke English. She needed a lot of reassurance that her problem was understood and could be helped, and that she would be listened to respectfully. She could then be referred to the local 'African women's clinic' for treatment. There are several such clinics in the UK, run by female staff with special expertise and understanding in helping women who have problems after FGM. In another example, a woman from Egypt refused a smear test as she was embarrassed and worried about being 'reported to the authorities' due to her FGM.

Although many women and organisations campaign against FGM, there are some women who press for more understanding and value the cultural elements of the practice as part of girls' initiation into adulthood (Ahmadu and Shweder, 2009). Ahmadu, who herself had the procedure in her home country of Sierra Leone, claims it is a myth that it causes sexual dysfunction, and also objects to women from these cultures being described as mutilated. Certainly, it should be of concern to health professionals that women could be made to feel 'mutilated' or inferior by the reactions of their doctors or midwives to the appearance of their genitals. It is also concerning that recent attention to the risk to children in the UK may make this a difficult issue for women to discuss with health care professionals due to the fear of being reported (McCartney, 2015). It is unclear whether recent changes to the law requiring mandatory reporting will be helpful in preventing FGM in girls, or harmful, by making it more difficult for women who have had this procedure to access health care with confidence.

Refugees and asylum seekers

There are particular health care issues that affect refugees and asylum seekers and other forced migrants, such as those who have been trafficked. Such issues can be complex and may include the after-effects of experiencing or witnessing torture, rape and violence (Adams, Gardiner and Assefi, 2004). There can also have been traumatic events during the journey to seek refuge, which can be compounded by traumatizing experiences in detention centres in the UK (Arnold, 2007). Those seeking asylum and undocumented migrants can also be haunted by insecurity and the fear of being sent back.

Many refugees have lost touch with significant family members, while some do not know if their family are dead or alive. Families may be scattered and contact may be difficult with family members left in a war-afflicted country, or in a refugee camp. There may be anxiety regarding the safety of family left behind (Fang et al., 2015). New arrivals are often traumatized, isolated and insecure regarding status. They may also have problems with housing, benefits and access to education or employment. High levels of stress, language barriers, experience of prejudice, worry about confidentiality, and lack of knowledge of the new health care system can all lead to difficulties accessing health care (Fang et al., 2015). Undocumented migrants may also struggle to access care due to lack of documents such as proof of address; however, GPs are able to register such patients at their discretion. For example, our practice does not require proof of address in order to facilitate registration of vulnerable or homeless patients.

These vulnerable patients' needs for health care can be complex: physical care for injuries, infections and untreated chronic illness, and mental health care for after-effects of trauma, particularly post-traumatic stress disorder (Adams, Gardiner and Assefi, 2004). Refugees' needs may be compounded by lack of access to health care in the past. For example, children may not have had any childhood immunizations, or records may be missing; women may suffer the after-effects of poor care in childbirth; and bullets or shrapnel may still be present in the body after injuries. There may also be an increased prevalence of infectious diseases such as tuberculosis (TB), Hepatitis B and HIV, depending on the country of origin.

Lack of health care for chronic disease can have serious consequences. For example, Makemba arrived in the UK aged 17 as an asylum seeker, in very poor health, malnourished, with kidney failure and nearly blind. This was a result of previous lack of access to medication and support for her insulin-dependent type 1 diabetes. Although she could now access appropriate help in the UK, much of the damage was irreversible. Jamil, who had escaped from Iraq in difficult circumstances, suffered from severe back and leg pain, anxiety and difficulty sleeping. He was reluctant to talk about his past, asking only for medication. His GP only found out about the torture Jamil had suffered when his solicitor asked for a medical report for his asylum claim. He was then able to refer Jamil for support from an appropriate service.

Patients who have come to the UK as refugees are particularly likely to have widely dispersed families. This can lie behind some difficulties: for example, Rashid, a Sudanese man in his forties, contacted his GP in great distress. He had recently been seen urgently at the hospital with chest pain, but had been reassured there was nothing wrong with his heart. The GP couldn't see why he would be distressed, especially as the pain was gone. Rashid explained that he had become ill at work, and he feared he would lose his job. This terrified him, as he not only supported his wife and children, but 10 members of his extended family in various Middle Eastern and African countries.

When extended family is not available for support, health care professionals may find themselves drawn into patients' lives as 'stand in' family. For example, a retired university professor from Iran felt lucky to have escaped, but was sad that his adult children had gone to Canada and the USA. As his health deteriorated, he often asked his GP (who was around the same age as his children) for her general advice, saying 'I think of you as my daughter'. Another patient, Ahmet, from Turkey, brought regular presents to his practice nurse whenever he had a diabetic check-up, remarking: 'You are my family'.

GPs can help forced migrants by making a holistic assessment of the situation of the patient and family, registering patients without documentation, and providing interpreters as required. Assessments should include considering acute medical health care needs, care for chronic diseases, mental health care, catching up on missing immunizations and screening, and referral for help with immigration status, housing, education and benefits. Therefore, the health care professional's role, as well as health care, may also include writing medical reports for immigration, housing and benefits claims, or to avoid detention (Arnold, 2007). Until patients' needs for security in legal status and housing are met, they are often unable to engage meaningfully in health care, psychological treatment or education. Unfortunately, the complex needs of refugees, and other forced migrants, are rarely matched by the increased funding and training needed for service providers.

Language barriers

Many migrants have language barriers to cope with. Some patients do not speak sufficient English to access medical care safely without help from an interpreter; some speak moderately well but with an increased chance of misunderstanding, and others speak English perfectly but with such a different accent that understanding is still challenging. Working with these different groups requires particular communication skills from practitioners – working with interpreters (whether informal or skilled professionals) either in person or by telephone. They need the skill to create mutual understanding with patients with limited English or a very different accent. The ability to speak other languages is, of course, very helpful, and at least being able to say 'good morning' or 'welcome' in local community languages helps to create rapport and is welcomed by patients.

Health care professionals who are themselves migrants, or from migrant families, and who have an additional home language may be greatly valued by patients from their country of origin. Some doctors gather a large following of patients who appreciate being able to consult in their most comfortable language. Patients may also feel that a doctor from their home country will have a greater understanding of their cultural background, beliefs and family life. However, patients may alternatively choose to avoid doctors from their own cultural background, due to fears about lack of confidentiality within a small community, or perceived criticism of not living within cultural norms. Professionals may also face challenges from feeling too drawn in to helping patients with whom they share a language, risking blurring professional boundaries (Costa, 2014).

For many migrant patients, interpreters will be required for safe and effective communication. However, working with interpreters has its own challenges for professionals, for patients and for the interpreters themselves, and is not always a simple solution to communication difficulties. Some issues are practical and require good organization: making sure the correct interpreter is present (Hadziabdic et al., 2011). There may be problems with dialects within languages, for example. Furthermore, different political groups sharing the same language can also be an issue. For example, a Kurdish refugee felt that his Turkish interpreter was unsympathetic about his history of torture by the Turkish police. Indeed, the interpreter told the doctor that the patient could not be telling the truth and was insulting his State. Alternatively, if the interpreter is seen to be linked with the patients' local community, patients may have concerns about confidentiality (Fang et al., 2015). Some patients are not aware of the availability of professional interpreting and so bring an informal interpreter when they would prefer a professional (Barron, Holterman and Shipster, 2010).

Telephone interpreting services can overcome some practical difficulties of pre-booking face-to-face interpreting, as it can be available at short notice; however many people find them too impersonal, and technical problems or background noise can cause poor audibility, and lines can cut off. Problems of different accents or dialects between patient and interpreter are also much more difficult to overcome without the added help of non-verbal communication. For example, the Portuguese Language line interpreter (from Portugal) clearly struggled to understand the Portuguese-speaking patient from Guinea Bissau. The patient illustrated her concern to the doctor by coughing and pointing at her chest, while the telephone interpreter said her trouble was constipation. Accuracy can be a problem with telephone interpreting, with some studies finding a high level of discrepancies (Lor and Chewning, 2015). However, some patients do value the confidentiality of telephone interpreting, compared with having another person present.

Often patients prefer an interpreter of the same gender, especially if sensitive issues such as sex or contraception need to be discussed. This can also be an issue for the interpreter: for example, the female Bengali interpreter explained to the nurse that she could not ask the young male patient questions about his sex life, as this was culturally inappropriate for her, particularly since she was known in the local community.

Despite having the appropriate interpreter, there may still be cultural issues that make dialogue difficult. For example, a doctor needed to interview a Japanese student who had recently taken an overdose, to assess for future suicide risk. His mother had flown over from Japan and was with him, along with a female Japanese interpreter. When the doctor asked the student 'How do you feel now about ending your life?' the interpreter covered her mouth with her hand and laughed. The doctor's immediate response was one of annoyance, as suicide is no laughing matter. However, the doctor then recalled that laughing can be a Japanese indication of embarrassment or anxiety, and not humour. The interpreter explained that she could not ask this question in front of the mother, as it was disrespectful. To avoid this type of culture clash, the doctor could have first discussed with the interpreter this sensitive topic of enquiry and agreed a way to perform a risk assessment without breaking cultural proprieties.

Patients frequently use family or other informal interpreters. This is often their preference, rather than involving a stranger in their consultation, and may also be more convenient than booking a professional interpreter. In practice, the pragmatic use of family members is rarely a problem, if patients are happy with this; and when a carer is interpreting for a frail or unwell relative it can be particularly helpful that they can advocate for the patient's problems and are aware of the diagnosis and treatment plan. Indeed, Greenhalgh, Robb and Scambler (2006), in a qualitative analysis, found that, contrary to policy makers' preference for professional interpretation, family interpreters shifted the power balance in favour of the patient, and were trusted by patients, shared their agenda and could advocate for their concerns. Leanza, Boivin and Rosenberg (2010) also found that professional interpreters interrupted the patient's illness stories more than family interpreters, but family interpreters were more likely to take control of the agenda from the patient. When sensitive issues such as a sexual history, domestic abuse or a serious diagnosis need to be discussed, using family interpreters can become inappropriate.

For example, on meeting a patient on the ward the night before surgery, a junior doctor became aware that the elderly Chinese patient did not even know she had cancer, as she pointed to her breast and said 'infection?'. The patient had been given her diagnosis with her daughter as interpreter. The daughter later explained that she had not felt able to tell her mother she had cancer, as it would be too distressing. In their culture it was normal not to tell family members any serious diagnosis; it was felt that knowing a diagnosis would lead the patient to give up and die. However, this cultural practice directly clashes with doctors' legal duty to have fully informed consent prior to surgery. This makes it very important for a professional interpreter to attend for obtaining informed consent for treatment. The patient's family can then attend to offer support and advocacy, without having the responsibility of breaking bad news to their relative. Whether we are thereby causing harm by breaking cultural norms through discussion of serious diagnoses with patients, who may not wish this, is difficult to know.

When children are called upon to interpret for adult family members, further issues arise. Children may have to assume an adult role they are not emotionally ready for, as advocate for their family's problems, or be kept out of school to help. In many families and cultures, it is not considered appropriate to discuss intimate issues such as sex or periods in front of children and so parents may avoid these areas (Barron, Holterman and Shipster, 2010). For example, a Somali mother of eight attended for a postnatal check, bringing her 12-year-old son, out from school, to interpret for her. The doctor needed to ask about her delivery and offer contraception advice, and concluded that the son's help was inappropriate. Fortunately, a female interpreter was available by telephone so that the clinical issues could be addressed, along with a discussion about the availability of professional interpreting in the future. Providing professional interpreters can help avoid children being called on in this way.

Many migrant patients do not need, or do not want, an interpreter, but prefer to speak English with their doctor or nurse, and many have sufficient, or perfect, English. However, for more delicate or emotional issues, it is worth bearing in mind that speaking in an acquired language, rather than a mother tongue, may alter what can be said, both through lack of knowledge of the subtleties of language and the way the language itself allows, or does not allow, things to be expressed (Burck, 2005). Different languages may have different concepts and allow the expression of ideas and issues in different ways: for example, there is no direct equivalent Bengali word for 'depression'. For complex issues or mental health care, with the need to express sensitive and complicated ideas, it can be helpful to ask even patients who speak good English if they would feel more comfortable speaking in their own language, with an interpreter, or, if possible, with a professional who speaks their language.

Often the greatest practical difficulties are encountered when patients have quite a limited grasp of English but an interpreter is not available or is declined, which quite commonly happens in practice. As an example, the practice nurse wanted the new patient to bring a urine specimen for testing; however, he didn't understand the term urine, or wee, so she asked him to bring a specimen of his water and he appeared to understand this. The patient then brought the specimen pot in full of tap water from home. This caused some hilarity in the practice, but was embarrassing and confusing for the patient.

When an interpreter is not available, or is declined, a possible fall back is online translation such as provided by Google Translate, currently covering some 90 languages. Research suggests that it is not yet reliable enough for some medical terminology. Gibson et al. (2014) found 53% of paragraphs of written information were translated completely accurately with 18% having major errors. Patil and Davies found similar results (2014). However, Khanna et al. (2010) found comparable adequacy although less fluency than professional translation. Nevertheless, it can be very useful in clinical practice for translating simple words such as 'urine' or short, simple sentences such as 'take one tablet twice a day'. There is also a speaker function for some languages, which can be useful if the patient is partially sighted or illiterate. Some research suggests that it may be better with Western European languages (Patil and Davies, 2014). Google Translate can be particularly useful for patients with good English, but who don't know medical words such as 'larynx' or 'appendix'; and of course, patients often reach for their phones to use it themselves. The programme can be used in either direction, with patients invited to type in words they want to translate or the professional typing in and potentially printing out useful explanations or instructions for the patient. However, there can often be difficulty with words that have many meanings, such as 'coil', or 'fits', and care is needed. There is likely to be increasing use of this option in the future as it gains in accuracy; and of course it is highly convenient, confidential, portable (on mobile devices) and free. Indeed, professional interpreting is not 100% accurate either: one study found a similar level of discrepancies in a study of telephone interpreting, with a 45% level of omissions and 27% of substitutions (Lor and Chewning, 2015).

Other simple skills to enhance communication include speaking slowly and clearly but not more loudly; repeating and writing down key points and, where there is difficulty understanding, rephrasing with an alternative word or simpler choice of word. For example, a patient didn't understand instructions to apply a cream 'inside the nostrils' and didn't complete his treatment; 'in the nose' would have been easier to understand.

Non-verbal communication by patient and doctor can be particularly important when verbal communication is difficult. At the most simple level, patients simply pointing to body areas of concern can be very helpful in directing doctors' attention to the right place. Indeed, pain and distress are often better conveyed non-verbally than in words. However, there are many pitfalls, as body language is not universal, but culturally determined. This can cause confusion, as when a patient is nodding, which the doctor takes as understanding and agreeing but may be merely polite acknowledgement that they are listening. Difficulties can occur with simple differences, such as greeting by hand shaking, which is normal in the Netherlands, sometimes done in the UK, but may cause offence with people of the opposite gender from some cultures. Eye contact and personal space are other areas which differ from culture to culture. In the UK, doctors are taught that it is polite to make eye contact with their patients and that patients who have minimal eye contact may be depressed or have other mental health problems. However, not making eye contact may, in many cultures, be a sign of respect. Clearly, it is not possible for professionals to be familiar with the different body language of many different cultures, only to remain alert for differences and take nothing for granted.

Health care professionals also need to consider their own use of non-verbal communication with patients. When there are challenges with language, backing up words with pointing, acting, diagrams, drawings or charts can be helpful, always checking the patient's understanding of this. For example, complex diagrams or charts may not be helpful to patients who have had no access to formal education in their country of origin. A shared sense of humour can help: on one occasion when an interpreter was not available, a young female GP and a similar age Ukrainian woman managed a consultation about a vaginal thrush infection and how to use a pessary treatment, almost entirely through acting and signs. Having an interpreter would certainly have been more convenient, but not as funny. This shared experience helped to create a warm, ongoing doctor–patient relationship.

Cultural sensitivity

In order to work effectively with patients from different countries and cultures, practitioners need attitudes and abilities which allow them to take into account patients' individual social, cultural and linguistic background, and communicate effectively with them. Unfortunately, many health professionals have had little training in this area. As Jenny Altschuler points out in Chapter 4, the concept of 'cultural competence' began to be more widely introduced into training only from the late 1990s, well after many current health care professionals qualified. However, in my experience, doctors training now have still had little, if any, education in this area and often identify it as a learning need.

There are many different ideas about what 'cultural competence' involves. In his research in Ireland, O'Hagan found patients who felt practitioners were culturally competent through the use of simple courtesies such as making an effort to pronounce patients' names correctly and addressing them respectfully (O'Hagan, 2001). Other studies emphasize practitioners' knowledge of different cultural and religious practices, and indeed there are many books and pamphlets aimed at health care professionals to help them be more knowledgeable about different groups. One example of this is the book *Caring for Muslim Patients* (Sheik and Gatrad, 2000), which can illuminate health issues: for example, around fasting for Ramadan or travel for the Hajj. For example, a frail, elderly Bengali lady with diabetes and heart disease was determined to fast for Ramadan. Her practice nurse was able to advise her about taking her tablets before sunrise and after sunset, instead of three times daily, but also to remind her that her religion advised her not to fast when it risked making her unwell. This practice nurse also organized an annual travel clinic for patients travelling to the Hajj.

There are potentially serious drawbacks, however, to relying on a knowledge-based approach to culture. Firstly, the idea of 'cultural competence' may imply that culture can be reduced to an area of technical expertise. This is a reductionist approach which can lead to a stereotyped approach to patients such as 'all Muslims don't drink alcohol, all Jews don't eat pork' (Kleinman and Benson, 2006). Individual patients may not conform to cultural norms or stereotypes: for example, the nurse carefully gave diet advice to a diabetic patient from the Caribbean, to find out later that he only ate Chinese food at home. A further problem with a purely knowledge-based approach is the variety of different cultural backgrounds found in modern practice. Currently, in Islington, London, there are over 150 languages used. Although it is certainly useful to gather information on commonly held cultural views in groups of patients that are seen frequently, it is quite impossible to cover all there is to know about different cultures. Furthermore, there are many factors other than culture that contribute to patients' concerns. The term 'cultural sensitivity' may be preferable as it suggests a state of mind more than a learned set of information.

Instead of a knowledge-based approach, the basic position of respectful interest and curiosity about other belief systems and cultural and family norms can be helpful. It is hard for health care practitioners, especially doctors, to take up a position of 'not knowing' as family therapists advo-cate (White and Epston, 1990) after training for so many years to be knowledgeable and to get things right. Health care professionals have a duty to give correct medical advice and treatment. This can lead to a situ-ation where doctors, sure they are 'right', forget to listen respectfully to patients' differing views. It is quite a challenge for doctors to think 'with two heads', both biomedically in terms of what is 'right', while at the same time considering what the patient believes and understands about their own illness and situation.

As an example, Dritan, a young man from Albania, consulted his GP with episodes that sounded like epileptic fits. His doctor was keen for Dritan to start treatment promptly and attend hospital for tests. However, Dritan did not want to do this, as he felt the most likely cause of his prob-lem was black magic. The doctor instantly dismissed this as nonsense, thereby alienating her patient who left without treatment. Fortunately, he returned later and his GP listened respectfully to his concerns about black magic. After some discussion, Dritan agreed to take tablets, as they might prevent the black magic from causing fits. Although doctor and patient continued to disagree on the cause of the problem, they reached an agreed treatment plan. In order to achieve this, the doctor had to give up some of her need to be 'right' in order to allow a more shared perspective to develop.

Certainly, for doctors to be sensitive in considering other cultures, we first need to be aware that we ourselves have a culture. It is too easy to fall into the trap of thinking that one's own culture is somehow 'natural' and 'right' and that it is other people who have odd cultural beliefs. This is particularly an issue for doctors who have spent many years training intensively in a biomedical perspective and find it difficult to see beyond it or develop insight into their own cultural norms (Lupton, 1994).

Cultural 'competence' or sensitivity is an issue for organizations as well as individuals. Health care organizations can do much to help facilitate access by patients from different backgrounds. This can include ensuring provision of suitable, trained interpreters in community languages, the availability of written information in different languages, the recruit-ment of health care staff who speak community languages, and diversity training for staff. A welcoming environment could also include notices in different community languages and recognition of different community festivals (Sheikh, Gatrad and Dhami, 2008). Staff also need to be prepared to explain the health care system to new arrivals: for example, how to arrange an appointment, obtain a repeat prescription and access urgent care. This all helps to create an environment in which all patients can feel at home and cultural sensitivity can flourish.

Recommendations for practice

- Be prepared to explain your health care system, and how to use it, to newly arrived patients.

- Try to obtain written documents of medical history for new arrivals and have them translated.

- Be aware of cultural differences in illness experience.

- Ask your patient about their ideas, concerns and expectations (explanatory models) of their illness and its treatment.

- Ask patients about alternative or traditional treatments they are using.

- Listen respectfully even if their ideas seem unusual or difficult to understand from your cultural perspective.

- Be aware of possible trauma histories for forced migrants. Ask sensitively about their history when relevant.

- Be prepared to help forced migrants with their wider needs for support, not just medical needs.

- Have organizational systems to provide the correct interpreter.

- Advertise the availability of professional interpreters.

- Learn to work well with interpreters; discuss sensitive or difficult issues with them first when possible.

- When necessary, speak slowly and clearly, repeating key points in simple language.

- Back up key information in writing – in the correct language whenever possible.

8

INTERNATIONAL HEALTH CARE MIGRATION

The strengthening of global labour markets means that a considerable number of people who migrate are highly skilled professionals. Whilst doctors, nurses, physiotherapists, and other health care professionals represent a small proportion of this group, the migration of health care professionals has had a significant effect on the health care systems of 'destination'[29] as well as 'source'[30] countries, the countries in which professionals like myself were born, trained and decided or felt forced to leave (McElmurry et al., 2006; Ormond, 2013; Shah, 2013).

Many health professionals who migrate go on to develop successful careers and establish a comfortable life for themselves and their families. Indeed, a high proportion of people who reach the top of their field were born and trained outside of the UK. However, regardless of whether the move is permanent or temporary, it can be extremely difficult dealing with the 'double culture shock', with the excitement, anxiety, confusion and insecurity of having to adapt professionally as well as personally (Austin, 2005; Guru et al., 2012). For example, depending on the country one leaves and moved to, health professionals may be faced with bureaucratic and financial barriers to registration and requalification; real and perceived obstacles to employment, promotion and integration; language and cultural barriers; working in health care settings where the practices and paradigms of medical treatment are unfamiliar, and where racism, other forms of discrimination and differences in accent mean patients, their families and colleagues are more likely to question one's knowledge and clinical competence (Larsen, 2007; Ormond, 2013; Shiwani, 2006, 2010).

As mentioned earlier, Jung (1954) proposed that many of us are driven to heal others through a need to heal ourselves. This suggests that migrant health care professionals are likely to find it particularly difficult balancing the personal gains of migration with the sadness, guilt and discomfort of living in relative privilege when parents and siblings continue to face economic hardship and political turmoil. My own experience suggests that it can feel extremely uncomfortable to be caring for vulnerable members of other peoples' family when one's own parents and siblings are ill and it is impossible to provide the hands-on support that is needed other than on a short-term basis. Likewise, particularly where the health care services of the country one leaves is unable to meet the health care needs of the local population, it can feel uncomfortable 'abandoning' the country that invested considerable financial and professional resources in one's training.

As these issues have received little academic attention, particular attention is paid to the more problematic consequences of international health care worker migration. However, it is important to recognize the enormous benefits migrant health professionals bring to the countries they move to and from, and the personal and professional gains of working elsewhere on a temporary or permanent basis.

Scale and consequences for sending countries

In 2006, the World Health Organization (WHO) identified 57 countries as having a critical shortage of health workers, most of which were in the developing world, with 36 in the poorest regions (WHO, 2006). For example, sub-Saharan Africa has the lowest density of doctors and nurses despite having the highest disease burden (Crisp and Chen, 2014): even though life expectancy is much higher in the more developed countries, almost 25% of doctors trained in sub-Saharan Africa work outside the region. More than 50% of doctors trained in Ghana and Nigeria emigrate to work in richer countries (Hagopian et al., 2005; WHO, 2010). This is true of other developing countries as well. Similar concerns have been raised about the numbers of physicians who have left Columbia, India, Nigeria, Pakistan and the Philippines (Astor et al, 2006). Moreover, at a time when India was facing a significant increase in the numbers of people infected by HIV/AIDS, approximately 50% of graduates from two of the best nursing colleges left the country to work elsewhere (McElmurry et al., 2006).

Migrant professionals comprise a considerable proportion of the health care workforce in many of the more developed countries. In common with many other European countries, the UK has a long tradition of recruiting health care professionals from abroad on a permanent and temporary basis to combat shortfalls in meeting staffing and practice targets. Today, the NHS is one of the largest employers in Europe, providing training to, and benefiting from the services of internationally trained health care professionals (Shah, 2013). Figures produced by the Health and Social Care Information Centre (HSCIC, 2016) show that 11% of all staff working for the NHS and in community health services (for whom data was available) are not British. The proportion of foreign nationals increases to 14% for all professionally qualified clinical staff and even more so for doctors (26%). Currently, 39% of doctors on the specialist register were trained abroad, particularly in EU (European Union) countries and other English-speaking countries with ties to Britain through the Commonwealth: after Britain, India provides the highest number of professionally qualified clinical staff, doctors and consultants. The figure is even higher (66%) for doctors who were not working as GPs or specialist registrars, for example doctors working in locum or mid-level positions (NHS Workforce Statistics, 2014). Indeed, many NHS specialisms are dependent on doctors trained abroad, particularly in specialties where posts are difficult to fill, such as emergency care, haematology and geriatric psychiatry (Shah, 2013).

Recent data on nurses and midwives are more difficult to come by. However in 2008, 16% of new registrations to the Nursing and Midwifery Council were nurses trained in EEA[31] and Third World countries. Foreign-born nurses are significantly over-represented in older adult care as opposed to the better-paid and more prestigious positions in the NHS (Serco, 2014). For example, an extensive review of the care of older adults revealed that more than 60 per cent of care workers in London were migrants, primarily from Zimbabwe, Poland, Nigeria, the Philippines and India, with a disproportionate percentage working in the private sector rather than local authorities where wages would have been higher (Cangiano et al., 2009). This pattern is not particular to Britain but true of many other EU countries and the USA, attesting to the fact that many of the richer countries are benefiting from the investment poorer countries make in training health care professionals to work with local populations.

Attempts to analyse trends in health care worker migration have been hampered by insufficient and inaccurate data. This stems from inconsistencies in the ways different countries monitor migration, and difficulties in keeping an accurate record of the numbers and professional status of people who leave to work elsewhere. As many countries cannot afford the financial burden of producing reliable statistics, finding ways of reliably recording international movements and information on occupations (to identify the occupations of health personnel) is difficult. Moreover, providing evidence on the migration of health personnel requires the political will to strengthen the capacity to produce and use statistics. While the majority of the destination countries have fairly good statistical systems, many source countries struggle with insufficient staff and uncoordinated administration. Furthermore, because some professionals move on a temporary rather than permanent basis, the statistics produced are likely to underestimate the number of migrant health professionals (Diallo, 2004; Ormond, 2013; Shah, 2013). An added complication is that difficulties in re-qualifying and finding employment mean many health care professionals and other care workers are not employed in the public sector but in private and informal care settings (McElmurry et al., 2006; Stilwell et al., 2003; Shah, 2013).

Record keeping has been hampered further by questions of whether those who obtain citizenship should continue to be seen as migrants. The widespread use of blanket categories such as 'internationally trained', 'overseas qualified' and 'foreign' conceals and obscures the heterogeneity of different migrant groups. Likewise, ethnicity and migration-related issues tend to be conflated, confused and used inter-changeably with foreignness, otherness and 'race'. In addition, migrant, black and minority ethnic status are almost always treated as a potential source of difficulty rather than strength, reinforcing negative assump-tions and stereotypes (Humphrey et al., 2009). However, even if more accurate data were available, data that is collected for administrative pur-poses will never be able to capture the full complexity of the impact of migration on the health care system of source and destination countries, and the more personal challenges and benefits for health care profession-als and their families.

As with all forms of migration, a wide range of complex and often contradictory factors inform decisions to migrate, including the desire for improved working conditions, more rewarding work, professional devel-opment, a better quality of life and, for those from countries dominated by political conflict, freedom from violence and oppression (Wismar et al., 2011). Economic policies to promote free and equitable trade are also relevant (Cangiano and Walsh, 2014): the likelihood of moving on a temporary or permanent basis is influenced by trade agreements, national strategies to export or import health care providers, profit motives and individual factors. Indeed, some countries (including India and the Philippines) have embraced the phenomenon of health care migration, for example by training nurses for 'export' to countries like the UK and USA and supporting legislative changes to facilitate this practice (Harris Cheng, 2009; McElmurry et al., 2006; Ormond, 2013; Shah, 2013).

Nonetheless, reduced numbers of health care staff place increased pres-sure on those who remain, affecting motivation and leading to a higher staff turnover, with many neglecting public sector responsibilities to work in the private sector. Losing professionally trained staff can result in cutting services, limiting access to public health services and medica-tions, and expecting the remaining workforce to deliver services more commonly outside of their practice and expertise largely unsupervised. In many cases the professionals who move are not only highly skilled but have played a central role in nursing and medical training. Moreover, although it is possible to train other staff to take their place, this requires considerable time as well as financial and professional investment (Crisp and Chen, 2014; Shah, 2013; Stilwell et al., 2003). However, statistical analysis indicates that globally, the health sector needs for human resources exceed the numbers of immigrant health workers: this suggests that their migration is neither the main cause of, nor would its reduction be the solution to, the crisis in resources (Dumont and Zurn, 2007). Although Dumont and Zurn's analysis took place several years ago, the situation is unlikely to have improved as rates of migration have increased rather than decreased since then.

A number of innovative programmes have been introduced aimed at addressing key gaps in health care in low- and middle-income countries where clinical resources are scarce (Crisp and Chen, 2014). In areas of sub-Saharan Africa affected by the HIV/AIDS pandemic, many health care services have introduced a process of task shifting, of entrusting nurses and paramedical staff with tasks more usually the responsibility of doctors. This has helped to increase access to lifesaving treatment, improve the workforce skills mix and efficiency of the health system, reduce the consequences of attrition and international 'brain drain' and enhance the role of the community (Nair and Webster, 2013; Shah, 2013).

For example, in Mozambique, 'tecnicos do cirurgia', mainly nurses with extra training, perform nearly all caesarean sections and the outcomes have been as good as those performed by physicians, at much lower costs (Pereira et al., 1996). Elsewhere Pakistan's 'Lady Health Workers' have been effective in influencing health promotion and treatment in villages (Douthwaite and Ward, 2005), and in Bangladesh the engagement of community health workers has contributed to increasing child survival rates (Haines et al., 2007). Similarly, in sub-Saharan Africa, several non-governmental organizations (NGOs) working alongside national health care services to address key gaps in care have started to employ laypeople, including 'accompagnateurs' (Behforous, Framer and Mukherjee, 2004), community health workers and 'expert patients' (people who are themselves HIV positive) to take on administrative work and assist in supporting HIV-infected and -affected adults and children to free trained medical staff to focus all their energies on other clinical work (Terry et al., 2012). However, it is not only unethical but also impractical to expect relatively unqualified (and often underpaid) people to assume responsibility for tasks for which they have had no or little training. Indeed, initiatives like these can only be effective where there is access to skilled supervision (Zachariah et al., 2009).

As early as 1978, the desire to reduce structural inequities in health care resulted in the WHO developing the human rights-based *Primary Health*

Care Framework, and in 2010 the *Global Code of Practice on the International Recruitment of Health Personnel*, aimed at enshrining the human rights of all and access to equitable health care. However, whilst the founding basis for human rights might be cosmopolitan, the mechanism for their realization is state-based. Organizations like the WHO do not have the power to ensure that resolutions like these are implemented: this requires multi-sectorial decision making and a reorientation of national and local policy. Moreover, although the Department of Health introduced an ethical code for recruiting international health workers in 2004, this code restricts active recruitment but allows for passive recruitment and recruitment from countries with specific agreements with the UK.

In discussing the consequences of the 'brain drain' for resource-starved countries, it is important to respect the human rights of the health care professionals concerned, including their right to escape life-constraining circumstances (including political conflict, poor working conditions, low salaries and high rates of unemployment), and the right to further their career through training and working elsewhere (McElmurry et al., 2006; Shah, 2013). Moreover, even if stricter legislation was passed, once started migration pathways and social networks tend to stimulate further migrations (Chamberlain, 2006). Access to people from a similar ethnic community, particularly family and friends, and professional associations composed of people from the same country strengthen these networks, building a sense of professional community (McElmurry et al., 2006).

Furthermore, the decision to migrate is often a family strategy aimed at increasing the quality of life and chances of survival: the possibility of sending remittances to support those who stay at home means migration can enhance the living standard of families regardless of whether they accompany the professional or stay at home. Indeed, it has been argued that remittances are a better way of assisting economically deprived countries than traditionally organized aid, as in some countries these remittances are significant in boosting the economy (Record and Mohiddin, 2006; Shah, 2013).

Ironically, one of the main motivators underpinning the push-pull towards migrating is the same for source and destination countries: the inability of health care systems to retain their workforce (Kingma, 2006; Kline, 2003). There is a long tradition of doctors, nurses and other professionals leaving the UK on a temporary or permanent basis to further their career, better their financial prospects and establish a different lifestyle. However, figures compiled by the British Medical Association (BMA) indicate an increase in the numbers leaving the UK. This is particularly true of GPs: in the absence of official data, the number of CGSs (Certificates of Good Standing) issued by the GMC (General Medical Council) is the most reliable indicator of how many consider leaving each year. Since

2008, there has been a 39% increase in the numbers of GPs requesting a CGS (Kenny, 2015).

Every doctor who applies for this certificate does not leave the UK, and even if they do, many remain on the medical register or return subsequently. Nonetheless, these figures suggest that fuelled by the stresses of excessive demands and workload, financial incentives and a desire for a better work/life balance, significant numbers of doctors (and other health care professionals, particularly nurses) are being lost to the UK (and NHS), placing additional stress on the workforce who remain. As discussed in relation to health care professionals from less developed countries, reaching such a decision can be enormously difficult: in addition to leaving family and close friends, many have mixed feelings about their decision, including guilt about abandoning the NHS in which they trained, contributing to a worsening GP crisis and the potential impact for patients (O'Grady, 2014).

In an attempt to remove barriers for GPs who might want to return to practise in the UK, the Royal College of General Practitioners has suggested they should be able to have their annual appraisal whilst in another country via Skype. However, to make any real inroads into stemming this tide, there would need to be a significant change in the demands, expectations and context of work in the UK. Consequently, rather than attempting to restrict the movement of health care professionals, it might be more effective to consider ways of ensuring UK-based staff feel less need to leave the country and to compensate source countries for the costs of their education (Austin, 2005).

This seems improbable in the near future: currently, the government is planning to institute changes that will affect the working conditions and pay of junior doctors, increasing rather than decreasing the numbers likely to leave the health service. In an attempt to reduce immigration, new legislation is being introduced whereby people from outside the European Economic Area must be earning £35,000 or more in order to be allowed to stay in the UK after six years. The Royal College of Nursing (RCN) anticipates that this legislation will have a disproportionate impact on the retention and recruitment of nurses from outside Europe, forcing many to return to their home countries, leaving hospitals with nothing to show for the millions of pounds spent on their recruitment and training (RCN, 2015).

The benefits to health care systems

As reflected above, the NHS and private health care organizations have a long tradition of recruiting health care professionals to alleviate staff shortages in caring for ill, disabled and dying people in the UK. Studies of the earlier waves of exiles indicate that the disproportionately high percentage of refugees were doctors who went on to make substantial contributions to medicine and science in Britain (Berlin, Gill and Eversley, 1997). This continues to be the case: many go on to specialize and work in the more disadvantaged areas local professionals are less willing to consider.

This is particularly true of geriatric care (Serco, 2014). In the early days of the NHS, the care of older people with chronic conditions was little more than tending to basic needs and took place in the back wards of large municipal hospitals. The founders of the specialty of geriatrics were determined to change this, partly to provide a more humane approach to medical care in late life and partly in response to the demand to release hospital beds for use by other patients. A crisis of staffing from the 1960s meant that by 1974 over 60% of consultant geriatric posts were filled by overseas trained graduates, particularly South Asian doctors. In contrast, between 1964 and 1991 overseas trained non-white doctors made up 3% of consultants in general medicine and 9% of all NHS consultants. Restrictions to career progression in other areas mean that doctors who obtained their initial medical qualifications in South Asian countries including India, Bangladesh, Sri Lanka, Pakistan and Myanmar before moving to the UK have been central to the shift towards more humane care for the elderly. However, their contribution is rarely acknowledged (Bornat, Henry and Raghuram, 2008; Esmail, 2007).

In a recent series of interviews with internationally born and trained professionals (including a midwife from Ghana, the manager of a surgical ward from the Philippines, a psychiatrist from South Africa, a cardiologist from Egypt, a dentist from Pakistan, a nurse from India, a maxillofacial surgeon from Australia and a geriatrician from Spain), people emphasized the benefits of working and furthering their training in the UK where methods of assessment, treatment and the control of infectious diseases are more advanced; where a higher level of care, funding and routine screening mean more people are able to survive conditions that would have been terminal in their home country (including congenital heart conditions); where access to high level care free of charge means people seek care soon enough to prevent problems; where people have a right to question and discuss their options rather than having to accept what they are told; and for those from countries where women's roles and rights are more circumscribed, where women are encouraged to speak on their own behalf rather than relying on what is transmitted through fathers, husbands and brothers. Whilst some drew attention to unfavourable comparisons (for example, that access to free care meant people were less self-reliant and missed appointments, and restrictions to the amount of time relatives could spend with hospitalized patients), far more emphasis was placed on the benefits to themselves and the recipients of care (Fox and Ifould, 2015).

Likewise, in an extensive analysis of the views of providers and recipients of older adult care about employing staff who were born and/or trained elsewhere, some respondents mentioned constraints such as lack of knowledge about local customs (for example, in the preparation of food) and language barriers (including colloquialisms related to health and personal needs). However, a greater proportion of what was said focused on the benefits: internationally trained employees were described as having a 'good work ethic', a more respectful attitude to older people, greater motivation to learn new skills and certain nationalities were seen to be particularly skilled in caring for the elderly. In addition, where the quality of care was perceived to have improved, over 80 per cent of managers felt this was a direct result of employing migrants. However, several managers praised migrants' willingness to work hours and shifts that were unacceptable to locally born staff, attesting to the importance of creating working conditions that are fair and abide with legislation. Although it is important to ensure all employees have fair working conditions, this is particularly important for people who feel they have less of a voice to challenge inappropriate demands and expectations (Serco, 2014).

Indeed, with their wealth of international experience and transcultural expertise, health care professionals who work elsewhere on a permanent or temporary basis are forging new relationships of care and responsibility between their countries of origin and settlement, playing a professionally, socially and even politically important role in the development of the health care service of their country of origin, creating goodwill, correcting misconceptions and boosting its reputation (Ormond, 2013; Shah, 2013). Many return to offer training and facilitate the transfer of more highly skilled staff to areas where health care is less developed, as in transfer of staff and professional development in relation to paediatric HIV/AIDS in sub-Saharan Africa (www.teampata.org). Similarly, the promotion of India and the Philippines as destinations for medical migration owes a great deal to the diasporic professionals of these two countries (Bookman and Bookman, 2007; Harris Cheng, 2009; Pandey et al., 2004).

In an era of global tourism, the diagnostic skills of colleagues with experience of working elsewhere can play a crucial role in reducing delays in treatment and unnecessary tests in relation to conditions less prevalent in the UK, as with bilharzia, an easily treatable infection caused by parasites that live in rivers and lakes in subtropical and tropical regions which results in symptoms suggestive of more serious conditions, including blood in the urine and flu-like symptoms. In addition, health care professionals trained elsewhere have introduced methods of treatment that are proving effective for some chronic conditions, as with acupuncture, homeopathy, meditation and Ayurvedic medicine, attesting to the fact that the transfer of knowledge and skills is not necessarily one-way.

Countries like Britain where a significant proportion of people are first- or second-generation migrants have a great deal to learn from professionals with a history of migration. Imagine the surprise and relief of arriving for a hospital appointment in a foreign country to be greeted by a doctor from one's own country. Coming from the same country does not mean each person's experience and understanding will be the same. However, there is likely to be a similar understanding of the health care system and range of services available back home, expectations of family and gendered roles in situations of illness, attitudes to confidentiality, care of the elderly, sexuality, mental illness, and religious practices that can affect health care, including circumcision and dietary restrictions. People with a similar background are also likely to be aware of situations in which misunderstandings might arise, and when the concepts and methods of treatment that are mentioned might seem strange or even inappropriate. Likewise, where there are language barriers, even if there are regional differences in accent and dialect, being seen by someone who speaks the same language means it is possible to communicate without a translator, reducing the length of consultations, time wasted (for example, when an interpreter does not arrive or it is not clear ahead of time that their services were required), potential compromises to confidentiality and costs to the health system.

Moreover, even if professionals are from a different country, as 'the products of several interlocking histories, belonging at the same time to several homes' (Hall, 1993, p. 362), they are likely to have an insider understanding of the challenges migrants face, including those of coming to terms with deteriorating health without access to the practical and emotional support of close family, the desire to protect those who live elsewhere by withholding information about illness, delays in hearing someone is seriously ill or has died and what it is like to grieve from a foreign land where no one understands one's relationship with the deceased, including stories of having loved, fought and made up (Llerena-Quin, 2004).

They are also likely to be understanding of aspects of migration less obviously linked with illness that affect emotional wellbeing, including the difficulties of adapting to living in a context in which the dominant culture, food, dress and climate are very different, having to explain differences to oneself and others, and managing the mistrust and prejudice accorded to people deemed 'foreign'. Those who moved as children and grew up in the UK may have seen their parents struggle to survive, establish themselves in a new country without the support of an extended family network, and, where the outside world feels hostile, work towards ensuring home is a safe place.

Similarly, health professionals who fled countries dominated by political turmoil and an oppressive regime will have insider knowledge of the fear and powerlessness such situations tend to evoke, and the 'survivor guilt' of living in relative comfort knowing parents and siblings who stayed behind are at risk. Some are also likely to know what it means to be a refugee in the UK so are uniquely placed in understanding the implications this can have for clinical work. For example, based on his own experience as a refugee, Yesilyurt, a psychologist, argues that viewing refugees as passive victims who cannot help themselves underestimates their tenacity, capacity to survive and active participation and that this is not only inaccurate, it reduces their readiness to draw on psychological services when needed and opens the door to racism and xenophobia (quoted in Tribe and Patel, 2007).

People vary in the extent to which they hold on to or let go of cultural and religious traditions following migration. However, an insider experience of migration means that instead of trying to bypass what seem like cultural hindrances, one is likely to be more accepting of traditional cultural beliefs and constraints. Insider experiences of moving from one cultural context to another also means one can understand that even the most deeply held beliefs are more fluid and open to re-definition than outsiders realize (Malik and Mandin, 2012).

These commonalities suggest that migrants would be best served by seeing someone from the same country. However, this is not necessarily the case: where people are struggling financially, professionally and socially, being treated by an 'inside-outsider', by a person who is in some ways similar but appears to be part of the establishment, can arouse a complicated mixture of envy, regret and hope. Political divisions in one's country of origin and differences in the extent to which one abides by traditional beliefs and practices can mean that it is easier to trust a professional who is an outsider to one's country and culture. Likewise, differences in skin colour, accent, education and socio-economic position mean that some people are exposed to, and/or perceive, greater scrutiny and discrimination even if they are from the same place.

Moreover, although many professionals have an added investment in working with people from the same country and/or other migrants, this is not always the case. Factors such as internalized racism and the desire to fit in can lead to attempts to differentiate oneself from people deemed to be 'other': indeed, confining one's work to these groups of people can mean that this aspect of identity, 'foreignness', remains central to how one is seen and experiences oneself.

Professional challenges

Life is not necessarily easy for those who move. On arrival, it is not unusual to find out that registration and requalification are more difficult than one realized, that recruiters promised more than one is actually able to receive and underestimated the costs of living and its effect on salaries (Haour-Knipe, 2013; Shiwani, 2006).

Where one's qualifications are not recognized, the financial and emotional costs of the re-credential process and of learning, unlearning and relearning dormant information can be enormous (Bornat, Henry and Raghuram, 2008). There is often a long delay between exams, registration and obtaining work, limiting the possibility of maintaining confidence in one's sense of professional competence (Stewart, Clark and Clark, 2007). This is particularly difficult for refugees and asylum seekers as the delay between arrival, accreditation and working is even longer:

> Henri, a highly skilled physician, fled political turmoil in his country of origin. Although he was ultimately given leave to remain in the UK, he found it enormously distressing having to rely on welfare and living apart from his family. However, what he found even more distressing was that in the absence of a professional network it was difficult to maintain his knowledge, skills and professional identity.

Problems identified by other refugee doctors include isolation and the lack of appropriate information and a clear route through the system (Cohn et al., 2006). In view of the shortage of trained health care staff, the waste of human resources is extremely frustrating: many refugee doctors have years of medical experience, are highly skilled, motivated, hardworking and committed to re-entering their profession. As reflected in a study of refugees who fled from Bosnia-Herzegovina to Austria (Wenzel, 1999), refugee doctors and psychologists can play a significant role in alleviating the heavy stress experienced by the medical and psychological services of the country in which they and their compatriots take refuge. Engaging with the traumatic experiences of other people can re-evoke feelings related to one's own traumatic past. However, provided professionals have found a way of coming to terms with their own experience, with appropriate training, mentoring and support, insider experiences of war and forced migration mean they have a great deal to offer general practices and other health care services in countries like the UK where there are a large number of refugees and asylum seekers (Ong and Gayen, 2003; Steven, Oxley and Fleming, 2008).

Even when registered, difficulties in finding employment can lead to accepting work in unfavourable areas where one is forced to work overtime on a mandatory basis and take on additional duties or work that lie beyond one's expertise. As a consequence of the high costs of living and difficulties in finding work in one's area of specialty some people who move to further their training intending to return to enhance the quality of services in their country of origin find this is impossible (Shiwani, 2006). In other cases, the practical, bureaucratic and financial costs to obtaining recognition for qualifications and requalifying result in seeking employment as housekeepers, cleaners (particularly older nurses) or practising illegally on an unregistered basis.

Moreover, depending on the country one moves to or from, even if one does find appropriate work, there may also be discrepancies between the culture of medicine and methods of treatment and one's previous training and clinical experience, as where doctor–patient relationships, attitudes to truth-telling and gendered assumptions are very different to what had been regarded culturally appropriate and best clinical practice (Fox and Ifould, 2015). Likewise, there may be a gap between what one is told and needs to know in order to operate effectively in the hospital or clinic setting, for example how the internet system and referral procedure work, and the financial implications and availability of particular interventions. The desire to fit in and avoid being seen as inadequate mean it can be difficult to acknowledge what one does not know or ask more than once (Lillis, St George and Upsell, 2006). It is always important to ensure new staff members have a comprehensive introduction to the workplace and access to a mentor/buddy. However, as reflected above, this is particularly important for people who trained and worked abroad.

One of the other challenges many professionals face is that where fluency in English informed one's decision of where to move, difficulties in understanding abbreviated, colloquial, slang, and other non-medical words and interpreting bodily cues can mean one does not have the 'right' verbal and non-verbal skills to operate effectively (Lilles, St George and Upsell, 2006). Similarly, differences in accent can make it difficult to understand face-to-face and telephone conversations, affecting the accuracy of diagnosis and treatment and the possibility of establishing trust: where patients (or indeed colleagues) struggle to understand what is said all parties are likely to feel less satisfied with the encounter (McElmurry et al., 2006; Wilner and Feinstein-Whittaker, 2013).

A number of high profile cases of malpractice have contributed to fears about, and mistrust in, foreign doctors, particularly those who are not fluent in English. This view has been backed up by figures released by the GMC showing that three-quarters of the doctors struck off the register between 2008 and 2013 were foreign-trained (Donnelly and Knapton, 2014). No one would argue with the importance of ensuring health care professionals who qualified overseas are able to demonstrate that their clinical and language skills are of a high enough standard to practise in Britain and entrusting professional organizations like the GMC with the responsibility of protecting society from deficient practitioners. Another cause for concern is that health regulators in the UK are not automatically alerted when a doctor is struck off the medical register in another country. With this in mind, there have been calls for the NHS to work towards establishing an internationally agreed mechanism to assist health care services in checking whether potential employees have been involved in malpractice and struck off the register elsewhere.

However, one cannot discount reports of racial and ethnic-based discrimination, particularly in assessing clinical skills (Esmail and Roberts, 2013). International medical graduates and doctors from ethnic minorities have been found to experience discrimination at almost every stage of their medical careers, including at admission to medical school, in their career progression, endowment of distinction awards, and responses to complaints against them (Moberly, 2014). Although discrimination seems to occur across all specialties, particular concerns have been raised about disproportionately high failure rates of those who take the examination for membership of the Royal College of General Practitioners (MRCGP).

Similar concerns have been raised in relation to the nursing profession: research indicates that internationally trained nurses and other health care professionals are rarely given the recognition they deserve, that they receive lower salaries, have fewer opportunities for advancement and feel discriminated against by UK-born colleagues, managers and patients, and experiences of mentoring are often marred by mentors' lack of cultural awareness (Allan, 2010; Henry, 2006; Larsen, 2007; Tilke et al., 2007).

The numbers of foreign-born health care professionals working in the UK suggests that many British-born people would be used to, and comfortable with, being treated by Indian, African and other migrant doctors and nurses. Although this might be true of a certain proportion of the population, it does not fit with the experience of many professionals and care workers. In a study of the views of nurses and care staff working in older adult acute care, reports of discrimination ranged from overtly negative references to race, colour and nationality, to more covert references, and legitimate concerns about language skills and lacking knowledge of local customs. In turn, managers expressed concern about their lack of training in responding to situations of discrimination, for example how to balance the need to respect the older adults entrusted to their care with the need to avoid discriminating against a job applicant or employee: whether to move migrant staff when an older adult refuses to be looked after by them, expect them to continue working, or confront the elderly person concerned (Cangiano et al., 2009).

Indeed, despite attempts to reduce institutionalized racism in the NHS, recent research indicates that black and minority ethnic (BME) doctors who were born and trained outside the UK are less likely to be shortlisted or gain posts at the prestigious teaching hospitals and medical schools, and have to accept lower remuneration in order to support themselves and their families (GMC, 2015; McManus and Wakeford, 2014). Many BME doctors who grew up and trained in the UK face similar barriers, particularly around selection where candidates seem to be excluded on the basis of a foreign surname. An added complication is that racism and other forms of discrimination can mean one has less confidence to challenge or resist censure and/or feels forced to accept work in particularly difficult specialties in areas where access to professional support is limited (Humphrey et al., 2009).

Likewise, many of the health care professionals I supervise have raised concerns about discrimination when discussing their clinical dilemmas. For example, Katerina, a Czech-born palliative nurse who is fluent in English but speaks with a Czech accent, talked about feeling embarrassed and unable to hold on to her sense of professional competence when confronted with a terminally ill elderly man who refused to be seen by her because she was a 'stupid foreigner'. Similarly, Sara who was born in Israel and had been working in the UK for a relatively short period of time, said she felt devalued and unable to speak for fear of expressing a rage she would regret later when the daughter of a dying woman asked about her accent and questioned her capacity to work with their family.

It can be extremely difficult deciding when and how to confront discrimination, and whether references to one's accent arise from discrimination or curiosity, whatever the circumstances are. However, it is likely to be particularly difficult in relation to someone who is extremely vulnerable and entrusted to one's care. An added complication is that where one has not had time to rebuild a professional community in the country in which one works, encounters like these tend to compound one's own questions about professional competence.

My own experience suggests that it is more difficult confronting discrimination when this relates to one's personal position than that of another. I remember how, as a relatively inexperienced family therapy supervisor, I felt unable to say anything when a supervisee who did not realize I was a Jew made an anti-Semitic comment about her clients. I suspect I kept quiet because I did not trust myself to say anything without coming across as attacking or defensive. Fortunately, another member of the supervision group challenged what she had said. However, if he had not my silence would have conveyed the message that these thoughts were shared and acceptable.

In other cases, discrimination is more covert. Begum, a palliative care consultant who was born and did her initial training in India, felt she was subject to far more scrutiny than her white British-born colleagues and had to fight to be included in meetings her peers were invited to as a matter of course. However she was reluctant to challenge her colleagues for fear of drawing attention to her position as a 'foreigner'. She was also unsure whether her exclusion was based on doubts about her professional expertise, discrimination, or a heightened sensitivity to the possibility of being treated as a second-class citizen.

The dominance of white privilege and experiences of marginalization mean that it is possible to internalize the racism that informs the wider social context (Pyke, 2010). Discrimination does not only operate at an institutional or interpersonal level: it is a form of symbolic violence that affects one's sense of self. Du Bois used the term 'double-consciousness' in describing the discomfort 'of looking at one's self through the eyes of others, of measuring one's soul by the tape of a world that looks on in amused contempt and pity' (1989, p. 3). This sense of self-questioning, self-disparagement and measuring oneself through the real and/or imagined eyes 'of a world that looks on in amused contempt and pity' seemed to underpin the account Seda, a community nurse, gave of her difficulties in working with a man who, like herself, was from Turkey: despite living on benefits in the UK, he went back to seek private treatment in Turkey, returning with medication and scans she and his GP felt were not only unnecessary but inappropriate.

Most professionals find these situations extremely difficult as it takes time to re-establish trust and discuss the advantages and disadvantages of this new treatment regime (Ormond, 2013). However, this is likely to be particularly challenging when one is from the same country, identified with the same ethnic group, and sees these actions as not only inappropriate but an abuse of a free state-funded health care system. Likewise, although many professionals feel a particular commitment to working with people from their country of origin and/or a similar background, confining one's work to this population has the potential to frame oneself as 'other'; as discussed in relation to interpreters, personal–professional boundaries can become more difficult to maintain, pulling both parties into a pattern of over-identification (Akhtar, 2006; Antinucci, 2004; Costa, 2014).

In contrast, Leslie, a white British-born manager of a psychosocial team, used supervision to reflect on her difficulties in knowing how to respond to concerns about Rozhin, a counsellor who was born and had trained in Iran. Comments by Rozhin's patients and feedback from other staff members suggested that people found her authoritarian, brusque and far too formal. However, Leslie was unsure whether Rozhin's behaviour was an indication of a culturally different approach to interacting with patients, an attempt to cover up her lack of confidence or that, as a foreigner, she might feel added pressure to avoid acting in what could be seen as an overly familiar way. As importantly, Leslie was anxious to avoid being seen as racist. Consequently, in supervising Leslie it was important to disentangle concerns about Rozhin's interactions with patients and colleagues from Rozhin's, Leslie's and my own engagement with racism.

High quality care involves being able to take risks, challenge patients, carers and colleagues, and follow intuitive hunches. However, as Leslie's concerns indicate, fear and post-colonial guilt about triggering rage about white people's history of treatment of black people can limit one's readiness to take risks, watering down the 'intuitive precarious footwork' (Gunaratnam, 2013, p. 104) that is central to sensitive management as well as collaborative care. What makes this particularly complicated is that although there are some objective measures against which to assess the quality of clinical care, judgements are more subjective when it comes to assessing culturally responsive care, including whether or not responses are oppressive or violating, what needs to change to accommodate culturally different approaches and values, and how to balance drawing on one's professional and personal knowledge while remaining open to other perspectives.

Personal challenges of migrating

Young (2015) is not a health care professional. However, his call to recognize that 'it's not workers who migrate but people' is extremely pertinent to the positions of health care professionals. Drawing on his own experience he argues that 'although migrants tend to move with the future in mind, whenever they move they leave part of themselves behind [....] and the losses keep coming. Funerals, christenings, graduations and weddings missed – milestones you couldn't make because your life was elsewhere'. Despite choosing to leave and establishing a successful life in the US, there were times when he was confronted with what he had lost, with aspects of his previous life that had not been 'discarded but atrophied'.

As Young suggests, even where migration opens up opportunities for professional advancement and a better life for one's family, some sense of loss and cultural shock is almost inevitable, regardless of whether the move is temporary or permanent. In common with other migrants, it can be difficult coming to terms with living apart from family, friends, familiar surroundings and conveniences of home. For health care professionals who move with a partner, the time and financial commitments required to requalify and establish one's self professionally can mean it is difficult to provide one another the level of support needed in adjusting to life in a new context. This tends to be particularly challenging when one has young children and one cannot draw on the support of family who would have played a significant role in childcare if the couple had remained in their country of origin.

In other situations, practical restraints and commitments to vulnerable relatives mean partners and children stay behind, particularly where the intention is to return after furthering one's training or earning sufficient money to increase the family's standard of living. Even if the decision to work elsewhere is shared and families remain connected through emails, calls, Skype and regular visits back home, it can be difficult to make up for gaps in contact and experiences that are unwitnessed and unshared (Falicov, 2013).

One of the more distressing findings to arise from studies of international domestic labour is the pain so many domestic workers from Third World countries experience when economic hardship forces them to leave their children in the care of relatives in order to look after the children of parents in First World countries (Altschuler, 2005; Ames, 2002; Ehrenreich and Hochschild, 2003; Horton, 2008; Parrenas, 2014; Pollock, 1994). Although domestic workers are usually hired because they are sensitive to the needs of others, personal engagement tends to be seen as antithetical to paid domestic work. However, care work is inherently relational, regardless of whether it involves routine bodily care or emotional attachment, affiliation and intimate knowledge (Stone, 1998). As such, coupled with loneliness and distance from their own children, it is not unusual for domestic workers to develop a strong attachment to the children entrusted to their care (Pollock, 1994).

The positions of domestic workers and health care professionals are very different. However, it is surprising that there has been no parallel consideration of ways in which health care professionals respond to the intimacy that tends to arise from engaging with people at times of heightened intensity when one is lonely and unable to look to family or close friends for closeness. Likewise, it is surprising that, as far as I know, no attempts have been made to explore the challenges health care professionals face in caring for vulnerable members of other people's family when unable to offer a similar level of care to their own family. Although some people are able to return to care for loved ones at such times, taking additional compassionate leave (usually unpaid) can feel impossible when one is worried about finances, retaining one's job and the prospects of promotion.

As discussed in relation to all migrants, even if parents supported the decision to leave, and are financially dependent on remittances from abroad, illness and the threat of death can confront both parties with the disjunction between anticipated and lived experience, reawakening the longing for the life that might have been. Reflecting on her own decision to continue working with people facing illness and bereavement while her mother was dying a long distance away (albeit in the same country), Walsh, a family therapist with extensive clinical experience, urges health care professionals to take time out from other commitments for what may be the last opportunity to spend time with the dying, and after their death to mourn and experience the mutual support of people who have known the deceased and attend to one's sense of loss (Walsh and McGoldrick, 2004). However, this is not always feasible.

Regret about the consequences of leaving his elderly non-migrant parents dominated the account Jack,[32] a 70-year-old cardiologist who left South Africa in his early twenties, gave in reflecting on the effect of migration on his family. He began by speaking about his father and wondering whether his health deteriorated more rapidly because he was not there before going on to describe his last conversation with his mother:[33]

> Jack: It was – it was – it was hard – I mean my mother used to say to me 'You will come back – won't you?' and I said 'Yes – I will come back'. But once I got on the plane I thought to myself – I wonder – and I didn't. I was there when she died – at her bedside – and that was terrible – absolutely terrible cause she – had cancer and she was in extraordinary pain and she said to me 'Can't you do something for me?' and I said: 'I'm not your doctor' and she said: 'But you are my son and you are a doctor – can't you do something for me?'

The hesitancy of Jack's account suggest embarrassment about mentioning his own distress in the face of his mother's greater suffering, and ambivalence about reflecting on aspects of migration he finds uncomfortable. Although migration offered him access to professional and social opportunities that would have been unavailable if he had stayed, his account suggests that it compromised the care he was able to offer his parents. However, his decision to tell this story near the start of our interview suggests a desire to frame compromises to adult children's ability to care for elderly parents as an almost inevitable consequence of migration. Subsequent discussions about his children suggest that it was only when one of Jack's own children had moved abroad and he reached the age his parents had been when he left that he could appreciate how difficult his absence might have been for them.

The GMC cautions doctors like Jack against providing medical care to anyone with whom they have a close personal relationship (GMC, 2013). However, many doctors and relatives feel there is no one they would trust more. For example, reflecting on her experience of working with a population where a high percentage of people are first- and second-generation migrants (including refugees), Megan, a GP who works for a culturally diverse inner London primary health care practice, began with her own experience. When she was 6 her parents left Brazil to further their careers in the UK. Having lived in the UK for many years, her parents' longing for the people, climate and life they had left behind increased in later life and they returned to Brazil in the knowledge that Megan, their only child, would remain in the UK. When her father developed Alzheimer's disease, Megan (and her mother) felt that as a GP she should be able to ensure they received the best possible care. However, despite frequent visits, she was unfamiliar with the workings of the Brazilian health care system. She found this particularly painful because her decision to become a doctor was partly inspired by the desire to care for her parents.

Although this is not particular to health care professionals, tapping into the centrality of family experiences and the guilt many feel about migrating and leaving their families, several commercial organizations have begun promoting health care packages to non-residents to ensure that non-migrant family have access to high quality medical care (Ormond, 2013). For example, companies like Royal Medical Tours Mumbai (2011) offers non-resident Indians a 'Parents' Package of Care' aimed at alleviating the gaps that arise when children do not live in the same country, particularly in later life when parents are frail and at increased risk of becoming ill.

Health care professionals living in an area where there are many compatriots who do not speak English or know how the health care system operates are often asked to intervene when people feel misunderstood by locally trained staff or do not understand what they have been told. It can be deeply gratifying to feel one has the knowledge and skills to help others at times of distress. However, it can be difficult to draw a boundary between the personal and the professional, and feel sure one is giving the best clinical advice when one can be stopped at the supermarket or on the street with critically important questions about health.

Recommendations for practice

Regardless of whether professionals who were born and/or trained abroad remain or return home, many find the experience of working in the UK extremely valuable and are able to further their careers through exposure to different forms of health care. However, it can be extremely difficult living and working in an unfamiliar setting without the buffer of family and friends, and attending to the ill members of other people's family when unable to offer help to one's own. Difficulties in re-registering, finding employment, transitioning into a health care system where the practices and paradigms of treatment are different, and discrimination and impediments to promotion mean it is not uncommon for people to feel devalued and abused by the experience, but to tolerate this to maintain the right to remain in the country (Allan, 2010; Alexis, Vydelingum and Robbins, 2007).

In an attempt to address some of these challenges, the EU set out a framework that is more respectful of the rights of migrant health care professionals and other skilled workers entitled *Decent Work Across Borders*. Emphasis is placed on the importance of improving data collection and analysis of labour market information on the demand and supply of professionals and skilled personnel in health care in the EU, alternative destination countries and the employment prospects in the participating countries; fostering policy dialogue to better understand circular migration schemes that are aligned with the International Labour Organization's Decent Work Agenda and mitigate the risks of brain drain in a pro-active manner; and designing mechanisms to facilitate online registration, skills testing and certification, preparation and counselling, placements for European employment and, upon return, re-employment in the home country.

In line with these guidelines, my experience of clinical work and supervision suggests that greater attention needs to be paid to establishing data that is accurate, consistent and comparable, to assisting migrant health care professionals in transitioning into a potentially different health care and socio-cultural context and working towards reducing racism and other forms of discrimination with the NHS and private health care systems.

Establishing accurate, consistent and comparable data

In the absence of more accurate and consistent data, understanding the full scope of international migration, push-pull factors underpinning decisions to move, impact on the health care services of source and destination countries and the complex professional and more personal challenges health professionals and their families face remains problematic. Moreover, as reflected in current media and policy debates surrounding the reliance of internationally trained staff and desires to stem the tide of immigration for 'fortress Britain' (Geddes, 2003), migration information is considered sensitive: many governments do not collect or share data across different departments of administration. Similarly, those who left clandestinely and remain concerned about family living elsewhere are likely to have fears about how such information might be used.

Nonetheless, it would be helpful to work towards standardizing data, collecting and analysing this information on a more regular basis, and using data that does exist more effectively: even if many countries do not have accurate information on health personnel migration, they are likely to have other sources of data that offer some insights into health worker migration. It would also be important to improve the quality and comparability of data to ensure greater confidence in the information that is compiled. This requires increased networking between the various source and destination countries to harmonize data collection instruments so information can be compared using the same templates. It would also require international agreements on the basis of established principles and standardized methods, including agreements on the minimum data required to track the movements of specialist personnel. This is likely to mean offering input to enhance the capacity of developing countries with poor statistical systems (Diallo, 2004).

Transitioning into a different health care and social system

More bridging programmes are needed to assist health professionals in registering, retraining, and where required, improving their proficiency in English. Beyond the critically important challenges of registration, retraining, employment and language proficiency, additional attention needs to be paid to supporting internationally trained staff in transitioning into a new social and health care system, where the paradigms and practices of medicine are unfamiliar (Austin, 2005; Guru et al., 2012). This includes explicit and clear communication between employers and recruitment agencies to avoid contractual misunderstandings, a clear and comprehensive orientation to the workplace and access to a designated mentor. Likewise, additional attention needs to be paid to the more personal challenges of living apart from family and close friends and adjusting to living in an unfamiliar social context.

Change is already under way: in the UK, other countries across Europe and the USA, a wide range of innovative programmes have been established to ensure migrant doctors, nurses, pharmacists and allied health care professionals gain appropriate experience and where relevant requalify and register (Austin, 2005; Gerrish and Griffith, 2004; Higginbottom et al., 2011; Moberly, 2014; Ong and Gayen, 2003). For example, within the UK, the BMA provides information for refugees and asylum-seeker doctors who hope to establish careers in the UK, free subscription to the *British Medical Journal*, access to websites covering a range of medico-political and health stories, access to the BMA library and a confidential telephone counselling service. In addition, the BMA coordinates a Refugee Liaison Group which serves as a forum for networking, information exchange and, where possible, collective action, and, in collaboration with the Refugee Council, has set up a voluntary database of refugees and asylum-seeking doctors. This includes an online portal that provides information on the requirements for UK registration, as well as advice and resources to ensure health professionals meet the appropriate requirements to become safe practitioners in the UK (www. rose.nhs.uk).

In addition, the NHS is partnering the Refugee Council, London Metropolitan University and three London-based hospitals in a project entitled Building Bridges which offers refugee doctors help in refreshing medical knowledge and skills before taking the Professional Linguistic Assessment Board tests; information about language courses and tuition to help increase their proficiency in English to communicate effectively with patients; access to specialist careers advisers, up-to-date information and guidance on routes towards professional registration; information on paid and voluntary work in the health care sector; and practical employability workshops related to health sector work. In common with other initiatives, these programmes provide refugees and other migrant health care professionals with information about the context and ethos of health care in the UK. This includes the importance attached to patient-centred health care: patients' right to information about their health and diagnosis of any condition, their right to be involved in decisions about any treatment or care they may receive and to be given information about serious side effects; informed consent; and confidentiality and respect for the privacy and dignity of all patients, regardless of gender, age, sexuality and ethnicity.

Similar programmes have been developed in relation to other care professions: for example, the Royal College of Nursing and Midwifery, Refugee Nurses Task Force and Pan London NHS Refugee Allied Health Professionals Group provide guidelines for migrant, refugee and asylum seeker nurses, midwives and allied health care professionals including information on the NHS, the requirement to work in the various professional roles, the principles on which health care in the UK is based, advice on improving English language skills and opportunities for voluntary and paid work, the latter of which is not open to asylum seekers (Hakesley-Brown, 2006; Royal College of Nursing and Midwifery, 2010). Likewise, the British Dental Association offers information and advice to refugee and other internationally trained dental professionals and dentists, and through the Council for Assisting Refugee Academics (CARA) makes small grants to refugee academics to assist them in rebuilding their lives and careers in dentistry within the UK. Other organizations like Medicruit provide similar opportunities for dentists trained in other European countries. Whilst these initiatives are motivated by the desire to assist people in transitioning into a different social and health care system, they are also driven by concern about the shortage of trained health care professionals.

Racism and personal–professional resonances

It is also important to provide guidance and additional training on equal opportunity, cultural diversity and racism to ensure that migrants, their colleagues and managerial staff are better equipped to deal with the tensions that can arise where relationships of care are marked by the politics and histories of 'race'. This means promoting a culture that values diversity at all levels within the NHS as well as the private sector. However, the irrational and unconscious aspects of racial dynamics and other forms of prejudice cannot simply be countered by appeals to the rational (Gunaratnam and Lewis, 2001); this requires reflecting on one's own engagement with racism, including the potential to distance oneself from those deemed to be other.

Unconscious phenomena mean we can never be fully aware of the ways in which the experiences of the people we encounter resonate with our own experience. Nonetheless, reflecting on the possibility of a link on one's own or in supervision can alert us to situations when impressions about others, including migrant colleagues, relate to our own blind spots, including personal experiences of loss, trauma and illness as well as discrimination, migration, political oppression and legacies of colonization, and the reverse: when thoughts and feelings that seem to be personal are a reflection of the experiences of others.

9

CONCLUSION

Despite the introduction of increasingly restrictive policies, economic imbalances, political conflict, demographic patterns and international population mobility mean migration and its consequences for the health of migrants and their non-migrant relatives are facts of global life. However, discussions about the health care of migrants have the potential to unsettle understandings of nationhood and civil rights, touching on moral and political debates about responsibility of a nation state to provide equitable health care to everyone residing in that country. This includes debates about whether vulnerable people whose right to remain in the country is contested should have access to free medical care when they are unable to pay, whether the state should provide interpreters or require migrants to learn English, and anxiety about the increased prevalence of conditions like tuberculosis (TB), raising questions about how we think of 'them' and 'us', and the distribution of limited resources (Haour-Knipe, 2013).

This book has been written at a particular point in history, at a time when medical advances mean many people are able to live fulfilling lives following the diagnosis of conditions that were terminal until fairly recently, and people who are brain dead can be kept alive with the aid of life support equipment. Coupled with this is an almost moral imperative to keep well: underlying much of what is said about illness is the assumption that with the appropriate diet and lifestyle the capacity to remain healthy and 'fight' (Greer, 2000) disease lies within our control.

Moreover, at this point in time discussions about migration and the plight of refugees are more polarized than ever before. At one end of the continuum, media and political debates about the 'war on terror' are fuelling the flames of xenophobic fears about the need to protect the rights of ordinary citizens from 'others'. At the other end, there has been an outpouring of public support for refugees with calls to stand up and be counted, as reflected in the numbers of people protesting in front of Parliament and driving vans laden with food and clothing across the channel to refugee camps in Europe. I have just returned from Lesbos, a Greek island, where medical and non-medical volunteers are giving up their time to support the hundreds and often thousands of refugees fleeing political conflict and economic hardship in Syria, Iraq, Eritrea and Afghanistan. As most of the refugees will have spent hours or even days waiting for a boat or inflatable dinghy to take them from Turkey to Greece, many arrive suffering from hypothermia, panic attacks and numbness as a result of sitting cramped up with children on their laps and legs. Some face the additional trauma of burying loved ones who died during the crossing but not being able to spare the time to fulfil traditional mourning rituals in case neighbouring countries close their borders to refugees. Likewise, in Idomeni, a camp in Northern Greece where we have just set up a project offering psychosocial support to refugees and volunteers, many people are desperate, struggling to hold on to their sense of self and hopes for safety while children as young as 2 or 3 are running around, unsupervised, seeking the affection their traumatized parents cannot provide from strangers.

There are important parallels between illness and migration: both forms of experience have the potential to disrupt expectations of how life is, should and ought to be (Yngvesson and Mahoney, 2000), calling to mind Freud's (1919) notion of the 'uncanny', a sense of estrangement that does not derive its terror and discomfort from the externally alien but from the strangely familiar from which one cannot separate. Similarly, both forms of experience have the potential to disturb understandings of who one is and relationships with others, requiring a reworking of identity, embodiment and memory to re-establish some sense of continuity between the past, present and imagined future.

In addition, both forms of experience are informed by government policy, access to formal and informal services and the promotion or prohibition of certain kinds of behaviour. However, as important as these material realities are, experiences of illness and migration are also informed by the 'lurid metaphors' (Sontag, 1991) and discourses that dominate the wider context in which we live, including discourses pertaining to the foreigner, 'race', physical vulnerability, control of the body and physical sensations ranging from sex to breathing difficulties, impacting on the providers as well as recipients of health care. Indeed, it is not just enough to be in a place and feel we belong: to belong we need to fit in and in order to fit in we need to be seen as belonging by others (Anderson, 1983).

As the research and clinical examples discussed here illustrate, for many people migration has a beneficial effect on health. Living in a different geographical environment where particular communicable diseases are less prevalent, access to preventative programmes, including immunization, and advanced methods of health care increase the possibilities of maximizing health and, when faced with illness, disability and the threat of death, the possibility of receiving treatment that draws on cutting-edge developments in medical care. Likewise, access to opportunities that are less obviously related to health care can lead to a greater sense of empowerment with beneficial consequences for one's own health and the health of one's family, mitigating the potentially traumatizing consequences of exposure to adverse events, as for example with transformations in gendered roles and expectations, escape from situations of war, and access to better employment, professional, financial and educational prospects. In other situations the consequences are more problematic, impacting on the experiences of subsequent generations. Where migration has been traumatic, attempts to stave off the unknown and uncontainable have the potential to freeze relationships, interfering with the possibility of negotiating subsequent transitions in the life cycle. Moreover, the physical and mental fragmentation associated with experiences of illness and treatment can re-evoke feelings and memories related to prior experiences of trauma, and vice versa, even if this lies beyond consciousness.

Working with people who chose or were forced to migrate, in some cases under traumatic circumstances, can have a profound effect on UK-born and trained health care professionals, and the health care systems in which we work. The experience can open our eyes to alternate approaches to illness and treatment, responses to frailty, professional–patient interactions, expressions of distress, discrimination, factors that contribute to resilience, bravery and determination to survive. These encounters can lead to a different understanding of our own experience of culture, history of migration, prejudice, capacity to respond to difficulties and responses to confrontations with mortality, bringing issues that are relevant to many other members of the population into increased visibility. However, the stresses of trying to transcend cultural and language barriers in working with people whose lives have been disrupted by migration, trauma and are facing financial and other practical problems, can mean it is impossible to offer the sort of care one would like, giving rise to feelings of incompetence, powerlessness and, in some cases, secondary traumatization.

A wide number of national and international resolutions have been reached aimed at avoiding disparities in health status and access to services between migrants and the host population, limiting discrimination and stigmatization, reducing excess morbidity and mortality and minimizing the negative impact of the migration process on health outcomes (Jayaweera, 2014). Although the UK is striving to comply with international standards and services have improved in some areas, this is not true throughout the country. Likewise, despite the introduction of innovative programmes aimed at helping professionals transition into a new health care system, many feel unsupported and continue to face discrimination.

As outlined earlier, to move forward additional research is needed to ascertain the challenges particular migrant groups face and factors that contribute to resilience and best practice. This requires extending routine data collection to include country of birth and duration in the UK, within the private sector as well as the NHS. It was also suggested that to minimize inconsistencies and the risk of policies organized around the image of the foreigner as a threat, a focal point for migrant health should be set up within the Department of Health, with links to other relevant government organizations (Jayaweera, 2014).

What is also needed is additional training on culturally diverse responses to illness and ways of engaging with people whose experiences are very different to one's own, trainings that are not only academic but involve exploring one's own prejudices, vulnerabilities and sensitivities. This includes looking beyond labels and stereotypes. For example, migrant women are often presented as particularly vulnerable and heavy users of health and social care services, relying on social housing and additional welfare benefits (Hargreaves and Friedland, 2013). Although this might be true of women living in the most deprived circumstances, an increased percentage of women are the primary breadwinners for their family, many of whom work in the health services and education and look after the children of the population of the country to which they move (Anderson, 2001; Ehrenreich and Hochschild, 2003; Lutz, 2008). Moreover, many women who have the right to claim health and social care services do not easily access these services.

In conclusion, although migration and illness are not the only or main determinants of experience, exploring how experiences of illness, self, family and professional competence have been affected by migration opens up the possibility of considering complexities of experience that have a profound effect on responses to illness, disability and death but tend to be overlooked. This includes the longing for the familiar, the added desire to integrate the various aspects of one's life, questions of the possibility of a return, challenges to ethnic identity and exposure to racism. However, these explorations mean being ready to engage with what is similar as well as different, including incapacitating versions of the self, recognizing the 'precariousness of the other' (Butler, 2003) and that the other is as real, competent and vulnerable as ourselves.

NOTES

1 There are considerable differences between the positions of people who move within the same state or country (internal migration), leave one country for another (external migration or emigration), those who move to a different country (immigration), and movements that are temporary or permanent. However, in general this book uses the term migrant as many of the issues discussed here are relevant to all people located and dislocated through migration.

2 The terms used to designate those who remain when a close relative migrates are all negative and framed in terms of lack, as with 'non-migrant' and 'the left behind', and fail to take account of the positive and agentic aspects of this position. However, as the more accurate 'those who choose or are forced to remain when a close relative migrates' is unwieldy, 'non-migrant' is used here.

3 None of the terms used to designate the country to which migrants move embrace the full complexity of migrant positions: 'country of settlement' and 'destination' suggest that people remain in the country to which they move, paving the way towards citizenship and/or permanent residence, and 'host' and country of 'reception' suggest the position of a visitor. However, for consistency, in most cases the term country of settlement or destination is used.

4 Likewise, none of the more commonly used terms embrace the complexity of migrants' relationships to the country they leave: 'country of birth' and 'origin' do not take account of circular and oscillating migrations and 'country of migration' suggests a less central relationship than is true for many. However, for consistency, in most cases country of origin and migration is used here.

5 The UK legal system draws on Article 1, 1951 of the Geneva Convention Relating to the Status of Refugees (Article 1, 1951) in defining a refugee as a person who 'owing to a well-founded fear of being persecuted for reasons of race, religion, nationality, membership of a particular social group, or political opinion, is outside the country of his nationality, and is unable to or, owing to such fear, is unwilling to avail himself of the protection of that country'.

6 An asylum seeker is someone who has applied for asylum and is waiting for a decision as to whether they will be recognized as a refugee. In other words, they have applied to the Home Office for refugee status and are waiting to hear the outcome of their application.

7 European Economic Area

8 A pogrom is a violent riot aimed at massacre or persecution of an ethnic or religious group, more commonly used in relation to Jews.

9 Although anti-Semitic attacks have not been a common feature of life in Ireland, at the turn of the previous century many Jews left Limerick following an economic boycott that escalated into assaults, stone throwing and intimidation.

10 www.unesco.org/shs/migration/glossary, accessed 20 March 2016.

11 Traditionally, people travelled from less to more highly developed countries for treatment unavailable or illegal in their own communities. Currently, there is also a trend to travel from more developed to less developed countries with specialized medical services because of costs. Migrants' decisions to seek care 'back home' tend to be informed by failures of and disappointment in the health care system of the country in which one is living to meet the needs of migrants, and a desire to access more familiar health care, obtain the support of non-migrant family and, in the case of a rare genetic disorder, to obtain treatment where the condition is better understood.

12 May be charged and treated as a debt even if one cannot pay.

13 As for antenatal care.

14 www.nhs.uk/conditions/female-genital-mutilation/pages/introduction.aspx, accessed 5 March 2016.

15 Originally coined in relation to Holocaust survivors, survivor guilt refers to situations where a person feels they have done wrong by surviving a traumatic event when others did not.

16 Khat is an amphetamine-like stimulant which can exacerbate pre-existing mental health problems but is also used to escape or cover up mental health problems.

17 Recommendations draw on my own clinical experience, the research and clinical literature and reviews of current policy and services including Jayaweera (2014) and Gulushak, Pace and Weekers (2010).

18 To illustrate that the concept of race is socially constructed but has real effects, this book uses the terms racialization or 'race'.

19 The burkha and niqab are head and face coverings respectively, which are symbols of modesty and religious faith worn by observant Muslim women.

20 The kippah is a head covering worn by observant Jewish men signifying religious faith.

21 Questions drawn from Kleinman, Eisenberg and Good (2006) and clinical experience.

22 Adapted from Burnham (2012).

23 Draws on personal experience of post-conflict work in Kosovo.

24 Drawn from Falicov (2013, p. 23).

25 Anonymized references to the accounts of Mary and subsequently to Charlie, Alex, Ruth and Jack draw on the author's study of the white South African migration to the UK during apartheid (2008). As with clinical examples, details have been changed to preserve anonymity.

26 Endogamy is the practice of marrying within a specific ethnic group, class or social group and rejecting others as being unsuitable for marriage or for other close personal relationships.

27 The South African grandmother mentioned above.
28 As with the Write to Life groups run by the Medical Foundation for the Care of Victims of Torture.
29 Although country of settlement and destination do not take account of circular or oscillating migrations, they are used in preference to recipient, a term that implies one-way transfer of skills and experiences.
30 The more commonly used terms to portray the countries from which health care professionals move, including source, donor, sending, migration and origin, all carry particular meanings. Although source is more usually used for commodities, and country of origin and migration do not take account of temporary and oscillating migrations, source and country of origin are used here as donor and sending implies a more conscious wish to gift or support the decision to leave than is usually the case.
31 European Economic Area
32 This account draws on a study of the white South African migration to the UK during apartheid, in which several participants were health care professionals. As with examples drawn from supervision and clinical work, details have been changed to ensure anonymity.
33 Dash sign signifies a pause.

REFERENCES

Abas, M., Punguing, S., Jirapramukpitak, T. et al. (2009) Rural–urban migration and depression in ageing family members left behind. *British Journal of Psychiatry* 195, 1 54–60.

Abdullahi, A., Copping, J., Kessel, A., Luck, M. and Bonell, C. (2009) Cervical screening: perceptions and barriers to uptake among Somali women in Camden. *Public Health* 123, 10 680–685. doi: 10.1016/j.puhe.2009.09.011.

Abelzova, M., Nasritdinov, E. and Rahimov, R. (2009) *The Impact of Migration on Elderly People: Grandparent-headed households in Kyrgyzstan.* HelpAge International Central Asia/Social Research Center, American University of Central Asia, Bishkek.

Abraham, M., Auspurg, K. and Hinz, T. (2010) Migration decisions within dual-earner partnerships: a test of bargaining theory. *Journal of Marriage and Family* 72, 4 876–892.

Abubakar, I., Stagg, H. R., Cohen, T. et al. (2012) Controversies and unresolved issues in tuberculosis prevention and control: a low-burden-country perspective. *The Journal of Infectious Diseases* 205, 2 S293–300.

Adams, K. M., Gardiner, L. D. and Assefi, N. (2004) Healthcare challenges from the developing world: post-immigration refugee medicine. *BMJ* 328, 1548.

Adelman, S., Blanchard, M., Rait, G. et al. (2011) Prevalence of dementia in African–Caribbean compared with UK-born white older people: two-stage cross-sectional study. *British Journal of Psychiatry* 199 119–125.

Agyemang, C., Addo, J., Bhopal, R. et al. (2009) Cardiovascular disease, diabetes and established risk factors among populations of sub-Saharan African descent in Europe: a literature review. *Global Health* 5, 7.

Ahmadu, F. and Shweder, R. (2009) Disputing the myth of the sexual dysfunction of circumcised women. *Anthropology Today* 25, 6 14–17.

Ahmed, S. (2004) *Cultural Politics of Emotion.* London, Routledge.

Akhtar, S. (1995) A third individuation: immigration, identity and the psychoanalytic process. *Journal of the American Psychoanalytic Association* 43, 4 1051–1084.

Akhtar, S. (2006) Technical challenges faced by the immigrant psychoanalyst. *Psychoanalytic Quarterly* 75, 1 21–43.

Al-Ali, N. (2002) Gender relations, transnational ties and rituals among Bosnian refugees. *Global Networks* 2, 3 249–262.

Alayarian, A. (2015) Trauma, resilience and vulnerability: an intercultural view of working with refugees. *The Psychotherapist* 59 23–25.

Albarran, J. W. and Salmon, D. (2000) Lesbian, gay, and bisexual experiences within critical care nursing, 1988–1998: a survey of the literature. *International Journal of Nursing Studies* 37 445–455.

Alcaraz, C., Chiquiar, D. and Salcedo, A. (2012) Remittances, schooling and child labor in Mexico. *Journal of Development Economics* 97, 1 156–165.

Alexis, O., Vydelingum, V. and Robbins, I. (2007) Engaging with a new reality: experiences of overseas minority ethnic nurses in the NHS. *Journal of Clinical Nursing* 16, 2 2221–2228.

Allan, H. (2010) Mentoring overseas nurses: barriers to effective and non-discriminatory mentoring practices. *Nursing Ethics* 17, 5. doi:10.1177/096933010368747.

All-Party Parliamentary Group on Dementia (2013) Dementia does not discriminate: the experiences of black, Asian and minority ethnic communities. Accessed at: www.scie-socialcareonline.org.uk/dementia-does-not-discriminate-the-experiences-of-black-asian-and-minority-ethnic-communities/r/ on 24 April 2016.

Altschuler, J. (2005) Asymmetrical power relations: domestic labour in global perspective. *European Journal of Women's Studies* 1, 2 227–230.

Altschuler, J. (2008a) Migration, the family and apartheid: journeys across geographical space, the life course and responses to political change. *Open University unpublished thesis.*

Altschuler, J. (2008b) Re-remembering and re-imagining relational boundaries: sibling narratives of migration. *Annual Review of Critical Psychology* 6 22–24.

Altschuler, J. (2011) *Counselling and Psychotherapy in Times of Illness and Death.* Basingstoke, Palgrave.

Alvarez, M. (1999) The experience of migration: a relational approach in therapy. *Journal of Feminist Therapy* 11, 1 1–29.

Ames, F. (2002) *Mothering in an Apartheid Society.* Cape Town, Fine Line Printers.

Amris, K. and Williams, A. C. (2015) Managing chronic pain in survivors of torture. *Pain Management* 5, 1. doi: 10.2217/pmt.14.50.

Amsterdam Declaration Towards Migrant Friendly Hospitals in an Ethno-culturally Diverse Europe (2004) Migrant-friendly hospitals. Accessed at: www.mfh-eu.net on 18 March 2016.

Anderson, B. (1983) *Imagined Communities.* London, Verso.

Anderson, B. (2001) Just another job? Paying for domestic work. *Gender and Development* 9, 1 25–33.

Anderson, J. A., Chai, H., Claman, H. N. et al. (1986) Candidiasis hypersensitivity syndrome: statement approved by the executive committee of the American Academy of Allergy and Immunology. *Journal of Allergy and Clinical Immunology* 78, 2 271–273.

Anderson, W. T. (1997) Dying and death in intergenerational families (in) Hargrave, T. D. and Hanna, M. S. (eds) *The Aging Family: New Visions of Theory, Practice and Reality.* New York, Bruner/Mazel.

Annunziato, R. A., Rakatomihanmina, V. and Rubacka, J. (2007) Examining the effects of maternal chronic illness on child well-being in single parent families. *Journal of Developmental Pediatrics* 28, 5 386–391.

Antinucci, G. (2004) Another language, another place: to hide or to be found? *International Journal of Psychoanalysis* 85, 1157–1173.

Antman, F. M. (2011) The intergenerational effects of paternal migration on schooling and work: what can we learn from children's time allocations? *Journal of Development Economics* 96, 2 200–208.

Antman, F. M. (2012) Elderly care and intrafamily resource allocation when children migrate. *Journal of Human Resources* 47, 2 331–363.

Arad, D. (2004) If your mother was an animal, what animal would she be? Creating play stories in family therapy: the animal attribution story telling technique. *Family Process* 43, 2 249–263.

Ardenne, P. (2004) The couple sharing long-term illness. *Sexual Relationship Therapy* 19, 3 291–308.

Arnold, F. (2007) Detained asylum seekers may be being re-traumatised. *BMJ* 334 916.

Aronsson, G. and Gustafsson, K. (2005) Sickness presenteeism: prevalence, attendance- pressure factors, and an outline of a model for research. *Journal of Occupational & Environmental Medicine* 47, 9 958–66.

Asen, E. and Tomson, P. (1995) *Family Solutions in Family Practice,* Lancaster, Quay Publishing.

Asis, M. M. B. (2006) Living with migration. *Asian Population Studies* 2, 1 45–67.

Aspinall, P. J. (2009) Suicide rates in people of South Asian origin in England and Wales. *British Journal of Psychiatry* 194, 6 566–7.

Aspinall, P. J. (2010) Suicide amongst Britain's immigrant population: data sources, analytical approaches and main findings (in) Sher, L. and Vilens, A. (eds) *Immigration and Mental Health*. New York, Nova Science Publishers.

Aspinall, P. J. and Watters, C. (2010) Refugees and asylum seekers: a review from an equality and human rights perspective. *Research Report 52*. London, Equality and Human Rights Commission.

Astor, A., Akhtar, T., Matallana, M. A. et al. (2006) Physician migration: views from professionals from Columbia, Nigeria, Pakistan and the Philippines. *Social Science and Medicine* 61, 2492–2500.

Atri, J., Falshaw, M., Gregg, R. et al. (1997) Improving uptake of breast screening in multiethnic populations: a randomised controlled trial using practice reception staff to contact non-attenders. *BMJ* 315, 1356–1359.

Austin, Z. (2005) Mentorship and mitigation of culture shock: foreign-trained pharmacists in Canada. *Mentoring and Tutoring: Partnership in Learning* 13, 1 133–149.

Avigad, J. and Rahimi, Z. (2004) Impact of rape on the family (in) Peel, M. (ed.) *Rape as a Method of Torture*. London, Medical Foundation Publication.

Azam, N. (2007) *Evaluation Report of the Meri Yaadain Dementia Project*. Bradford, Girlington Advice and Training Centre.

Balarajan, R. (1996) Ethnicity and health: the challenges ahead. *Ethnicity and Health* 1, 1 3–5.

Balarajan, R. and Soni Raleigh, V. (1993) *Ethnicity and Health. A Guide for the NHS*. London, Department of Health.

Balint, M. (1957) *The Doctor, His Patient and the Illness*. London, Pitman.

Barakat, L. P., Kazak, A. E., Gallagher, P. R. et al. (2000) Posttraumatic stress symptoms and stressful life events predict the long-term adjustment of survivors of childhood cancer and their mothers. *Journal of Clinical Psychology in Medical Settings* 7, 4 189–196.

Barnes, J., Kroll, L., Burke, O., Lee, J., Jones, A. and Stein, A. (2000) Qualitative interview study of communication between parents and children about maternal breast cancer. *British Medical Journal* 321, 7259 479–482.

Barrera, M., Chung, J. Y. Y. and Fleming, C. F. (2004) A group intervention for siblings of pediatric cancer patients. *Journal of Psychosocial Oncology* 22, 2 21–39.

Barron, D. S., Holterman, C. and Shipster, P. (2010) Seen but not heard: ethnic minorities' views of primary healthcare interpreting provision: a focus group study. *Primary Health Care Research and Development* 11/2(132–141) 1463–4236.

Basch, L. G., Glick Schiller, N. and Blanc-Szanton, C. (1994) *Nations Unbound: Transnational Projects, Post-colonial Predicament, and Deterritorialized Nation-states*. Langhorne, Gordon and Breach.

Bhatia, R. and Wallace, P. (2007) Experiences of refugees and asylum seekers in general practice: a qualitative study. *BMC Family Practice* 8, DOI: 10.1186/1471-2296-8-48.

Beautrias, A. L. (2000) Risk factors for suicide and attempted suicide among young people. *Australian and New Zealand Journal of Psychiatry* 34, 3 420–436.

Beck, U. and Beck-Gernsheim, E. (2014) *Love at a Distance – The Chaos of Global Relationships*. Berlin, Suhrkamp Verlag.

Becker, G. (2002) Dying away from home: quandaries of migration for elders in two ethnic groups. *Journal of Gerontology: Social Sciences* 57, 2 S79–95.

Behforous, H. I., Framer, P. and Mukherjee, J. S. (2004) From directly observed therapy to *Accompagnateurs:* enhancing AIDS treatment outcomes in Haiti and in Boston. *Clinical Infections Disease* Supplement 5, 38 S429–236.

Belanger, D. and Linh, T. G. (2011) The impact of transnational migration on gender and marriage in sending communities of Vietnam. *Current Sociology* 59, 1 59–77.

Ben-Ezer, G. (2006) *The Migration Journey: The Ethiopian Jewish Exodus*. New Brunswick, NJ, Routledge.

Bengi-Arslan, L., Verhulst, F. C. and Crijnen, A. (2002) Prevalence and determinants of minor psychiatric disorder in Turkish immigrants living in the Netherlands. *Social Psychiatry and Psychiatric Epidemiology* 37, 3 118–124.

Benjamin, J. (1998) *Shadow of the Other: Intersubjectivity and Gender in Psychoanalysis*. London, Routledge.

Ben-Shlomo, Y., Evans, S., Ibrahim, F. et al. (2008) The risk of prostate cancer amongst Black men in the United Kingdom: The PROCESS Cohort Study. *European Urology* 53, 99–105.

Bennett, S. A. (1993) Inequalities in risk factors and cardiovascular mortality among Australia's immigrants. *Public Health Association of Australia* 17, 3 251–261.

Berlin, A., Gill, P. and Eversley, J. (1997) Refugee doctors in Britain: a wasted resource. *BMJ* 315, 264.

Berry, J. W., Phinney, K. S., Sam, D. L. et al. (2006) Immigrant youth: acculturation, identity, and adaptation. *Applied Psychology* 55, 3 303–352.

Betancourt, J. R., Green, A. R. and Carrillo, J. E. (2000) The challenges of cross-cultural care. *Bioethics Forum* 16, 3, 27–31.

Bhabha, H. (1994) *The Location of Culture*. London, Routledge.

Bhatia, R. and Wallace, P. (2007) Experiences of refugees and asylum seekers in general practice: a qualitative study. *BMC Family Practice* 8, 48. doi: 10.1186/1471-2296-8-48.

Bhopal, K. (1998) South Asian women in East London: motherhood and social support. *Women's Studies International Forum* 21, 5 485–492.

Bhopal, R. S. and Usher, J. (2002) Heterogeneity among Indians, Pakistanis, and Bangladeshis is key to racial inequities. *BMJ* 325, (7369): 903.

Bhugra, D. (2000) Migration and schizophrenia. *Acta Psychiatrica Scandinavica* Supplement s407, 68–73.

Bhugra, D. (2004) Migration and mental health. *Acta Psychiatrica Scandinavica* 109, 4 243–258.

Bhugra, D. and Becker, M. A. (2005) Migration, cultural bereavement and cultural identity. *World Psychiatry* 4, 1 18–24.

Bhui, K., Craig, T., Mohamud, S. et al. (2006) Mental disorders among Somali refugees. *Social Psychiatry and Psychiatric Epidemiology* 41, 5 400–408.

Bienvenue, O. J. and Neufeld, K. J. (2011) Post-traumatic stress disorder in medical settings: focus on the critically ill. *Current Psychiatric Report* 13, 1 3–9.

Bindel J. (2014) *An Unpunished Crime: The Lack of Prosecutions for Female Genital Mutilation in the UK*. London, New Culture Forum.

Blank, T., Asencio, M., Descartes, L. and Griggs, J. (2009) Intersection of older GLBT health issues. *Journal of GLBT Family Studies* 5, 9–34.

Bloch, A. (2011) Intimate circuits: modernity, migration and marriage among post-Soviet women in Turkey. *Global Networks* 11, 4 502–21.

Blumhagen, D. (1980) Hypertension: a folk illness with a medical name. *Culture Medicine and Psychiatry* 4, 197–227.

Bogic, M., Ajdukovic, D., Bremner, S. et al. (2012) Factors associated with mental disorders in long-settled war refugees: refugees from the former Yugoslavia in Germany, Italy and the UK. *British Journal of Psychiatry* 200, 3 216–223.

Bogner, D., Brewin, C. and Herlihy, J. (2010) Refugees' experiences of Home Office interviews: a qualitative study on the disclosure of sensitive personal information. *Journal of Ethnic and Migration Studies* 36, 3 519–535.

Bollini, P., Pampallona, S., Wanner, P. et al. (2009) Pregnancy outcome of migrant women and integration policy: a systematic review of the international literature. *Social Science and Medicine* 68, 3 452–61.

Bonilla-Silva, E. (2006) *Racism Without Racists* (2nd edition). Rowman and Littlefield.

Bonney, N., McCleery, A. and Forster, E. (2002) Migration, marriage and the life course: commitment and residential mobility (in) Boyle, P. J. and Halfacree, K. (eds) *Migration and Gender in the Developed World*. London, Routledge.

Bookman, M. Z. and Bookman, K. R. (2007) *Medical Tourism in Developing Countries*. New York, Palgrave Macmillan.

Bor, R., du Plessis, P. and Russell, M. (2004) The impact of disclosure of HIV on the index patient's self-defined family. *Journal of Family Therapy* 26, 167–192.

Borges, G., Breslau, J., Su, M. et al. (2009) Immigration and suicidal behavior among Mexicans and Mexican Americans. *American Journal of Public Health* 99, 4 728–733.

Bornat, J., Henry, L. and Raghuram, P. (2008) Overseas-trained South Asian doctors and the development of geriatric medicine. *Generations Review* 18, 3.

Bornstein, N. K. (2013) Psychological acculturation: perspectives, principles, processes and prospects (in) Gold, S. J. and Nawyn, S. J. (eds) *The Routledge International Handbook of Migration Studies*. London, Routledge Press.

Boss, P. (2006) *Loss, Trauma and Resilience: Therapeutic Work with Ambiguous Loss*. New York, WWW Norton & Co.

Boss, P. and Carnes, D. (2012) Myth of closure. *Family Process* 51, 456–469.

Bourdieu, P. (1991) *Language and Symbolic Power*. Oxford, Polity Press.

Bowlby, J. (1969/1999) *Attachment: Attachment and Loss* (vol. 1) (2nd ed.) New York, Basic Books.

Boyarin, D. and Boyarin, J. (1993) Diaspora: generation and the ground of Jewish identity. *Critical Inquiry* 19, 4 693–725.

Boyle, P. J., Kulu, H., Cooke, T. et al. (2008) Moving and union dissolution. *Demography* 45, 1 209–222.

Braga, L. L., Mello, F. M. and Fiks, J. F. (2012) Transgenerational transmission of trauma and resilience: a qualitative study with Brazilian offspring of Holocaust survivors. *BMC Psychiatry* 12, 134. doi: 10.1186/1471-244X-12-134.

Bragg, L. (2013) Vulnerable migrant women and charging for maternity care in the UK: advocating change (in) Thomas, F. and Gideon, J. (eds) *Migration, Health and Inequality*. London, Zed Books.

Brah, A. (1996) *Cartographies of Diaspora: Contesting Identities*. London, Routledge.

Braziel, J. E. and Mannur, A. (2003) Nation, migration, globalization: points of contention in diaspora studies (in) Braziel, J. E. and Mannur, A. *Theorizing Diaspora: A Reader*. Oxford, Blackwell Publishing.

British Medical Association (2012, 1 November) *Access to Health Care for Asylum Seekers and Refused Asylum Seekers – Guidance for Doctors*. British Medical Association.

Brody, H. (1999) The biopsychosocial model, patient-centred care, and culturally sensitive practice. *Journal of Family Practice* 48, 8 585–587.

Brom, D. and Kleber, R. (2009) Resilience as the capacity for processing trauma (in) Brom, D., Pat-Horenczyk, R. and Ford, J. D. (eds) *Treating Traumatized Children*. London, Routledge.

Broom, M. E. and Powell Stuart, W. (2006) Interventions with families of an acutely ill child (in) Crane, D. R. and Marshall, E. S. (eds) *Handbook of Families and Health*. London, Sage.

Brown, E. (2013) *Tackling Female Genital Mutilation: Summary of Peer Research*. Options UK, Trust for London, Esmee Fairburn Foundation and Rosa UK Fund for Women and Girls.

Bryant, R., Sutherland, K. and Guthrie, R. M. (2007) Impaired specific autobiographical memory as a risk factor for posttraumatic stress after trauma. *Journal of Abnormal Psychology* 116, 4 837–841.

Brydon, L., Walker, C., Wawrzyniak, A. J. et al. (2009) Dispositional optimism and stress-induced changes in immunity and negative mood. *Brain Behaviour Immunity* 23, 6 810–816.

Buchbinder, A., Casillias, J. and Zelzter, L. (2011) Meeting the psychosocial needs of sibling survivors. *Journal of Pediatric Oncology Nursing* 28, 3 123–136.

Budtz-Lilly, A., Vestergaard, M., Fink, P., Carlsen, A. H. and Rosendal, M. (2015) Patient characteristics and frequency of bodily distress syndrome in primary care: a cross-sectional study. *Journal of the Royal College of General Practitioners* 65, 638, 617.

Burck, C. (2005) *Multilingual living: Explorations of Language and Subjectivity.* Houndmills, Palgrave Macmillan.

Burnett, A. (2002) *Meeting the Health Needs of Refugee and Asylum Seekers in the UK. An Information and Resource Pack for Health Workers.* London, Department of Health.

Burnham, J. (2015, October) *Overcoming Problems – Creating Possibilities Through … Wrestling with Restraints and Embracing Resources in Therapy and Supervision.* Unpublished presentation: Manchester Association of Family Therapy, 23rd October 2015.

Burns, F. M., Imrie, J. Y., Nazroo, J. et al. (2007) Why the(y) wait? Key informant understandings of factors contributing to late presentation and poor utilization of HIV health and social services by African migrants in Britain. *AIDS Care* 19, 102–108.

Burns, F. M., Mercer, C. H., Evans, A. R. et al. (2009) Increased attendances of people of eastern European origin at sexual health services in London. *Sexually Transmitted Infections* 85, 1 75–78.

Bursztein Lipsicas, C. and Makinen, I. H. (2010) Immigration and suicidality in the young. *Canadian Journal of Psychiatry* 55, 5 274–281.

Bursztein Lipsicas, C., Makinen, I. H., Apter, A. et al. (2012) Attempted suicide among immigrants in European countries: an international perspective. *Social Psychiatry and Psychiatric Epidemiology* 47, 1 241–251.

Burton, C., McGorm, K., Weller, D. and Sharpe, M. (2011) Depression and anxiety in patients repeatedly referred to secondary care with medically unexplained symptoms: a case-control study. *Psychological Medicine* 41, 3 555–563.

Bury, M. (1982) Chronic illness as biographical disruption. *Sociology of Health and Illness* 4, 2 167–182.

Butler, J. (2003) *Precarious Life: The Powers of Mourning and Violence,* London, Verso.

Butler, M., Warfa, N., Khatib, Y. et al. (2015) Migration and common mental disorder: an improvement in mental health over time? *International Review of Psychiatry* 27, 1 51–63.

Byng-Hall, J. (1995) *Rewriting Family Scripts.* New York, Guilford Press.

Byrne, A. (2000) Researching one an-other (in) Byrne, A. and Lentin, R. (eds) *(Re)searching Women.* Dublin, Institute of Public Administration.

Cacioppo, J. T., Hughes, M. E., Waite, L. J. et al. (2006) Loneliness as a specific risk factor for depressive symptoms: cross-sectional and longitudinal analyses. *Psychology and Aging* 21, 1 140–151.

Campbell, C. M. and Edwards, R. R. (2012) Ethnic differences in pain and pain management. *Pain Management* 2, 3 219–230.

Candib, L. (2002) Truth telling and advance planning at the end of life: problems with autonomy in a multicultural world. *Families, Systems and Medicine* 20, 213–228.

Cangiano, A., Shutes, I., Spencer, S. and Leeson, G. (2009) *Migrant Care Workers in Aging Societies Research Findings in the United Kingdom*. Compass ESRC Centre on Migration, Policy and Society.

Cangiano, A. and Walsh, K. (2014) Recruitment processes and immigration regulations: the disjointed pathways to employing migrant carers in ageing societies. *Employment and Society* 28, 3 372–389.

Cano, A., Johansen, A. B. and Geisser, M. (2004) Spousal congruence on disability, pain, and spouse responses to pain. *Pain* 109, 3 258–265.

Cantor-Graae, E. and Selten, J. P. (2005) Schizophrenia and migration: a meta analysis and review. *American Journal of Psychiatry* 162, 1 12–24.

Cantrell, M. A. (2011) A narrative review summarizing the state of the evidence on the health-related quality of life among childhood cancer survivors. *Journal of Pediatric Oncology Nursing* 28, 2 75–82.

Carballo, M. and Mboup, M. (2005) *International Migration and Health*. A paper prepared for the Policy Analysis and Research Programme of the Global Commission on International Migration.

Carballo, M. and Nerukar, A. (2001) Migration, refugees, and health risks. *Emerging Infectious Disease* 7, 3 556–560.

Carling, J. (2008) The human dynamics of transnationalism. *Ethnic and Racial Studies* 31, 4 1452–1477.

Carter, R. T. (2007) Racism and psychological and emotional injury: recognizing and assessing race-based traumatic stress. *Counseling Psychologist* 35, 13–105. doi: 10.1177/0011000006292033.

Carter, B. and McGoldrick, M. (1999) *The Expanded Family Lifecycle. Individual Family and Social Perspectives* (Third edition). Boston, Allyn & Bacon.

Castro, A. and Farmer, P. (2005) Understanding and addressing AIDS-related stigma: from anthropological theory to clinical practice in Haiti. *American Journal of Public Health* 95, 1 53–59.

Ceuterick, M., Vandebroek, I. and Pieroni, A. (2011) Resilience of Andean urban ethnobotanies: a comparison of medicinal plant use among Bolivian and Peruvian migrants in the United Kingdom and in their countries of origin. *Journal of Ethnopharmacology* 136, 1 27–54.

Challiol, H. and Mignonac, K. (2005) Relocation decision-making and couple relationships: a quantitative and qualitative study of dual earner couples. *Journal of Organic Behaviour* 26 247–274.

Chamberlain, M. (2003) Rethinking Caribbean families: extending the links. *Community, Work & Family* 6, 1 63–76.

Chamberlain, M. (2006) *Family Love in the Diaspora: Migration and the Anglo-Caribbean Experience*. Edison, NJ, Transaction Publishers.

Chamberlain, M. and Leydesdorff, S. (2004) Transnational families: memories and narratives. *Global Networks* 4, 3 227–241.

Chao, R. and Tseng, V. (2002) Parenting of Asians (in) Bornstein, M. H. (ed.) *Handbook of Parenting: Volume 4 Social Conditions and Applied Parenting*. Lawrence Erlbaum Associates.

Chase, E. (2013) Unaccompanied young asylum seekers in the UK: mental health and rights (in) Thomas, F. and Gideon, J. (eds) *Migration, Health and Inequality*. London, Zed Books.

Cheng, J. and Sun, Y. H. (2014) Depression and anxiety among left-behind children in China: a systematic review. *Child: Care, Health and Development.* doi:10.1111/cch.1221.

Cheung, M. (2008) Resilience of older immigrant couples long-term marital satisfaction as a protective factor. *Journal of Couple & Relationship Therapy: Innovations in Clinical and Educational Interventions* 7, 1 19–38.

Chochinov, H. M., Tataryn, D., Clinch, J. J. et al. (1999) Will to live in the terminally ill. *Lancet* 354, 816–819.

Chow, E. O. W. (2015) Narrative therapy an evaluated intervention to improve stroke survivors' social and emotional adaptation. *Clinical Rehabilitation* 9, 315–326.

Clark, C. J., Everson-Rose, S. A., Suglia, S. F. et al. (2010) Association between exposure to political violence and intimate-partner violence in the occupied Palestinian territory: a cross-sectional study. *Lancet* 375, 310–316.

Clarke, M., Finlay, I. and Campbell, I. (1991) Cultural boundaries in care. *Palliative Medicine* 5, 63–5.

Clifford, J. (1997) *Routes: Travel and Translation in the Late Twentieth Century.* Cambridge, MA, Harvard University Press.

Cline, T., Crafter, S. and Prokopiou, E. (2014) Child language brokering in schools: a discussion of selected findings from a survey of teachers and ex-students. *Educational and Child Psychology* 31, 2 34–45.

Cochrane, R. and Bal, S. S. (1987) Migration and schizophrenia: an examination of five hypotheses. *Social Psychiatry* 22, 180–191.

Cohen, S., Moran-Ellis, J. and Smaje, C. (1999) Children as informal interpreters in GP consultations: pragmatics and ideology. *Sociology of Health and Illness* 2, 2 163–186.

Cohn, S., Alenya, J., Murray, K. et al. (2006) Experiences and expectations of refugee doctors: qualitative study. *British Journal of Psychiatry* 189, 74–78.

Coles, R. L. (2001) Elderly narrative reflections on the contradictions in Turkish village family life after migration of adult children. *Journal of Aging Studies* 15, 383–406.

Combrinck-Graham, L. A. (1985) A developmental model for family systems. *Family Process* 24, 3 139–150.

Connelly, N. A., Guy, F. and Rudiger, N. A. (2006) Older refugees in the UK: a literature review. *A Refugee Council Working Paper for the Older Refugees Programme.* Accessed at: www.refugeecouncil.org.uk/assets/0001/7053/Older_refugees_workingpaper.pdf on 18 March 2016.

Connolly, N. L., Forsythe, L. and Njike, G. (2015) *Older Refugees in the UK: A Literature Review A Refugee Council Working Paper for the Older Refugees Programme.* Refugee Council, Age Concern and Association of Greater London Women.

Cooper, B. (2005) Schizophrenia, social class and immigrant status: the epidemiological evidence. *Epidemiologia e Psichiatria Sociale* 14, 3 137–144.

Costa, B. (2014) You can call me Betty. *Healthcare Counselling and Psychotherapy Journal* 14, 4 20–25.

Crafter, S., O'Dell, L., de Abreu, G. and Cline, T. (2009) Young peoples' representations of 'atypical' work in English society. *Children and Society* 23, 176–188.

Craig, T. (2007) Mental distress and psychological interventions in refugee populations (in) Bhugra, D., Craig, T. and Bhui, K. (eds) *Mental Health of Refugees and Asylum Seekers*. Oxford, Oxford University Press.

Creed, F., Henningsen, P. and Funk, P. (2011) *Medically Unexplained Symptoms, Somatization and Bodily Distress: Developing Better Clinical Services*. Cambridge, Cambridge University Press.

Cremeans-Smith, J. K., Parris Stephens, M. A., Franks, M. M. et al. (2003) Spouses' and physicians' perceptions of pain severity in older women with osteoarthritis: dyadic agreement and patients' well-being. *Pain* 106, 27–34.

Crisp, N. and Chen, L. (2014) Global supply of health professionals. *New England Journal of Medicine* 370, 950–957.

Crooks, V. A., Kingsbury, P., Snyder, J. and Johnston, R. (2010) What is known about the patient's experience of medical tourism? A scoping review. *BMC Health Services Research* 10, 1 266.

Cross, T. L. (1988) *Cultural Competence Continuum Focal Point Bulletin*. Portland State University, The Research and Training Centre on Family Support and Children's Mental Health.

Curtis, E. A. and Dixon, M. S. (2005) Family therapy and systemic practice with older people: where are we now? *Journal of Family Therapy* 27, 43–64.

Cuthbertson, S., Goyder, E. and Poole, J. (2009) Inequalities in breast cancer at diagnosis in the Trent region and implications for the breast screening service. *Journal of Public Health* 31, 3 398–405.

Czarnoka, J. and Slade, P. (2000) Prevalence and predictors of post-traumatic stress symptoms following childbirth. *J Psychology of Clinical Psychology* 39, 35–51.

Dale, A. (2008) *Migration, Marriage and Employment Amongst Indian, Pakistani and Bangladeshi Residents in the UK*. University of Manchester, CCSR Working Paper.

Danese, A., Moffitt, T. E., Harrington, H. et al. (2009) Adverse childhood experiences and adult risk factors for age-related disease. *Archives of Pediatrics and Adolescent Medicine* 163, 12 1135–1143.

Daniels, G. (2012) With an exile's eye: developing positions of cultural reflexivity (with a bit of help from feminism) (in) Krause, I.-B. (ed.) *Culture and Reflexivity in Systemic Psychotherapy*. London, Karnac Books.

Darling, N. (1999) *Parenting Style and its Correlates*. ERIC Clearinghouse on Elementary and Early Childhood Education: ED427896, 1999-03-00.

Davey, M. P., Askew, J. and Godette, K. (2003) Parent and adolescent responses to non-terminal parental cancer. *Families, Systems and Health* 21, 3 245–258.

Davies, A. A., Basten, A. and Frattini, C. (2009) *Migration: A Social Determinant of the Health of Migrants*. Background paper developed within the framework of the IOM project 'Assisting Migrants and Communities'. Geneva, International Organization for Migration.

Davies, M. M. and Bath, P. A. (2001) The maternity information concerns of Somali women in the United Kingdom. *Journal of Advanced Nursing* 36, 2 237–245.

Davies, S. and Nolan, M. (2003) 'Making the best of things': relatives' experience of decisions about care-home entry. *Ageing and Society* 23, 4 429–450.

Deboosere, P. and Gadeyne, S. (2005) Adult migrant mortality advantage in Belgium: evidence using census and register data. *Population* 60, 200. doi: 10.3917/popu.505.0765.

de Graaf, F. M. and Francke, A. L. (2009) Barriers to home care for terminally Ill Turkish and Moroccan Migrants. *BioMed Central Palliative Care* 8, 3.

Denborough, D. (2008) *Collective Narrative Practice: Responding to Individuals, Groups and Communities Who Have Experienced Trauma*. Adelaide, Dulwich Centre Publications.

Department for Education and Skills (DfES) (2004) Aiming high: guidance on supporting the education of refugee and asylum seeking children. DfES/0287/2004.

Department of Health (2015) Guidance on implementing the overseas visitor hospital changing regulations. Accessed at: www.gov.uk/government/uploads/system/uploads/attachment_data/file/496951/Overseas_visitor_hospital_charging_accs.pdf on 20 March 2016.

Derluyn, I. and Brockaet, E. (2008) Unaccompanied refugee children and adolescents: the glaring contrast between a legal and psychological perspective. *International Journal of Law and Psychiatry* 31, 319–330.

Derrida, J. (1988) The original discussion of '*Differance*' (in) Wood, D. and Bernasconi, R. (eds) *Derrida and Difference*. Evanstone, Northwestern University Press.

Derrida, J. (2000) Foreigner question (in) Dufourmantelle, A. and Derrida, J. (eds) *Of Hospitality*. Stanford, Stanford University Press.

Diallo, K. (2004) Data on the migration of health-care workers: sources, uses, and challenges. *Bulletin World Health Organization* 82, 8 601–607.

Diareme, D., Tsiantis, J., Romer, G. et al. (2007) Mental health support for children of parents with somatic illness: a review of the theory and intervention concepts. *Families, Systems and Health* 25, 1 98–118.

Dixon-Woods, M., Cavers, D., Agarwal, S. et al. (2006) Conducting a critical interpretive review of the literature on access to health care by vulnerable groups. *BMC Medical Research Methodology* 6, 35 doi:10.1186/1471-2288-6-35.

Doerfler, L. A., Paraskos, A. and Piniarski, L. (2005) Relationship of quality of life and perceived control with posttraumatic stress disorder symptoms three to six months after myocardial infection. *Journal of Cardiopulmonary Rehabilitation* 25, 166–172.

Doka, K. J. (1999) Disenfranchised Grief. *Bereavement Care* 18, 3 37–39.

Donnelly, L. and Knapton, S. Doctors from India more likely to be struck off. *Telegraph*. Accessed at: www.telegraph.co.uk/news/health/news/10809221/Doctors-from-India-more-likely-to-be-struck-off.html on 26 March 2016.

Dorner, L. M., Orellana, M. F. and Jiménez, R. (2008) 'It's one of those things that you do to help the family': language brokering and the development of immigrant adolescents. *Journal of Adolescent Research* 23, 5 515–543.

Doron, A. and Broom, A. (2011) *Health, Culture and Religion in South Asia: Critical Perspectives*. London, Routledge.

Douthwaite, M. and Ward, P. (2005) Increasing contraceptive use in rural Pakistan: an evaluation of the Lady Health Worker Programme. *Health Policy Plan* 20, 2 117–123.

Doyle, L. and McCorriston, M. (2008) Beyond the school gates: supporting refugee and asylum seeking children in secondary school. London, Refugee Council.

Dreyer, G., Hull, S., Aitken, Z. et al. (2009) The effect of ethnicity on the prevalence of diabetes and associated chronic kidney disease. *Quarterly Journal of Medicine* 102, 261–269.

Duarte, S. (2008) Small arms and their effect on children in armed conflict *Conflicts of Interest Children in Zones of Instability*. Panel Discussion, United Nations.

Du Bois, W. E. (1898) The study of the Negro problems. *The Annals of the American Academy of Political and Social Science*, 11 1–23.

Duldulao, A. A., Takeuchi, D. T. and Hong, S. (2009) Correlates of suicidal behavior among Asian Americans. *Archives of Suicide Research* 13, 277–290.

Dumont, J. C. and Zurn, P. (2007) Immigrant health workers in OECD countries in the broader context of highly skilled migration. *International Migration Outlook*, Sopemi 2007.

Dumper, H. (2002) *Refugee Needs and Gaps in Services – Portsmouth*. London, Refugee Action.

Dumper, H. (2005) *Refugee Council: Making Women Visible – Strategies for a More Woman-Centred Asylum and Refugee Support*. London, Refugee Council.

Dustman, C., Frattini, T. and Theodoropoulos, N. (2010) Ethnicity and second generation immigrants (in) Gregg, P. and Wadsworth, J. (eds) *The Labour Market in Winter: The State of Working Britain*. London, The Work Foundation.

Edwards, R., Hadfield, J., Lucey, H. and Mauthner, M. (2006) *Sibling Identity and Relationships: Sisters and Brothers*. London, Routledge.

Ehlers, A., Hackman, A. and Michael, T. (2004) Intrusive reexperiencing in post-traumatic stress disorder: phenomenology, theory, and therapy. *Memory* 12, 4 403–415.

Ehrenreich, B. and Hochschild, A. R. (2003) Introduction *Global Woman: Nannies, Maids and Sex Workers in the New Economy*. New York, Metropolitan Books.

Ekblad, S., Marttila, A. and Emilsson, M. (2000) Cultural challenges in end-of-life care: reflections from focus groups' interviews with hospice staff in Stockholm. *Journal of Advanced Nursing* 31, 1 623–630.

Elander, J., Beach, M. C. and Haywood, C. (2011) Respect, trust, and the management of sickle cell disease pain in hospital: comparative analysis of concern-raising behaviors, preliminary model, and agenda for international collaborative research to inform practice. *Ethnicity and Health* 16, 4–5 405–421.

Elkeles, T. and Seifert, W. (1996) Immigrants and health: unemployment and health-risks of labour migrants in the Federal Republic of Germany, 1984–1992. *Social Science and Medicine* 43, 7 1035–1047.

Englund, H. (1998) Death, trauma and ritual: Mozambican refugees in Malawi. *Social Science and Medicine* 46, 9 1165–1174.

Escandell, X. and Tapias, M. (2010) Transnational lives, travelling emotions and idioms of distress among Bolivian migrants in Spain. *Journal of Ethnic and Migration Studies* 120, 809–816.

Escobar, J., Hoyos, N. C. and Gara, M. A. (2000) Immigration and mental health: Mexican Americans in the United States. *Harvard Review of Psychiatry* 8, 2 64–72.

Esmail, A. (2007) Asian doctors in the NHS: service and betrayal. *British Journal of General Practice* 7, 543 827–834.

Esmail, A. and Roberts, C. (2013) Academic performance of ethnic minority candidates and discrimination in the MRCGP examinations between 2010 and 2012: analysis of data. *BMJ* 347. doi: http://dx.doi.org/10.1136/bmj.f5662.

ESRC (2012) *How has Ethnic Diversity Grown?* 1991-2001-2011 ESRC Centre on Dynamics of Ethnicity. Accessed at: www.ethnicity.ac.uk/medialibrary/briefings/dynamicsofdiversity/how-has-ethnic-diversity-grown-1991-2001-2011.pdf on 4 March 2015.

Fadiman, A. (1997) *The Spirit Catches You and You Fall Down.* New York, Farrar, Straus and Giroux.

Fagundes, C. P., Berg, C. A. and Wiebe, D. J. (2012) Intrusion, avoidance, and daily negative affect among couples coping with prostate cancer: a dyadic investigation. *Journal of Family Psychology* 26, 246–253.

Falicov, C. (2007) Working with transnational immigrants: expanding meanings of family, community and culture. *Family Process* 46, 156–171.

Falicov, C. J. (2013) *Latino Families in Therapy* (2nd edition). New York, Guilford Press.

Fang, M. L., Sixsmith, J., Lawthom, R. et al. (2015) Experiencing 'pathologized presence and normalized absence'; understanding health related experiences and access to health care among Iraqi and Somali asylum seekers, refugees and persons without legal status. *BMC Public Health* 15, 1 1–12.

Fazel, M., Reed, R. V., Panter-Brick, C. and Stein, A. (2011) Mental health of displaced and refugee children resettled in high-income countries: risk and protective factors. *The Lancet* 379, 9812 266–282.

Fearon, P., Kirkbride, J. B., Morgan, C. et al. (2006) Incidence of schizophrenia and other psychoses in ethnic minority groups: results from the MRC AESOP study. *Psychological Medicine* 36, 1541–1550.

Fedorocicz, Z. and Walczyk, T. D. (2006) A trisomial concept of sociocultural and religious factors in health care decision-making and service provision in the Muslim world (in) Papadopoulos, I. (ed.) *Transcultural Health and Social Care: Developing Culturally Competent Practitioners.* Oxford, Elsevier.

Feldman, R. (2006) Primary health care for refugees and asylum seekers: a review of the literature and framework for services. *Public Health* 120, 809–816.

Feldman, R (2013) When maternity doesnt matter: dispersing pregnant women seeking asylum refugeecouncil.org.uk/maternity on 12th May, 2016

Fennelly, K. (2005) The healthy migrant effect. *Healthy Generations* 5, 3 1–3.

Figueiras, M. J. and Weinman, J. (2003) Do similar patient and spouse perceptions of myocardial infarction predict recovery? *Psychology and Health* 18, 2 201–216.

Fisher, L. (2006) Research on the family and chronic disease among adults: major trends and directions. *Family Systems and Health* 24, 4 373–380.

Fisher, S. B. (2014) *Neurofeedback in the Treatment of Developmental Trauma.* New York, WW Norton.

Fitzpatrick, R., Hinton, J., Newman, S. et al. (1984) *The Experience of Illness.* London, Tavistock.

Flores, G. (2000) Culture and the patient-physician relationship: achieving cultural competency in health care. *Journal of Pediatrics* 136, 1 14–23.

Flores, G. (2005) The impact of medical interpreter services on the quality of health care: a systematic review. *Medical Care Research and Review* 62, 255–99.

Fobair, P., O'Hanlon, K., Koopmans, C. et al. (2001) Comparison of lesbian and heterosexual women's response to newly diagnosed breast cancer. *Psycho-Oncology* 10 40–51.

Forray, A., Mayes, L. C., Magriples, U. and Epperson, C. N. (2014) Prevalence of post-traumatic stress disorder in pregnant women with prior pregnancy complications. *Journal of Maternal Fetal Neonatal Medicine* 22, 6 522–527.

Fortier, A. M. (2000) *Migrant Belongings: Memory, Space, Identity*. Oxford, Berg.

Fortuna, L. R., Perez, D. J., Canino, G. et al. (2007) Prevalence and correlates of lifetime suicidal ideation and suicide attempts among Latino subgroups in the United States. *Journal of Clinical Psychiatry* 68, 572–581.

Foster, T. L., Gilmer, M. J. and Venatta, K. (2012) Changes in siblings after the death of a child from cancer. *Cancer Nursing* 35, 5 347–354.

Fox, G. and Ifould, R. (2015, 10 October) NHS workers from abroad: I don't think people appreciate what they have. *Guardian Weekend*.

Frank, A. (1995) *The Wounded Story Teller: Body, Illness and Ethics*. Chicago, The University of Chicago Press.

Franklin, P., Crombie, A. and Boudville, N. (2003) Live related renal transplantation: psychological, social, and cultural issues. *Transplantation* 76, 8 1247–1252.

Fredman, G., Christie, D. and Bear, N. (2007) Reflecting teams with children: the bear necessities *Clinical Child Psychology and Psychiatry* 12, 2 211–222.

Freud, S. (1912) The dynamics of the transference. *Standard Edition* 12, 99–108.

Freud, S. (1917) *Mourning and Melancholia XVII* (2nd edition, 1955). London, Hogarth Press.

Freud, S. (1919/2003) *The Uncanny*, trans McClintock, D. London, Penguin.

Friedlmeier, W., Corapci, F. and Cole, P. M. (2011) Socialization of emotions in cross-cultural perspective. *Social and Personality Psychology Compass* 5, 410–427.

Gabriels, R. L., Wamboldt, D. R., McCormick et al. (2000) Children's illness drawing and asthma symptom awareness. *Journal of Asthma* 3, 7 565–574.

Gagnon, M. (2010) Managing the other within the self: bodily experiences of HIV/AIDS (in) Rudge, T. and Holmes, D. (eds) *Abjectly Boundless: Boundaries, Bodies and Health Work*. Farnham, Surrey, Ashgate Publication.

Galanti, G.-A. (2015) *Caring for Patients From Different Cultures* (5th edition). Philadelphia, University of Pennsylvania Press.

Gao, Y., Li, L. P., Kim, J. H. et al. (2010) The impact of parental migration on health status and health behaviours among left behind adolescent school children in China. *BMC Public Health* 10, 56.

Gardner, K. and Grillo, R. (2002) Transnational households and ritual: an overview. *Global Networks* 2, 3 179–190.

Gaudion, A., McLeish, J. and Homeyard, C. (2006) Access to maternity care for 'failed' asylum seekers. *International Journal of Migration, Health and Social Care* 2, 2. doi: 10.1108/17479894200600012.

Geddes, A. (2003) *The Politics of Migration and Immigration in Europe*. London, Sage.

General Medical Council (GMC) (2013) *Good Medical Practice*. Accessed at: www.gmc-uk.org/guidance on 26 March 2016.

General Medical Council (GMC) (2015) *Interactive reports to investigate factors that affect progression of doctors in training* Accessed at: www.gmc-uk.org/Briefing_note__Exams_and_recruitment_outcome_reports.pdf_60060997.pdf_60086828.pdf on 26 March 2016.

Gerhardt, C., Vernatta, K., McKellop, M. et al. (2003) Comparing family functioning, parental distress and the role of social support of care givers with and without a child with juvenile rheumatoid arthritis *Journal of Pediatric Psychology* 28 5–15.

Gerrish, K. and Griffith, V. (2004) Integration of overseas registered nurses: evaluation of an adaptation program. *Journal of Advanced Nursing* 45, 6 579–587.

Gibson, L., Ow, D., Sliwinski, A., Izquierdo, L., Bolton, D. M., Lawrentschuk, N. (2014) An evaluation of internet-based language translation software as a health communication tool with non-English speaking patients. *BJU International* 113, 80 1464–4096.

Giddens, A. (1991) *Modernity and Self-Identity. Self and Society in the Late Modern Age*. Cambridge, Polity.

Gideon, J. (2013) Access versus entitlements: the health seeking for Latin American migrants in London (in) Thomas, F. and Gideon, J. (eds) *Migration, Health and Inequality*. London, Zed Books.

Gilbert, R. L., Antoine, D., French, C. et al. (2009) The impact of immigration on tuberculosis rates in the United Kingdom compared with other European countries. *International Journal of Tuberculosis and Lung Disease* 13, 645–651.

Giles, J. and Mu, R. (2005) Elder parent health and the migration decision of adult children: evidence from rural China. *IZA DP* 2333, 1–56.

Gilligan, C. and Brown, L. M. (1993) Meeting at the crossroads: women's psychology and girls' development. *Feminism Psychology* 3, 1 11–35.

Golding, J. M. and Burnam, M. A. (1990) Immigration, stress, and depressive symptoms in a Mexican-Americans community. *Journal of Nervous Mental Disorder* 178, 161–171.

Good, B. (1977) The heart of what's the matter – the semantics of illness in Iran. *Culture, Medicine and Psychiatry* 1, 25–58.

Graham, E., Jordan, L. P. and Yeoh, B. S. A. (2014) Parental migration and the mental health of those who stay behind to care for children in South-East Asia. *Social Science & Medicine* doi:10.1016/j.socscimed, 2014.10.060.

Granger, E. and Baker, M. (2003) The role and experience of interpreters (in) Tribe, R. and Raval, H. (eds) *Working with Interpreters in Mental Health*. London, Bruner-Routledge.

Graves, J. (2002) *The Emperor's New Clothes: Biological Theories of Race at the Millennium*. Fayetteville, University of Arkansas Press.

Gray, W. N., Szulczewski, L. Z., Regan, S. M. P. et al. (2014) Cultural influences in pediatric cancer: from diagnosis to cure/end of life. *Journal of Pediatric Oncology Nursing* 31, 5 252–271.

Green, R. J. and Mitchell, V. (2008) Gay and lesbian couples in therapy: homophobia, relational ambiguity and social support (in) Gurman, A. S. (ed.) *Clinical Handbook of Couple Therapy* (4th edition). New York, Guilford Press.

Greenfield, P. M., Quiroz, B. and Raeff, C. (2000) Cross-cultural conflict and harmony in the social construction of the child (in) Harkness, S., Raeff, C. and Super, C. M. (eds) *Variability in the Social Construction of the Child New Directions in Child Development*. San Francisco, Jossey-Bass.

Greenhalgh, T., Robb, N. and Scambler, G. (2006) Communicative and strategic action in interpreted consultations in primary health care: a Habermasian perspective. *Social Science and Medicine* 63, 1170–1187.

Greer, S. (2000) Fighting spirit in patients with cancer. *The Lancet* 335, 9206 847–848.

Grillo, R. (2011) Marriages, arranged and forced: the UK debate (in) Kofman, E., Kohli, M., Kraler, A. et al. (eds) *Gender, Generations and the Family in International Migration*. Amsterdam, Amsterdam University Press.

Grinberg, L. and Grinberg, R. (1984) *Psychoanalytic Perspectives on Migration and Exile*. London, Yale University Press.

Grove-White, R. (2014, 27 May) Immigration Act 2014: what next for migrants' access to NHS care? *Migrant Rights Network*.

Gunaratnam, Y. (2013) *Death and the Migrant: Bodies, Borders and Care*. London, Bloomsbury.

Gunaratnam, Y. and Lewis, G. (2001) Racialising emotional labour and emotionalising racialized labour: anger, fear and shame in social welfare. *Journal of Social Work Practice* 15, 2 131–148.

Guregard, S. and Seikkula, J. (2014) Establishing therapeutic dialogue with refugee families. *Contemporary Family Therapy* 36, 51–57.

Guru, R., Sadiqqe, M. A., Ahmed, Z. and Khan, A. A. (2012) Effects of culture shock on foreign health care professionals. *Journal of Environmental Science* 1, 1 53–62.

Guruge, S., Shirpak, K. R., Hyman, I. et al. (2010) A meta-synthesis of post-migration changes in marital relationships in Canada. *Canadian Journal of Public Health* 101, 4 327–331.

Gushulak, B., Pace, P. and Weekers, J. (2010) Migration and health of migrants (in) Koller, T. (ed.) *Poverty and Social Exclusion in the WHO European Region: Health Systems Respond*. Copenhagen, WHO Regional Office for Europe.

Haagsman, K. and Mazzucato, V. (2014) The quality of parent–child relationships in transnational families: Angolan and Nigerian migrant parents in the Netherlands. *Journal of Ethnic and Migration Studies* 40, 11 1677–1696.

Habermas, J. (1989) *The Theory of Communicative Action Vol 2: The Critique of Functionalist Reason*. London, Polity Press.

Hadziabdic, E., Heikkilä, K., Albin, B. et al. (2011) Problems and consequences in the use of professional interpreters: qualitative analysis of incidents from primary healthcare. *Nursing Inquiry* 1320–7881.

Hagedoorn, M., Sanderman, R., Bolks, T. N. et al. (2008) Distress in couples coping with cancer: a meta-analysis and critical review of role and gender effects. *Psychological Bulletin* 134, 1 1–30.

Hagopian, A., Ofosu, A., Fatusi, A. et al. (2005) The flight of physicians from West Africa: views of African physicians and implications for policy. *Social Science and Medicine* 61, 8 1750–1760.

Haines, A., Sanders, D., Lehmann, U. et al. (2007) Achieving child survival goals: potential contribution of community health workers. *Lancet* 369, 9579 2121–2131.

Hakesley-Brown, R. (2006) *A Guide for Refugee Nurses and Midwives*. London, Employability Forum Praxis.

Halford, W. K., Scott, J. L. and Smythe, J. (2000) Couples and coping with cancer: helping each other through the night (in) Schmaling, K. G. and Sher, T. J. G. (eds) *The Psychology of Couples and Illness: Theory, Research and Practice*. Washington, DC, American Psychological Association.

Hall, S. (1993) Culture, community, nation. *Cultural Studies* 7, 3 349–363.

Hamilton, J. G., Lobel, M. and Moyer, A. (2009) Emotional distress following genetic testing for hereditary breast and ovarian cancer: a meta-analytic review. *Health Psychology* 28, 4 510–518.

Hamilton, R. and Moore, D. (2006) *Educational Interventions for Refugee Children: Theoretical Perspectives and Implementing Best Practice*. Abingdon, Routledge.

Hammerton, J. (2004) The quest for family and the mobility of modernity in narratives of postwar British emigration. *Global Networks* 4, 3, 271–284.

Handlin, O. (1973) *The Uprooted: The Epic Story of the Great Migrations that made the American People*. Boston, Little, Brown & Company.

Haour-Knipe, M. (2013) Context and perspectives: who migrates and what are the risks? (in) Thomas, F. and Gideon, J. (eds) *Migration, Health and Inequality*. London, Zed Books.

Hard, D. L., Myers, J. R. and Gerberich, S. G. (2002) Traumatic injuries in agriculture. *Journal of Agricultural Safety and Health* 8, 1 51–65.

Harding, S. and Rosato, M. (1999) Cancer incidence among first generation Scottish, Irish, West Indian and South Asian migrants living in England and Wales. *Ethnicity and Health* 4, 1 83–92.

Harding, S., Rosato, M. and Teyhan, A. (2009) Trends in cancer mortality among migrants in England and Wales, 1979–2003. *European Journal of Cancer* 45, 12 2168–2179.

Hargreaves, S. and Friedland, J. S. (2013) Impact on and use of health services by new migrants in Europe (in) Thomas, F. and Gideon, J. (eds) *Migration, Health and Inequality*. London, Zed Books.

Hargreaves S., Holmes, A. H., Saxena, S. et al. (2008) Charging systems for migrants in primary care: the experiences of family doctors in a high-migrant area of London. *Journal of Travel Medicine* 15, 1 13–18.

Harris, D. (2009) The paradox of expressing *speechless terror*: ritual liminality in the creative arts therapies' treatment of posttraumatic distress. *The Arts in Psychotherapy* 36, 2 96–101.

Harris Cheng, M. (2009) The Philippines' health worker exodus. *The Lancet* 373, 9658 111–112.

Hatzidimitriadou, E. and Cahir, C. S. (2013) Post-migration wellbeing, community activism and empowerment: the case of Turkish-speaking women in London (in) Thomas, F. and Gideon, J. (eds) *Migration, Health and Inequality*. London, Zed Books.

Hawkins, O. (2015) *Migration Statistics* House of Commons Briefing Paper SN06077 3 December, 2015.

Hawkley, L. C., Thisted, R. A., Masi, C. M. and Cacioppo, J. T. (2010) Loneliness predicts increased blood pressure: 5-year cross-lagged analyses in middle-aged and older adults. *Psychology and Aging* 25, 1.

Health Protection Services (2011) *Migrant Health: Infectious diseases in non-UK born populations in the United Kingdom: An update to the baseline report*. London, HPA.

Health and Social Care Information Centre (HSCIC) (2016) *NHS Workforce Statistics – November 2015, Provisional statistics* 23 February 2016. Accessed at: www.hscic.gov.uk/searchcatalogue?productid=20107&returnid=1907 on 26 March 2016.

Heeren, M., Mueller, J., Ehlert, U. et al. (2012) Mental health of asylum seekers: a cross-sectional study of psychiatric disorders. *BMC Psychiatry* 12, 114 doi:10.1185/1471-244X-12-114.

Helgeson, V. S., Cohen, S. and Fritz, H. (1998) Social ties and cancer (in) Holland, J. C. and Breitbart, W. (eds) *Psycho-Oncology*. New York, Oxford University Press.

Helman, C. (1981) Disease versus illness in general practice *Journal of the Royal College of General Practitioners* 31 548–552.

Helman, C. (1985) Communication in primary care: the role of patient and practitioner–explanatory models. *Social Science and Medicine* 20, 9 923–931.

Helman, C. (2007) *Culture, Health and Illness* (5th edition). New York, Hodder Arnold Publication.

Helps, S. and Shepherd, N. (2014) Developing ways of working with parents and their infants to improve the core deficits of autism. *The Social World Around the Baby* 2, 3 21–25.

Henry, L. (2006) Institutional disadvantage: old Ghanaian nurses and midwives reflections on career progression and stagnation in the NHS. *Journal of Clinical Nursing Special Issue* 16, 12 2196–2203.

Henwood, A. and Ellis, M. (2015) Giving a voice to people with dementia. *The Psychologist* 28, 976–979.

Herbert, E. and Carpenter, B. (2007) Fathers – the secondary partners: professional perceptions and a father's recollections. *Children and Society* 8, 1 31–41.

Herman, J. L. (1997) *Trauma and recovery: the aftermath of violence from domestic abuse to political terror*. New York, Basic Books.

Hernandez, D. J., Denton, N. A. and Macartney, S. E. (2007) Family circumstances of children in immigrant families (in) Landsford, J. E., Deater-Deckard, K. and Bornstein, M. H. (eds) *Immigrant Families in Contemporary Society*. New York, Guilford Press.

Hernandez, M. and McGoldrick, M. (1999) Migration and the life cycle (in) Carter, B. and McGoldrick, M. (eds) *The Changing Family Life Cycle*. Boston, Allyn and Baker.

Hickling, F. W. (2005) The epidemiology of schizophrenia and other common mental health disorders in the English-speaking Caribbean. *Pan American Journal of Public Health* 18, 4–5 256–262.

Hicks, M. and Bhugra, D. (2003) Perceived causes of suicide attempts by UK South Asian women. *American Journal of Orthopsychiatry* 73, 4 455–462.

Higginbottom, G. M. A., Richter, M. S., Mogale, R. S. et al. (2011) Identification of nursing assessment models/tools validated in clinical practice for use with diverse ethno-cultural groups: an integrative review of the literature. *BMC Nursing* 201110, 16 doi: 10.1186/1472-6955-10-16.

Hirsch, M. (1999) Projected memory: holocaust photographs in personal and public fantasy (in) Bal, M., Crewe, J. and Spitzer, L. (eds) *Acts of Memory: Cultural Recall in the Present.* Hanover, University Press of New England.

Hirsch, J. S. (2003) *A Courtship after Marriage: Sexuality and Love in Mexican Transnational Families.* Berkeley, University of California Press.

Holmes, J. (2001) *The Search for a Secure Base: Attachment Theory and Psychotherapy.* Hove, Brunner-Routledge.

Hondagneu-Sotelo, P. (2007) *Domestica: Immigrant Workers Cleaning and Caring in the Shadows of Affluence.* Berkeley, University of California Press.

Hondagneu-Sotelo, P. and Messner, M. (1994) Gendered displays and men's power: the 'new' man and the Mexican immigrant (in) Brod, H. and Kaufman, M. (eds) *Theorizing Masculinities.* Thousand Oaks, Sage.

Hopkins, P. E. and Hill, M. (2008) Pre-flight experiences and migration stories: the accounts of unaccompanied asylum-seeking children. *Children's Geographies* 6, 3 257–268.

Horton, S. (2008) A mother's heart is weighed down with stones: a phenomenological approach to the experience of transnational motherhood. *Cultural Medical Psychiatry.* doi 10.1007/s11013-008-9117-z.

Hubard, G., Kidd, L. and Kearney, N. (2010) Disrupted lives and threats to identity: the experiences of people with colorectal cancer within the first year following diagnosis. *Health* 14, 2 131–146.

Huemer, J., Karnik, N. S. and Steiner, H. (2009) Mental health issues in unaccompanied refugee minors. *Child and Adolescent Psychiatry and Mental Health* 3, 13.

Hughes, G. (2014) Finding a voice through 'the tree of life': a strength-based approach to mental health for refugee children and families in schools. *Clinical Child Psychology and Psychiatry* 19, 1 139–153.

Hultsjo, S. and Hielm, K. (2005) Immigrants in emergency care: Swedish health care staff's experiences. *International Nursing Review* 53, 4 278–285.

Humphrey, C. et al. (2009) *Challenges encountered by ethnic minority and migrant doctors, healthcare workers and related groups and the implications for performance regulation.* Full Research Report, ESRC RES-153-25-0102, Swindon: ESRC.

Hunter, R., Noble, S., Lewis, S. et al. (2015) Post-traumatic stress disorder in medical settings: a focus on venous thromboembolism (VTE). *Health Psychology Update* 24, 2 17–24.

Hyman, I., Guruge, S. and Mason, R. (2008) The impact of migration on marital relationships. *Journal of Comparative Studies* 39, 1 149–163.

Ide, N., Kõlves, K., Cassaniti, M. et al. (2012) Suicide of first-generation immigrants in Australia, 1974–2006. *Social Psychiatry and Psychiatric Epidemiology* 47, 12 1917–1927.

Iliceto, P., Pompili, M., Candilera, G. et al. (2013) Suicide risk and psychopathology in immigrants: a multi-group confirmatory factor analysis. *Social Psychiatry and Psychiatric Epidemiology* 48 1105–1114.

Illich, I. (1991) *Limits to Medicine*. London, Penguin.

Iliffe, S. D. and Manthorpe, J. (2004) The debate on ethnicity and dementia: from category fallacy to person-centred care? *Aging & Mental Health* 8, 4. doi: 10.1080/13607860410001709656.

Ineichen, B. (2008) Suicide and attempted suicide among South Asians in England: who is at risk? *Mental Health Family Medicine* 5, 3 135–138.

International Organization for Migration (IOM) (2013) *World Migration Report*.

Jaremka, L. M., Andrige, R. R., Fagundes, C. P. et al. (2014) Pain, depression, and fatigue: loneliness as a longitudinal risk factor. *Health Psychology* 33, 9 948–957.

Jaremka, L. M., Fagundes, C. P., Bennett, J. M. et al. (2013) Loneliness promotes inflammation during acute stress. *Psychological Science* 24, 7 1089–1097.

Jaremka, L. M., Fagundes, C. P., Glaser, R. et al. (2013) Loneliness predicts pain, depression, and fatigue: understanding the role of immune dysregulation. *Psychoneuroendocrinology* 38, 8 1310–1317.

Jarvis, E. (1998) Schizophrenia in British immigrants: recent findings, issues and implications. *Transcultural Psychiatry* 35, 1 39–74.

Jayaweera, H. (2014) *Health of Migrants in the UK: What Do We Know?* Migration Observatory Briefing, University of Oxford.

Jayaweera, H. and Quigley, M. (2010) Health status, health behaviour and healthcare use among migrants in the UK: evidence from mothers in the Millennium Cohort Study. *Social Science & Medicine* 71, 1002–1010.

Jeon, H. J., Lee, J. Y., Lee, Y. M. et al. (2010) Lifetime prevalence and correlates of suicidal ideation, plan, and single and multiple attempts in a Korean nationwide study. *The Journal of Nervous and Mental Disease* 198, 643–646.

Jivraj, S. and Simpson, L. (2015) How has ethnic diversity grown? (in) Jivraj, S. and Simpson, L. (eds) *Ethnic Identity and Equality in Britain*. Bristol, Policy Press.

Johnson, M. (2006) Integration of new migrants (in) Spencer, S. (ed.) *Refugees and Other New Migrants: A Review of the Evidence on Successful Approaches to Integration*. University of Oxford: COMPAS.

Johnson, H. and Thompson, A. (2008) The development and maintenance of post-traumatic stress disorder (PTSD) in civilian adult survivors of war trauma and torture: a review. *Clinical Psychology Review* 28, 1 36–47.

Joseph, S., Williams, R. and Yule, W. (1997) *Understanding Posttraumatic Stress: A Psychosocial Perspective on PTSD and Treatment*. Chichester, Wiley.

Juckett, G. (2005) Cross-cultural medicine. *American Family Physician* 1, 72, 11 2267–2274.

Juhász, J., Makara, J. and Taller, A. (2010) Possibilities and limitations of comparative research on international migration and health. *PROMINSTAT Working Paper* 9.

Jung, C. (1954/1985) *The Practice of Psychotherapy: Essays on the Psychology of the Transference and Other Subjects*. Princeton University Press.

Kagawa-Singer, M. and Backhall, L. (2001). Negotiating cross-cultural issues at end of life: 'You got to go where he lives'. *Journal of American Medical Association* 286, 2993–3001.

Kai, J. (2013) Enhancing consultations with interpreters: learning more about how. *British Journal of General Practice* 63, 607 66–67.

Kai, J., Beavan, J. and Faull, C. (2011) Challenges of mediated communication, disclosure and patient autonomy in cross-cultural cancer care. *British Journal of Cancer* 105, 7 918–924.

Kangas, M., Henry, J. L. and Bryant, R. A. (2002) Posttraumatic stress disorder following cancer: A conceptual and empirical review. *Clinical Psychology Review* 22, 4 499–524.

Karbani, G., Lim, J. N. W., Hewison, J. et al. (2011) Culture, attitude and knowledge about breast cancer and preventative measures: a qualitative study of South Asian breast cancer patients in the UK. *Asian Pacific Journal Cancer Prevention* 12, 6 1619–1626.

Karr-Morse, R. (2012) *Scared Sick: The Role of Childhood Trauma in Adult Disease.* Philadelphia, Basic Book.

Kayser, K., Watson, L. E. and Andrade, J. L. (2007) Cancer as a 'we-disease': examining the process of coping from a relational perspective. *Family Systems and Health* 25, 4 404–418.

Kelley, N. and Stevenson, J. (2006) First do no harm: denying healthcare to people whose claims have failed. Refugee Council. Accessed at: www.refugeecouncil.org.uk/policy/position/2006/healthcare on 7 March 2016.

Kelly, R., Morrell, G. and Sriskandarajah, D. (2005) Migration and health in the UK. Accessed at: www.ippr.org/research/files/team19/project158/FFHealthFinal2%20_2_.pdf on 26 March 2016.

Kenny, C. (2015, 23 March) 5,000 doctors a year considering leaving the UK to emigrate abroad. *Pulse.*

Khanna R., Eck, M., Koenig C., Karliner, L. and Fang, M. (2010) Accuracy of Google Translate TM for medical educational material. *Journal of Hospital Medicine* 5, 41, 1553–1592.

Kholi, N. and Dalal, A. K. (1998) Psychological recovery of women with cervical cancer: The role of cultural beliefs (in) Lonner, J. W., Dinnel, D. L., Forgays, D. K. and Hayes, S. (eds) *Merging Past, Present, and Future in Cross-cultural Psychology.* Lisse, the Netherlands, Swets & Zeitlinger.

Khoo, S. W. and Zhao, Z. (2001) A decomposition of immigrant divorce rates in Australia. *Journal of Population Research* 18, 1 68–77.

Kia Keating, M. and Ellis, B. H. (2007) Belonging and connection in resettlement: young refugees, school belonging and psychosocial adjustment. *Clinical Child Psychology and Psychiatry* 12, 1 29–43.

Kim, Y., Carver, C. S., Spillers, R. L. et al. (2012) Dyadic effects of fear of recurrence on the quality of life of cancer survivors and their caregivers. *Quality of Life Research,* 21, 517–525.

Kingma, M. (2006) *Nurses on the Move: Migration and the Global Health Care Economy.* New York, Cornell University Press.

Kirkcaldy, B. D., Siefen, R. G., Wittig, U. et al. (2005) Health and emigration: subjective evaluation of health status and physical symptoms in Russian-speaking migrants. *Stress and Health* 21, 5 295–309.

Kirkbride, J. B. and Jones, P. B. (2011) Epidemiological aspects of migration and mental health (in) Bhugra, D. and Gupta, S. (eds) *Migration and Mental Health.* Cambridge, Cambridge University Press.

Kirmayer, L. J., Narasiah, L., Munoz, M. et al. (2011) Common mental health problems in immigrants and refugees: general approach to the patient in primary care. *Canadian Medical Association Journal* 183, 12 E959–E967.

Kissane, D. W., Grabsch, B., Clarke, D. M. et al. (2007) Supportive-expressive group therapy for women with metastatic breast cancer: survival and psychosocial outcome from a randomized controlled trial. *Psycho-Oncology* 16, 4 277–286.

Klasen, F., Oettingen, G., Daniels, J. et al. (2010) Posttraumatic resilience in former Ugandan child soldiers. *Child Development* 81, 4 1096–1113.

Klein, M. (1975) *Envy and Gratitude and Other Works.* New York, Delta.

Kleinman, A. (1978) Clinical relevance of anthropological and cross-cultural research: concepts and strategies. *American Journal of Psychiatry* 135, 4 427–431.

Kleinman, A. (1980) *Patients and Healers in the Context of Culture.* Berkeley, University of California Press.

Kleinman, A. (1988) *The Illness Narratives.* New York, Basic Books.

Kleinman, A. (2006) Culture, moral experience and medicine. *Mount Sinai Journal of Medicine* 11, 73 6 834–839.

Kleinman, A. and Benson, P. (2006) Anthropology in the clinic: the problem of cultural competency and how to fix it. *PLoS Med* 3, 10 e294.

Kleinman, A., Eisenberg, L. and Good, B. (2006) Culture, illness, and care: clinical lessons from anthropologic and cross-cultural research. *FOCS* 4 140–149.

Kline, D. S. (2003) Push and pull factors in international nurse migration. *Journal of Nursing Scholarship* 35, 2 107–111.

Knodel, J. E. and Saengtienchai, C. (2007) Rural parents with urban children: social and economic implications of migration for the rural elderly in Thailand. *Population Space and Place* 13, 3 193–210.

Koch, S. C. and Weidinger-von der Recke, B. (2009) Traumatized refugees: an integrated dance and verbal therapy approach. *The Arts in Psychotherapy* 36, 5 289–296.

Koenig, H. G. (2009) Research on religion, spirituality, and mental health a review. *Canadian Journal of Psychiatry* 54, 5 283–289.

Kramer, B., Boelk, A. Z. and Auer, C. (2006) Family conflict at the end of life: lessons learned in a model program for vulnerable older adults. *Journal of Palliative Medicine* 9, 3 791–801.

Krause, I.-B. (1989) Sinking heart: a Punjabi communication of distress. *Social Science and Medicine* 29, 4 563–575.

Krause, I.-B. (2002) *Culture and Family Therapy.* London, Karnac Books.

Kreuter, M. W. and McClure, S. M. (2004) The role of culture in health communication. *Annual Review of Public Health* 25, 439–455.

Kubler-Ross, E. (1970) *On Death and Dying.* London, Tavistock.

Kuhn, R. (2006) The effects of fathers' and siblings' migration on children's pace of schooling in rural Bangladesh. *Asian Population Studies* 2, 1 69–92.

Kymlicka, W. (2001) *Politics in the Vernacular: Nationalism, Multiculturalism and Citizenship.* Oxford, Oxford University Press.

Labree, L. J. W., van de Mheen, H., Rutten, F. et al. (2011) Differences in overweight and obesity among children from migrant and native origin: a systematic review of the European literature. *Obesity Reviews* 12, 5 e535–e547.

La Plante, W. A., Lobato, D. and Engel, R. (2001) Review of group interventions for pediatric chronic conditions. *Journal of Pediatric Psychology* 26, 7 435–453.

Laoire, C. N. (2001) A matter of life and death? men, masculinities and staying 'behind' in rural Ireland. *Sociologia Ruralis* 41, 2 220–236.

Larsen, J. A. (2007) Embodiment of discrimination and overseas nurses' career progression. *Journal of Clinical Nursing* 16, 12 2187–2195.

Lau, A. S., Jernewall, N. M., Zane, N. and Myers, H. F. (2002) Correlates of suicidal behaviors among Asian American outpatient youths. *Cultural Diversity & Ethnic Minority Psychology* 8, 199–213.

Launer, J. (1995) A social constructionist approach to family medicine. *Family Systems Medicine* 13, 3/4 379–389.

Launer, J. (1996) Towards systemic general practice. *Context* 26 Spring 42–45.

Launer, J. (2002) *Narrative-based Primary Care: A Practical Guide.* Oxford, Radcliffe.

Lavee, Y. and May-Dan, M. (2003) Patterns of change of marital relationships among parents of children with cancer. *Health Social Work* 28 255–263.

Law, S. and Liu, P. (2008) Suicide in China: unique demographic patterns and relationship to depressive disorder. *Current Psychiatry Reports* 10, 1 80–86.

Lawler, M., Selby, P., Aapro, M. S. and Duffy, S. (2014) Ageism in cancer care. *BMJ* 348:g1614.

Leanza, Y., Boivin, I. and Rosenberg, E. (2010) Interruptions and resistance: a comparison of medical consultations with family and trained interpreters. *Social Science & Medicine* 70,12 1888–1895.

Lee, E. and Chan, J. (2004) Mourning in Chinese culture (in) Walsh, F. and McGoldrick, M. (eds) *Living Beyond Loss* (2nd edition). London, WW Norton and Company.

Lee, R. E. and Dwyer, T. (1995) Co-constructed narratives around being 'sick': a minimalist model. *Contemporary Family Therapy* 17, 1 65–82.

Le Shan, L. (1989) *Cancer as a Turning Point: A Handbook for People with Cancer, Their Families and Health Professionals.* New York, Penguin.

Lester, D. (2006) Suicide and Islam. *Archives of suicide research: official journal of the International Academy for Suicide Research* 10, 1 77–97.

Levinas, E. (1994) *Nine Talmudic Readings* (trans. Aronowicz, A.). Bloomington, Indiana University Press.

Levine, P. S. and Kline, M. (2007) *Trauma Through a Child's Eyes: Awakening the Ordinary Miracle of Healing.* Berkeley, North Atlantic Books.

Lewis, G. (2011) Saving Mothers Lives 2006–2009. *British Journal of Obstetrics and Gynaecology* 118, Sup 1 1–203.

Lievesley, N. (2010) *The Future Ageing of the Ethnic Minority Population of England and Wales.* London, Runnymede and the Centre for Policy on Ageing.

Lillis, S., St George, I. and Upsell, R. (2006) Perceptions of migrant doctors joining the New Zealand medical workforce. *New Zealand Medical Journal* 119, 1229:U1844.

Little, M., Paul, K., Jordens, C. F. C. and Sayers, E. J. (2002) Survivorship and discourses of identity. *Psycho-Oncology* 11, 170–178.

Llerena-Quinn, R. (2004) Naming the tears: the multiple contexts of loss (in) Walsh, F. and McGoldrick, M. (eds) *Living Beyond Loss: Death in the Family* (2nd edition). New York, WW Norton & Company.

Longhurst, R. (2010) Infant oral mutilation. *British Dental Journal* 209, 12 591–592.

Lor, M. and Chewning, B. (2015), Telephone interpreter discrepancies: videotapes of Hmong medication consultations. *International Journal of Pharmacy Practice* doi: 10.1111/ijpp.12206.

Lucassen, L. and Laarman, C. (2009) Immigration, intermarriage and the changing face of Europe in the post war period. *History of the Family* 14, 52–68.

Lupton, D. (1994) *Medicine as Culture*. London, Sage.

Lutz, H. (2008) *Migration and Domestic Work: A European Perspective on a Global Theme*. Aldershot, Ashgate.

MacFarlane, A. and Dorkenoo, E. (2014) *Female Genital Mutilation in England and Wales: Updated statistical estimates of the numbers of affected women living in England and Wales and girls at risk Interim report on provisional estimates*. London, City University, Equality Now and Home Office.

MacGrath, P., Vun, M. and McLeod, L. (2001) Needs and experiences of non-English-speaking hospice patients and families in an English-speaking country. *American Journal of Hospice & Palliative Care* 18, 305–312.

Maciel, J. A., van Putten, Z. and Knudson-Martin, C. (2009) Gendered power in cultural contexts. *Family Process*. Part 1: Immigrant couples 48, 9–23.

Maitra, B. and Krause, I.-B. (2015) *Culture and Madness: A Training Resource, Film and Commentary for Mental Health Professionals*. London, Jessica Kingsley.

Malik, R. and Mandin, P. (2012) Engaging within and across culture (in) Krause, I-B. (ed.) *Culture and Reflexivity*. London, Karnac Books.

Mallon, G. P. (2013) Social work practice with gay men and lesbian women (in) Mallon, G. P. (ed.) *Foundations of Social Work Practice with Lesbian and Gay Persons*. Bingham, NY, Hayworth Press.

Manderson, L. and Allotey, P. (2003) Story telling, marginality and community in Australia: how immigrants position their difference in health care settings. *Medical Anthropology* 22, 1–21.

Manley, J. J. and Mayeaux, R. (2004) Ethnic differences in dementia and Alzheimer's disease (in) Anderson, N. B., Bulatao, R. A. and Cohen, B. (eds) *Critical Perspectives on Racial and Ethnic Differences in Health in Later Life*. Washington, National Academies Press.

Mann, S. and Russell, S. (2002) Narrative ways of working with women survivors of childhood sexual abuse. *International Journal of Narrative Therapy and Community Work* 3, 3–21.

Manne, S., Ostroff, J., Rini, C. et al. (2004) The interpersonal process model of intimacy: the role of self-disclosure, partner disclosure and partner responsiveness in interactions between breast cancer patients and their partners. *Journal of Family Psychology* 18, 589–599.

Marchetti-Mercer, M. C. (2012) Those easily forgotten: the impact of emigration on those left behind. *Family Process* 51, 3 376–390.

Marlow, L. A. V., Wardle, J. and Waller, J. (2015) Understanding cervical screening non-attendance among ethnic minority women in England. *British Journal of Cancer* 113, 5 833–839.

Marmot, M. J., Allen, J., Goldblatt, R. et al. (2010) Fair society, healthy lives. *The Marmot Review*, London.

Marshall, H., Woollett, A. and Dosanjh, N. (1998) Researching marginalized standpoints: some tensions around plural standpoints and diverse 'experiences' (in) Henwood, K., Griffin, C. and Phoenix, A. (eds) *Standpoints and Differences: Essays in the Practice of Feminist Psychology*. London, Sage.

Martinson, I. M. and Yee, K. H. (2003) Parental involvement in restoring the health of a child with cancer in Hong Kong. *Journal of Pediatric Oncology Nursing* 20, 5 233–244.

Massey, D. (1991) A global sense of place. *Marxism Today* 38, 24–29.

Masterson, A. R., Usta, J., Gupta, J. and Ettinger, A. S. (2014) Assessment of reproductive health and violence against women among displaced Syrians in Lebanon. *BMC Women's Health* 14, 25 1–8.

Mattingly, C. F. (1998) *Healing Dramas and Clinical Plots: The Narrative Structure of Experience*. Cambridge, Cambridge University Press.

Mauthner, M. (2003) *Sistering: Power and Change in Female Relationships*. Basingstoke, Palgrave Macmillan.

Mazzucato, V., Cebotar, V., Veale, A. et al. (2014) International parental migration and the psychological well-being of children in Ghana, Nigeria, and Angola. *Social Science & Medicine* 13 18–30.

McBrien, J. L. (2011) The importance of context. Vietnamese, Somali and Iranian refugee mothers discuss their settled lives and involvement in their children's schools. *Compare: A Journal of Comparative and International Education* 41, 1 75–90.

McCann, D. (2014) Responding to the clinical needs of same-sex couples (in) Scharff, D. and Scharff, J. S. (eds) *Psychoanalytic Couple Therapy*. London, Karnac Books.

McCartney, M. (2015) Breaching trust won't stop FGM. *BMJ* 351, h5830.

McColl, H., McKenzie, K. and Bhui, K. (2008) Mental healthcare of asylum-seekers and refugees. doi:10.1192/PT.BP.107.005041.

McDonald, J. T. and Kennedy, S. (2004) Insights into the 'healthy immigrant effect': health status and health service use of immigrants to Canada. *Social Science and Medicine* 59, 8 1613–1627.

McElmurry, B. J., Solheim, F. K., Hishi, R. et al. (2006) Ethical concerns in nurse migration. *Journal of Professional Nursing* 22 226–235.

McGoldrick, M., Shlesinger, J. M., Lee, E. et al. (2004) Mourning in different cultures (in) Walsh, F. and McGoldrick, M. (eds) *Living Beyond Loss: Death in the Family* (2nd edition). New York, WW Norton & Company.

McKay, L., Macintyre, S. and Ellaway, A. (2003) *Migration and health: a review of the international literature*. Occasional Paper 12, Medical Research Council, Social and Public Health Sciences Unit. MRC Social & Public Health Sciences Unit publication.

McKay, S., Craw, M. and Chopra, D. (2006) *Migrant Workers in England and Wales: An Assessment of Migrant Worker Health and Safety Risks*. London, Health and Safety Executive.

McLamara, R. (2013) Addressing the psychological impact of BRCA testing Oncology Nurse Advisory, 29 October 29. Accessed at: www.oncologynurseadvisor.com/breast-cancer/addressing-the-psychological-impact-of-brca-testing/article/318416/ on 18 March 2016.

McLoyd, V., Cauce, A. M., Takeuchi, D. and Wilson, L. (2000) Marital processes and parental socialization in families of color: a decade review of research. *Journal of Marriage and the Family* 62, 4 1070–1093.

McManus, I. C. and Wakeford, R. (2014) PLAB and UK graduates' performance on MRCP (UK) and MRCGP examinations: data linkage study. *British Medical Journal* 348, 2621.

McPherson, M., Arango, P., Fox, H., Lauver, C., McManus, M., Newacheck, P. W. et al. (1998) A new definition of children with special healthcare needs. *Pediatrics* 102, 137–140.

Mendoza, F. S., Javier, J. R. and Burgos, A. E. (2007) The health of children in immigrant families (in) Lansford, J. E., Deater-Deckard, K. and Bornsten, M. H. (eds) *Immigrant Families in Contemporary Society*. New York, Guilford Press.

Meyerstein, I. (2015) The 'healing' pillow: a practical spiritual tool for coping with illness. *International Journal of Emergency Mental Health and Human Resilience* 17, 2 552–554.

Michel, G., Rebholz, C. E., von der Weid, N. X. et al. (2010) Psychological distress in adult survivors of childhood cancer: the Swiss childhood cancer survivor study. *Journal of Clinical Oncology* 28, 10 1740–1748.

Migerode, L. and Hooghe, A. (2012) High conflict divorced couples: combining systemic and psychodynamic perspectives. *Journal of Family Therapy* 34, 4 387–402.

Miles, S. H. (2006) *Oath Betrayed: Torture, Medical Complicity and the War on Terror*. New York, Random House.

Miltiades, H. B. (2002) The social and psychological effect of an adult child's emigration on non-immigrant Asian Indian elderly parents. *Journal of Cross-Cultural Gerontology* 17, 33–55.

Mitchell, J. (2003) *Siblings, Sex and Violence*. Cambridge, Polity Press.

Mitchell, B. L. and Mitchell, L. C. (2009) Review of the literature on cultural competence and end-of-life treatment decisions: the role of the hospitalist. *Journal National Medical Association* 101, 9 920–926.

Mizrahi, I., Kaplan, G., Milshtein, E. et al. (2008) Coping simultaneously with 2 stressors: immigrants with ovarian cancer. *Cancer Nursing* 31, 126–133.

Moberly, T. (2014) Minority report: how the UK's treatment of foreign and ethnic minority doctors needs to change. *BMJ* 22, 348 doi:10.1136/bmj.g2839.

Modell, B., Darlison, M., Birgens, H. et al. (2007) Epidemiology of haemoglobin disorders in Europe. *Scandinavian Journal of Clinical and Laboratory Investigation* 67, 1 39–69.

Moller, T., Anderson, H., Aareleid, T. et al. (2003) Cancer prevalence in Northern Europe: the EUROPREVAL study. *Annals of Oncology* 14, 946–957.

Montgomery, E. and Patel, N. (2011) Torture rehabilitation: reflections on outcome studies. *Torture* 21, 2 141–145.

Mooney, A. and Statham, J. (2002) *The Pivot Generation Informal Care and Work After Fifty*. London, The Policy Press and the Joseph Rowntree Foundation.

Morales, A. and Hanson, W. (2005) Language brokering: an integrative review of the literature. *Hispanic Journal of Behavioral Sciences* 27, 4 471–503.

Moriarty, J., Sharif, N. and Robinson, J. (2011) *Black and Minority Ethnic People With Dementia and Their Access to Support and Services.* Research briefing. London, Social Care Institute for Excellence.

Mu, P. F., Ma, F. C., Ku, S. M. et al. (2001) Families of Chinese children with malignancy: the factors impact on mother's anxiety. *Journal of Pediatric Nursing* 16, 4 287–295.

Mu, P. F., Ma, F. C., Hwang, B. and Chao, Y. M. (2002) Families of children with cancer: the impact on anxiety experienced by father. *Cancer Nursing* 25, 1 66–73.

Mulder, C. H. and Cooke, T. J. (2009). Family ties and residential locations. *Population, Space and Place* 15, 299–304.

Munet-Vilaro, F. (2004) Delivery of culturally competent care to children with cancer and their families—the Latino experience. *Journal of Pediatric Oncology Nursing* 21, 3 155–159.

Nair, C., Nargundkar, M., Johansen, H. and Stracha, J. (1990) Canadian cardiovascular disease mortality: first generation immigrants versus Canadian born. *Health Reports* 2, 3 203–228.

Nair, M. and Webster, P. (2013) Health professionals' migration in emerging market economies: patterns, causes and possible solutions. *Journal of Public Health* 35, 1 157–163.

National Cancer Intelligence Network and Cancer Research UK (2009) *Cancer Incidence and Survival by Major Ethnic Group, England 2002–2006.*

National Health Service (2015) *The National Health Service (Charges to Overseas Visitors) Regulations 2015 238.* Accessed at: www.legislation.gov.uk/uksi/2015/238/pdfs/uksi_20150238_en.pdf on 20 March 2016.

NCAT/FIS (2012) Cancer and the Irish community. *National Cancer Action Team/Federation of Irish Societies* Health Supplement 2, London.

Ncube, N. (2006) The tree of life project: using narrative ideas in work with vulnerable children in Southern Africa. *The International Journal of Narrative Therapy and Community Work* 1, 3–16.

Nelson, S. C., Hackman, H. W., O'Conner, T. G. and Scott, B. C. (2013) Race matters: perceptions of race and racism in a sickle cell center. *Pediatric Blood Cancer* 60, 3 451–454.

Neyzi, L. (2004) Fragmented in space: the oral history narrative of an Arab from Antioch, Turkey. *Global Networks* 4, 3 285–297.

Noh, S. and Kaspar, V. (2003) *Diversity and Immigrant Health.* Toronto, University of Toronto.

Norredam, M., Mygind, A. and Krasnick, A. (2006) Access to health care for asylum seekers in the European Union – a comparative study of country politics. *European Journal of Public Health* 16, 3 285–290.

Nutkiewicz, M. (2007) Chronic pain patients and torture survivors: intersecting lines and lines of demarcation. *Newsletter of the IASP Special Interest Group on Pain from Torture, Organized Violence and War.*

O'Brien, I., Duffy, A., Nicholl, H. (2009) Impact of childhood chronic illnesses on siblings: a literature review. *British Journal of Nursing* 18, 22 1360–1364.

O'Conner, T. G. and Scott, B. C. (2007) *Parenting and Outcomes for Children.* Joseph Rowntree Foundation. Accessed at: www.jrf.org.uk/bookshop/ on 26 March 2016.

Ødegaard, Ø. (1932) Emigration and insanity. *Acta Psychiatrica Neurologica Scandinavica* Suppl 4, 1–206.

O'Donnell, C. A., Higgins, M., Chauhan, R. et al. (2008) Asylum seekers' expectations of and trust in general practice: a qualitative study. *British Journal of General Practice* 58, 557 870–876.

Office for National Statistics (2014) *Migration Statistics Quarterly Report*. Accessed at: www.ons.gov.uk/ons/rel/migration1/migration-statistics-quarterly-report/index.html on 20 March 2016.

O'Grady, P. (2014, 28 July) I feel guilty about leaving but it's becoming harder to do the job. *Pulse.*

O'Hagan, K. (2001) *Cultural Competence in the Caring Professions*. London, Jessica Kingsley Publishers.

O'Leary, J. (2004) Grief and its impact on prenatal attachment in the subsequent pregnancy. *Archives of Womens Mental Health* 1–12.

Oliver, C. (2013) Country case study on the impacts of restrictions and entitlements on the integration of family migrants: qualitative findings, the United Kingdom. Oxford, *COMPAS* University of Oxford.

Oliver, D., Foot, C. and Humphreys, R. (2014) *Making Our Health and Care Systems Fit For an Aging Population*. London, Kings Fund publication.

Olwig, F. K. (2002) A wedding in the family: home making in a global kin network. *Global Networks* 2, 3 205–281.

Ong, Y. L. and Gayen, A. (2003) Helping refugee doctors get their first jobs: the pan-London clinical attachment scheme. *Hospital Medicine* 64, 8 488–490.

Ormond, M. (2013) Harnessing 'diasporic' medical mobilities (in) Thomas, F. and Gideon, J. (eds) *Migration, Health and Inequality*. London, Zed Books.

Orton, L., Griffiths, J., Maia, G. et al. (2012) Resilience among asylum seekers living with HIV. *BMC Public Health* 12, 926 doi:10.1186/1471-2458-12-926.

Pachter, L. M. et al. (1992) Clinical implications of a folk illness: empacho in mainland Puerto Ricans. *Medical Anthropology* 13, 4 285–299.

Packman, W., Horsley, H., Davies, B. and Kramer, R. (2006) Sibling bereavement and continuing bonds. *Death Studies* 30, 817–841.

Palriwala, R. and Uberoi, P. R. (2008) Exploring the links: gender issues in marriage and migration (in) Palriwala, R. and Uberoi, P. R. (eds) *Marriage, Migration and Gender*. New Delhi, Sage.

Pande, R. (2014) Geographies of marriage and migration: arranged marriages and South Asians in Britain. *Geography Compass* 8, 2 75–86.

Pandey, A., Aggarwal, R., Devane, R. and Kuznetsov, Y. (2004) *India's Transformation to Knowledge-based Economy – Evolving Role of the Indian Diaspora*. Evaluserve, 21 July. Accessed at: http://info.worldbank.org/etools/docs/library/152386/abhishek.pdf on 26 March 2016.

Panter Brick, C., Grimon, M. P., Kalin, M. and Eggermann M. (2015) Trauma memories, mental health and resilience. *J Child Psychology and Psychiatry* 56, 7 814–825.

Papadopoulos, I. and Lay, M. (2006) Culturally competent health promotion for minority ethnic groups, refugees, Gypsy travellers and New Age travellers in the UK (in) Papadopoulos, I. (ed.) *Transcultural Health and Social Care: Developing Culturally Competent Practitioners*. Oxford, Elsevier.

Papadopoulos, I., Lees, S., Lay, M. and Gebrehiwot, A. (2004) Ethiopian refugees in the UK: migration, adaptation and settlement experiences and their relevance to health. *Ethnicity and Health* 9, 1 55–73.

Papadopoulos, I., Tilki, M. and Taylor, G. (1998) *Transcultural Care: A Guide for Health care Professionals*. Wiltshire, Quay Books.

Papadopoulos, R. (2007) Refugees, trauma and adversity-activated development. *European Journal of Psychotherapy and Counselling* 9, 3 301–312.

Papastergiadis, N. (2000) *The Turbulence of Migration*. Cambridge, Polity Press.

Parrenas, R. S. (2005) *Children of Global Migration: Transnational Families and Gendered Woes*. Stanford, CT, Stanford University Press.

Parrenas, R. S. (2014) Migrant domestic workers as 'one of the family' (in) Anderson, B. and Shutes, I. (eds) *Migration and Care Labour*. Basingstoke, Palgrave.

Patel, N., Kellezi, B. and Williams, A. C. (2014) Psychological, social and welfare interventions for psychological health and well-being of torture survivors. *Cochrane Common Mental Disorders Group* doi: 10.1002/14651858.CD009317. pub2.

Pat-Horenczyk, R., Rabinowitz., R. G., Rice, A. and Tucker-Levin, A. (2009) The search for risk and protective factors in childhood PTSD (in) Brom, D., Pat-Horenczyk, R. and Ford, J. D. (eds) *Treating Traumatized Children*. London, Routledge.

Patil, S. and Davies, P. (2014) Use of Google Translate in medical communication: Evaluation of accuracy. *BMJ* 349 0959-8146 1756–1833.

Pereira, C., Bugalho, A., Bergstrom, S. et al. (1996) A comparative study of caesarean deliveries by assistant medical officers and obstetricians in Mozambique. *British Journal of Obstetric Gynaecology* 103, 508–512.

Perez Foster, R. (2001) When immigration is trauma: guidelines for the individual and family clinician. *American Journal of Orthopsychiatry* 71, 2 153–170.

Phillimore, J. et al. (2010) *Delivering in an Age of Super-Diversity: West Midlands Review of Maternity Services for Migrant Women*. Department of Health and University of Birmingham.

Phillips, D. (2015) Segregation, mixing and encounter (in) Vertovic, S. (ed.) *International Handbook of Diversity Studies*. Abingdon, Routledge.

Phinney, J. S. and Ong, A. (2007) Conceptualization and measurement of ethnic identity: current status and future directions. *Journal of Counseling Psychology* 54, 3, 271–281.

Phoenix, A. (2004) Extolling eclecticism: language, psychoanalysis and demographic analysis in the study of 'race' and racism (in) Bulmer, M. and Solomos, J. (eds) *Researching Race and Racism*. London, Routledge.

Phoenix, A. and Husain, F. (2007) *Parenting and Ethnicity*. York, Joseph Rowntree Foundation.

Pipher, M. (1999) *Another Country*. New York, Riverhead Books.

Pinto, R., Ashworth, M. and Jones, R. (2008) Schizophrenia in black Caribbeans living in the UK: an exploration of underlying causes of the high incidence rate. *British Journal of General Practice* 58, 551 429–434.

Pollock, G. (1994) Territories of desire: reconsiderations of an African childhood (in) Robertson, G., Mash, M., Tickner, L. et al. (eds) *Travellers' Tales*. London, Routledge.

Pont, K., Ziviani, J., Wadley, D. et al. (2009) Environmental correlates of children's active transportation: a systematic literature review. *Health & Place* 15, 849–862.

Portelli, A. (1990) Uchronic dreams: working-class memory and possible worlds (in) Samuel, R. and Thompson, P. (eds) *The Myths We Live By*. London, Routledge.

Portes, A. and Rumbaut, R. (2001) *Legacies: The Story of the Immigrant Second Generation*. Berkeley, University of California Press.

Pottie, K., Greenaway, C., Feightner, J. et al. (2011) Evidence-based clinical guidelines for immigrants and refugees. *CMAJ* 183. E824–925 doi:1503/cmaj.090313.

Pottie, K., Dahal, G., Georgiades, K. et al. (2014) Do first generation immigrant adolescents face higher rates of bullying, violence and suicidal behaviours than do third generation and native born? *Journal of Immigrant and Minority Health* doi 10.1007/s10903-014-0108-6.

Powell, J., Kitchen, N. and Heslin, N. (2002) Psychosocial outcome at three and nine months after good neurological recovery from aneurismal subarachnoid haemorrhage: predictors and prognosis. *J Neurological Neurosurgical Psychiatry* 72, 772–781.

Pratt Ewing, J. K. (2008) *Stolen Honour: Stigmatizing Muslim Men in Berlin*. Stanford, Stanford University Press.

Price, M. A., Tennant, C. C., Butow, P. N. et al. (2001) The role of psychosocial factors in the development of breast carcinoma: part II life event stressors, social support, defense style, and emotional control and their interactions. *Cancer*, 91 4 686–697.

Priebe, S., Sandhu, S., Dias, S. et al. (2011) Good practice in health care for migrants: views and experiences of care professionals in 16 European countries. *BMC Public Health* 11, doi: 10.1186/1471-2458-11-187.

Probyn, E. (2004) Everyday shame. *Cultural Studies*, 18, 2/3 328–349.

Pyke, K. D. (2010) What is internalized racial oppression and why don't we study it? Acknowledging racism's hidden injuries. *Sociological Perspectives* 53, 4 551–572.

Radley, A. (1994) *Making Sense of Illness*. London, Sage.

Raftery, J., Jones, D. R. and Rosato, M. (1990) The mortality of first and second generation Irish immigrants in the UK. *Social Science & Medicine* 31, 5 557–584.

Rathbone, J. (2009) Living with terminal illness. *Context* 101, 18–19.

Ratkowska, L. and De Leo, D. (2013) Suicide in immigrants: an overview. *Scientific Research* 2, 3 124–133.

Rauf, A. (2011) *Caring For Dementia: Exploring Good Practice on Supporting South Asian Carers Through Access to Culturally Competent Service Provision*. Bradford, Meri Yaadain Dementia Team.

Razum, O., Zeeb, H., Akgun, S. and Yilmaz, S. (1998) Low overall mortality of Turkish residents in Germany persists and extends into a second generation: merely a healthy migrant effect? *Tropical Medicine & International Health* 3, 4 293–303.

Razum, O., Zeeb, H. and Rohrmann, S. (2000) The 'healthy migrant effect' – not merely a fallacy of inaccurate denominator figures. *International Journal of Epidemiology* 21, 199–200.

Rechel, B., Mladovsky, P., Ingleby, D. et al. (2013) Migration and health in an increasingly diverse Europe. *Lancet* 381, 9874 1235–1245.

Record, R. and Mohiddin, A. (2006) An economic perspective on Malawi's medical 'brain drain'. *Globalization and Health* 2, 12 doi:1186/17744-8603-2-12.

Redshaw, M. and Keikkila, K. (2011) Ethnic differences in women's worries about labour and birth. *Ethnicity and Health* 16, 3 213–223.

Refugee Council (2015) *Children in the Asylum System.*

Renzaho, A. M. N., Green, J., Mellor, D. and Swinburn, B. (2010) Parenting, family functioning and lifestyle in a new culture: the case of African migrants in Melbourne, Victoria, Australia. *Child and Family Social Work* 16, 2 228–240.

Renzaho, A. M. N., Swinburn, B. and Burns, C. (2008) Maintenance of traditional cultural orientation is associated with lower rates of obesity and sedentary behaviours among African migrant children to Australia. *International Journal of Obesity* 32, 4 594–600.

Richards, H., Reid, M. and Watt, G. (2003) Victim blaming revisited: a qualitative study of beliefs about illness causation, and responses to chest pain. *Family Practice* 20, 711–716.

Richardson, A., Thomas, V. N. and Richardson, A. (2006) 'Reduced to nods and smiles': experiences of professionals caring for people with cancer from black and ethnic minority groups. *European Journal of Oncology Nursing* 10, 2 93–101.

Rickard, J. (2011) *Torn Apart: United by Love, Divided by Law.* Scotland, Findhorn Press.

Rober, P. and De Haene, L. (2014) Intercultural therapy and the limitations of a cultural competency framework: about cultural differences, universalities and the unresolvable tensions between them. *Journal of Family Therapy* 36, 3–20.

Robinette, J. W. and Charles, S. T. (2014) Age, rumination, and emotional recovery from a psychosocial stressor. *Journals of Gerontology, Series B: Psychological Sciences and Social Sciences* 1–9.

Rochelle, T. L. and Marks, D. F. (2010) Medical pluralism of the Chinese in London: an exploratory study. *British Journal of Health Psychology* 15, 715–728.

Roehlkepartian, E. G., King, E. G., Wagener, L. and Benson, P. L. (2006) *Handbook of Spiritual Development in Childhood and Adolescence.* London, Sage.

Roizblatt, A., Biederman, N. and Brown, J. (2011) Extreme traumatization in Chile: the experience and treatment of families. *Journal of Family Therapy* 36, 1 24–38.

Rolland, J. (1994) *Families, Illness, and Disability: An Integrative Treatment Model.* New York, Basic Books.

Romer, G., Barkmann, C., Thomalla, G. et al. (2002) Children of somatically ill parents: a methodological review. *Clinical Child Psychology and Psychiatry* 7, 1 17–38.

Roose, S. and Neimeyer, R. A. (2007) Reauthoring the self: chronic sorrow and posttraumatic stress following the onset of CID (in) Martz, E. and Livneh, H. (eds) *Coping With Chronic Illness and Disability.* New York, Springer.

Rosaldo, R. (1989) *Culture and Truth: The Remaking of Social Analysis*. Boston, Beacon Press.

Rousseau, C. and Guzder, J. (2008) School-based prevention programs for refugee children. *Child and Adolescent Psychiatric Clinics of North America* 17, 3 533–49.

Royal College of Nursing and Midwifery (2010) *A Practical Guide and Information for Refugee Midwives*. NHS Employers.

Royal College of Obstetricians and Gynaecologists (2004) *Why Mothers Die: Confidential Enquiry into Maternal and Child Health*.

Royal Medical Tours, Mumbai Pvt Ltd (2016) *Parents' Care package*. Accessed at: www.medicaltourindia.com/parents-health-care-package.asp on 7 March 2016.

Ruiz, P., Maggi, I. C. and Yusim, A. (2011) Impact of acculturation stress on mental health of migrants (in) Bhugra, D. and Gupta, S. (eds) *Migration and Mental Health*. Cambridge, Cambridge University Press.

Rumbaut, G. (1997) Paradoxes (and orthodoxies) of assimilation. *Sociological Perspectives* 40, 3 483–511.

Russell, C., White, M. B. and White, C. P. (2006) Why me? Why now? Why multiple sclerosis? Making meaning and perceived quality of life in a Midwestern sample of patients with multiple sclerosis. *Families, Systems, & Health* 24, 1 65–81.

Russell, S. T., Crockett, L. J. and Chao, R. K. (2010) Asian American parenting and parent-adolescent relationships. *Journal of Youth Adolescence* 40, 245–247.

Rutter, J. and Andrews, H. (2009) *Home Sweet Home? The nature and scale of British remigration to the UK*, London: Age Concern. Accessed at: www.ippr.org/images/media/files/project/2011/12/home_sweet_home.pdf on 7 March 2016.

Rutter, M. (2012) Resilience as a dynamic concept. *Developmental Psychopathology* 24, 335–344.

Said, E. (1978) *Orientalism*. New York, Vintage Books.

Said, E. W. (2002) *Reflections on Exile and Other Essays*. Cambridge, Mass, Harvard University Press.

Saile, R., Neuner, F., Ertl, V. and Cantani, C. (2013) Prevalence and predictors of partner violence against women in the aftermath of war: a survey among couples in northern Uganda. *Social Science and Medicine* 86, 17–25.

Sallfors, C. and Hallberg, L. R. M. (2003) A perspective on living with a chronically ill child. *Family Systems and Health* 21, 2 193–204.

Salway, S., Barley, R., Allmark, P. et al. (2011) *Ethnic Diversity and Inequality: Ethical and Scientific Rigour in Social Research*. York, Joseph Rowntree Foundation.

Sanghere, S. (2009) *The Boy with the Topknot: A Memoir of Love, Secrets and Lies in Wolverhampton*. Penguin.

Scheppers, E., van Dongen, E., Dekker, J. et al. (2006) Potential barriers to the use of health services among ethnic minorities: a review. *Family Practice* 233 325–348.

Seale, C., Rivas, C. and Kelly, M. (2013) The challenge of communication in interpreted consultations in diabetes care: a mixed methods study. *British Journal of General Practice* 63, 607 125–133.

Segal, L. (2013) *Out of Time: The Pleasures and the Perils of Ageing*. London, Verso.

Selten, J. P., Cantor-Graae, E. and Khan, R. S. (2003) Migration and schizophrenia. *Current Opinion Psychiatry* 20, 2 111–115.

Serco Commission. (2014) *Commission on Hospital Care For Frail Older Adults*. Accessed at: www.hsj.co.uk/frail-older-people on 26 March 2016.

Shah, R. (2013) International health care worker migration (in) Thomas, F. and Gideon, J. (eds) *Migration, Health and Inequality*. London, Zed Books.

Shapiro, F. and Laliotis, D. (2010) EMDR and the adaptive information processing model: integrative treatment and case conceptualization. *Clinical Social Work Journal* 39, 2 191–200.

Sharpe, D. and Rossiter, L. (2002) Siblings of children with a chronic illness: a meta-analysis. *Journal of Pediatric Psychology* 8, 699–710.

Shavit, A. (2013) *My Promised Land*. New York, Spiegl and Grau.

Sheikh, A. and Gatrad, A. R. (eds) (2000) *Caring for Muslim Patients*. Abingdon, Radcliffe Medical Press.

Sheikh, A., Gatrad, S. and Dhami, R. (2008) Consultations for people from minority groups. *British Medical Journal* 337, a273.

Shen, Y., Kim, S. Y. and Chao, R. Y. W. (2014) Language brokering and adjustment among Chinese and Korean American adolescents: a moderated mediation model of perceived maternal sacrifice, respect for the mother, and mother–child open communication. *American Journal of Psychology* 5, 2 86–95.

Shirpak, K. R., Maticka-Tyndale, E. and Chinichian, M. (2011) Post migration changes in Iranian immigrants' couple relationships in Canada. *Journal of Comparative Family Studies* 40, 6 51–75.

Shiwani, M. H. (2006) Plight of immigrant doctors in the UK: grass is not that green. *Journal of the Pakistan Medical Association* 56, 6 151–152.

Shiwani, M. H. (2010) Prospects for trainees from Pakistan: time to streamline the links ith UK. *Journal of the College of Physicians and Surgeons* 20, 11 707–708.

Shortall, C., McMorran, J., Taylor, K. et al. (2015) Experiences of pregnant migrant women receiving ante/peri and postnatal care in the UK. *A Doctors of the World Report on the Experiences of attendees at their London Drop-In Clinic*. Accessed at: http://b.3cdn.net/droftheworld/08303864eb97b2d304_lam6brw4c.pdf on 7 March 2016.

Shotter, J. (1994) *Conversational Realities: Constructing Life through Language*. London, Sage.

Shoval, G., Schoen, G., Vardi, N. and Zalsman, G. (2007) Suicide in Ethiopian immigrants in Israel: a case for study of the genetic-environmental relation. *Archives of Suicide Research* 11, 3 247–253.

Silove, D., Steel, Z., McGorry, P. et al. (2002) The impact of torture on post-traumatic stress symptoms in war-affected Tamil refugees and immigrants. *Comprehensive Psychiatry* 43, 1 49–55.

Simpson, J., Robson, K., Creighton, S. M. and Hodes, D. (2012) Female genital mutilation: the role of health professionals in prevention, assessment, and management. *BMJ* 344 doi: http://dx.doi.org/10.1136/bmj.e1361.

Singh, G. K. and Hiatt, R. A. (2006) Trends and disparities in socioeconomic and behavioural characteristics, life expectancy, and cause-specific mortality of native-born and foreign-born populations in the United States, 1979–2003. *International Journal of Epidemiology* 35, 4 903–919.

Singh, G. K. and Miller, B. A. (2004) Health, life expectancy, and mortality patterns among immigrant populations in the United States. *Canadian Journal of Public Health* 95, 3 1–15.

Singh, G. K. and Siahpush, M. (2002) Ethnic-immigrant differentials in health behaviors, morbidity, and cause-specific mortality in the United States: an analysis of two national data bases. *Human Biology* 74:83–109.

Skovdal, M. and Daniel, M. (2012) Resilience through participation and coping-enabling social environments: the case of HIV-affected children in sub-Saharan Africa. *Africa Journal of AIDS Research* 11, 3 153–164.

Slaughter, V. and Griffiths, M. (2007) Death understanding and fear of death in young children. *Clinical Child Psychology and Psychiatry* 12, 4 525–535.

Sluzki, C. E. (1979) Migration and family conflict. *Family Process* 18, 4 379–390.

Sluzki, C. E. (1993) Towards a model of family and political victimization: implications for treatment and recovery. *Psychiatry*, 56 178–187.

Smith, A., Lalonde, R. N. and Johnson, S. (2004) Serial migration and its implications for the parent–child relationship: a retrospective analysis of the experiences of the children of Caribbean immigrants. *Cultural Diversity and Ethnic Minority Psychology* 10, 2 107–122.

Smith, S. K., Zimmerman, S., Williams, C. S. et al. (2011) Post-traumatic stress symptoms in long-term non-Hodgkin's Lymphoma survivors: does time heal? *Journal of Clinical Oncology* doi: 10.1200/JCO.2011.37.2631.

Solomon, A. (2012) *Far From the Tree: Parents, Children and the Search For Identity.* UK, Simon and Schuster.

Song, M. (1997) 'You're becoming more and more English': investigating Chinese siblings' cultural identities. *New Community* 23, 3 343–362.

Sontag, S. (1991) *Illness as Metaphor and AIDS and its Metaphors.* London, Penguin Books.

Spector, A., Gardner, C. and Orrelle, M. (2011) The impact of Cognitive Stimulation Therapy groups on people with dementia: views from participants, their carers and group facilitators. *Aging and Mental Health* 15, 8 945–949.

Spiegel, D., Bloom, J. R., Kraemer, H. C. and Gottheil, E. (1989) Effect of psychosocial treatment on survival of patients with metastatic breast cancer. *Lancet* 14, 2 888–891.

Spiegel, D., Butler, L. D., Giese-Davis, J. et al. (2007) Effects of supportive-expressive group therapy on survival of patients with metastatic breast cancer: a randomized prospective trial. *Cancer* 110, 5 1130–1138.

Srivastana, R. (2007) *The Health Care Professional's Guide to Clinical Cultural Competence.* Toronto, Elsevier.

Steven, A., Oxley, J. and Fleming, W. G. (2008) Mentoring for NHS doctors: perceived benefits across the personal–professional interface. *Journal of Research Social Medicine* 101, 11 552–557.

Stewart, J., Clark, D. and Clark, P. F. (2007) *Migration and Recruitment of Healthcare Professionals: Causes, Consequences and Policy Responses*. Policy Brief 7, Focus Migration.

Stilwell, B., Diallo, K. and Zurn, P. (2003) Migration of health care workers from developing countries: strategic approaches to its management. *Bulletin of the World Health Organization* 82, 8 595–600.

Stirbu, I., Kunst, A. E., Vlems, F. A. et al. (2006) Cancer mortality rates among first and second generation migrants in the Netherlands: convergence toward the rates of the native Dutch population. *International Journal of Cancer* 19, 11 2265–2272.

Stone, D. (1998) *Valuing 'Caring Work': Rethinking the Nature of Work in the Human Sciences*. Radcliffe Public Policy Institute.

Stoppelbein, L. and Greening, L. (2007) Brief report: the risk of posttraumatic stress disorder in mothers of children with pediatric cancer and Type I Diabetes. *Journal of Pediatric Psychology* 32, 2 223–229.

Suárez-Orozoco, C. and Suárez-Orozoco, M. M. (2001) *Children of Immigration*. Cambridge, Mass, Harvard University Press.

Suarez-Orozco, C., Rhodes, C. and Milburn, M. (2009) Unraveling the immigrant paradox. *Youth and Society* X 1–33.

Suarez-Orozco, C., Todorovo, I. L. G. and Louie, J. (2002) Making up for lost time: the experience of separation and reunion amongst immigrant families. *Family Process* 41 625–643.

Sundquist, J., Bayard-Burfield, L., Johansson, L. M. et al. (2000) Impact of ethnicity, violence and acculturation on displaced migrants: psychological distress and psychosomatic complaints among refugees in Sweden. *Journal of Nervous & Mental Disease* 188, 6 357–365.

Surbone, A., Kagawa-Singer, M., Terret, C. and Baider, L. (2006) The illness trajectory of elderly cancer patients across cultures: SIOG position paper. *Annals of Oncology* 18, 4 633–638.

Swoboda, D. (2006) Embodiment and the search of illness legitimacy among women with contested illnesses. *Michigan Feminist Studies* 19.

Syal, M. (2015) Growing up between cultures is tough – until you realise it's a creative blessing. *Guardian Immigration Special* 25th March.

Szczepura, A., Price, C. and Gumber, A. (2008) Breast and bowel cancer screening uptake patterns over 15 years for UK South Asian ethnic minority populations, corrected for differences in socio-demographic characteristics. *BMC Public Health* 8 346 doi:10.1186/1471-2458-8-346.

Takeuchi, D. T., Chun, C., Gong, F. et al. (2002) Cultural expressions of distress. *Health* 6, 2 221–236.

Tellez-Giron, P. (2007) Providing culturally sensitive end-of-life care for the Latino/a community. *Wisconsin Medical Journal* 106, 7 402–406.

Terry, B., Bisano, M., McNamara, M. et al. (2012) Task shifting: meeting the human resources needs for acute and emergency care in Africa. *African Journal of Emergency Medicine* 2, 4 182–187.

Thastum, M., Johansen, M. B., Gubba, L. et al. (2008) Coping, social relations, and communication: a qualitative exploratory study of children with cancer. *Clinical Child Psychology and Psychiatry* 13, 1 123–138.

Thibodeaux, A. and Deatrick, J. A. (2007) Cultural influence on family management of children with cancer. *Journal of Pediatric Oncology Nursing* 24, 4 227–233.

Thomas, F. and Gideon, J. (2013) Introduction (in) Thomas, F. and Gideon, J. (eds) *Migration, Health and Inequality*. London, Zed Books.

Tickle, L. (2015, 26 September) No place to go: the unaccompanied children facing deportation from the UK. *Guardian Report.*

Tilke, M., Dye, K., Markey, K. et al. (2007) Racism: the implications for nursing education. *Diversity in Health and Social Care* 4, 4 303–312.

Tilki, M. (2006) Human rights and health inequalities: UK and EU policies and initiatives relating to the promotion of culturally competent care (in) Papadopoulos, I. (ed.) *Transcultural Health and Social Care: Developing Culturally Competent Practitioners*. London, Churchill Livingstone/Elsevier.

Tilki M., Ryan L., D'Angelo, A. et al. (2009) *The Forgotten Irish: Report of a Research Project Commissioned by Ireland Fund of Great Britain*. London. Ireland Fund of Great Britain Accessed at: http://eprints.mdx.ac.uk/6350 on 7 March 2016.

Tomm, C., Hoyt, M. and Madigan, S. (2001) Honoring our internalized others and the ethics of caring: a conversation with Carl Tomm (in) Hoyt, M. (ed.) *Interviews with Brief Therapy Experts* Philadelphia, Brunner-Routledge.

Tongomoo, O. (2015) Meeting with representatives of Congolese Support Group, 26 September 2015.

Tribe, R. and Patel, N. (2007) *The Psychologist* 20, 3 149–151.

Tse, C. Y., Chong, A. and Fok, S. Y. (2003) Breaking bad news: a Chinese perspective. *Palliative Medicine* 17, 4 339–343.

Ujcic-Voortman, J. K., Bann, C. A., Seidell, J. C. and Verhoef, A. P. (2012) Obesity and cardiovascular disease risk among Turkish and Moroccan migrant groups in Europe: a systematic review. *Obesity Review* 13, 1 2–16.

UK Government (2015) Statement opposing female genital mutilation. Accessed at: www.gov.uk/government/publications/statement-opposing-female-genital-mutilation on 7 March 2016.

Ullman, E., Barthel, A., Licino, J. et al. (2013) Increased rate of depression and psychosomatic symptoms in Jewish migrants from the post-Soviet-Union to Germany in the 3rd generation after the Shoa. *Translational Psychiatry* 3, 3 e241.

Umberson, D. (2003) *Death of a Parent*. Cambridge, Cambridge University Press.

Ummel, D., Achille, M. and Mekkelholt, J. (2011) Donors and recipients of living kidney donation: a qualitative metasummary of their experiences. *Journal of Transplantation* ID 626501 http://dx.doi.org/10.1155/2011/626501.

United Nations (2003) *International Convention on the Rights of and the Protection of The Rights of All Migrant workers and Member of their Families*. United Nations Treaty Collection.

Valtorta, N. and Hanratty, B. (2012) Loneliness, isolation and the health of older adults: do we need a research agenda? *Journal of the Royal Society of Medicine* 105 518–522.

van Bergen, D. D., Smit, J. H., Kerkhof, A. J. F. M. et al. (2006) Gender and cultural patterns of suicidal behavior: young Hindustani immigrant women in the Netherlands. *The Journal of Crisis Intervention and Suicide Prevention* 27, 4 181–188.

van den Muisjenburgh, M., van Weel-Baumgarten, E., Burns, N. et al. (2013) Communication in cross-cultural consultations in primary care in Europe: the case for improvement. *Primary Health Care Research and Development* 1–12.

van der Feltz-Cornelis, C. M., Hoedeman, R., Keuter, E. J. and Swinkels, J. A. (2012) Presentation of the multidisciplinary guideline Medically Unexplained Physical Symptoms (MUPS) and Somatoform Disorder in the Netherlands: disease management according to risk profiles. *Journal of Psychosomatic Research* 72, 2 168–169.

van der Geest, A. M., Mui, A. and Vermuelen, H. et al. (2004) Linkages between migration and the care of frail older people: observations from Greece, Ghana and the Netherlands. *Ageing and Society* 24, 3 431–450.

Victor, C. R., Burholt, V., Visser, M. W. et al. (2012) Loneliness and ethnic minority elders in Great Britain: an exploratory study. *Journal of Cross Cultural Gerontology* 27, 1 doi:10.1007/s1082-012-9161-6.

Visser, A., Huizinga, G. A., Hoekstra, H. J. et al. (2005) Emotional and behavioural functioning of children of a parent diagnosed with cancer: a cross-informant perspective. *Psycho-Oncology* 14 746–758.

Voracek, M. and Loibi, M. (2008) Consistency of immigrant and country-of-birth suicide rates: a meta-analysis. *Acta Psychiatrica Scandinavica* 118, 4 259–271.

Vullnetari, J. and King, R. (2008) 'Does your granny eat grass?' On mass migration, care drain and the fate of older people in rural Albania. *Global Networks* 8, 2 139–171.

Walker, G. (1983) The pact: The caretaker-parent/ill-child coalition in families with chronic illness. *Family Systems Medicine* 1, 4 6–29.

Walker, G. (1991) *In the Midst of Winter*. New York, Norton.

Waller, J., Robb, K., Stubbings, S. et al. (2009) Awareness of cancer symptoms and anticipated help seeking among ethnic minority groups in England. *British Journal of Cancer* 101, Supplement 2, S24–S30.

Walsh, F. and McGoldrick, M. (2004) Loss and the family: a systemic approach (in) Walsh, F. and McGoldrick, M. (eds) *Living Beyond Loss*. London, Norton.

Walsh, S. D., Edelstein, A. and Vota, D. (2012) Suicidal ideation and alcohol use among adolescents in Israel. *European Psychologist* 17, 2 131–142.

Walters, W. H. (2002) Later-life migration in the United States: a review of recent research. *Journal of Planning Literature* 17, 1 37–66.

Wang, D. and Li, H. (2007) Nonverbal language in cross-cultural communication. *US-China Foreign Language* 5, 10 69.

Wang, Q. (2004) The cultural context of parent-child reminiscing: a functional analysis (in) Pratt, M. W. and Fiese, B. H. (eds) *Family Stories and the Life Course: Across Time and Generations*. Mahwah, NJ, Erlbaum.

Watson, M., Haviland, J., Davidson, J. and Bliss, J. (2000) Fighting spirit in patients with cancer. *The Lancet* 335, 84.

Webb, R., Richardson J., Esmail A. et al. (2004) Uptake for cervical screening by ethnicity and place of birth: a population based cross-sectional study. *Journal of Public Health* 24, 3 293–296.

Weingarten, K. (1991) The discourses of intimacy: adding a social constructionist and feminist view. *Family Process* 30, 285–306.

Weingarten, K. (1994) *The Mother's Voice: Strengthening Intimacy in Families.* Orlando, Harcourt Brace and Company.

Weingarten, K. (2013) The 'cruel radiance of what is': helping couples live with chronic illness. *Family Process* 52, 1 83–101.

Weingarten, K. and Worthen, M. E. (1997) A narrative approach to understanding the illness experience of a mother and daughter. *Family Systems and Health* 15, 1 41–54.

Weller, D., Coleman, D., Robertson, R. et al. (2007) The UK colorectal cancer screening pilot: results of the second round of screening in England. *British Journal of Cancer* 97, 1601–1605.

Wenger, G. C., Davies, R., Shahatahmasebi, S. and Scott, A. (1996) Social isolation and loneliness in old age: review and model refinement. *Ageing and Society,* 6, 333–358.

Wenzel, T. (1999) Refugee doctors can do valuable work in European host countries. *British Medical Journal* 16, 318 (7177): 196.

White, M. and Epston, D. (1990) *Narrative Means to Therapeutic Ends.* New York, WW Norton.

Wild, S. H., Fischbacher, C. M., Brock, A. et al. (2006) Mortality from all cancers and lung, colorectal, breast and prostate cancer by country of birth in England and Wales, 2001–2003. *British Journal of Cancer* 94, 1079–1085.

Wilkinson, S. and Kitzinger, C. (1996) Theorizing representing the other (in) Wilkinson, S. and Kitzinger, C. (eds) *Representing the Other: a Feminism and Psychology Reader.* London, Sage.

Williams, A. and van der Merwe, J. (2013) The psychological impact of torture. *British Journal of Pain* 7, 2 101–106.

Wilner, L. K. and Feinstein-Whittaker, M. (2013) Perspectives on Communication Disorders and Sciences in Culturally and Linguistically Diverse (CLD). *Populations* 20 90–100 doi:10.1044/cds20.3.90.

Wilson, J. (2005) Engaging children and young people (in) Vetere, A. and Dowling, E. (eds) *Narrative Therapies with Children and Their Families.* London, Routledge.

Wismar, M., Maier, C., Glinos, I. et al. (2011) *Health Professional Mobility and Health Systems: Evidence from 17 European Countries.* Brussels, WHO European Observatory.

Witty, K., Branny, K., White, A. et al. (2014) Engaging men with penile cancer in qualitative research: reflections from an interview-based study. *Nurse Researcher* 21, 3 13–19.

Wong, S., Bond, M. H. and Mosquera, R. (2008) The influence of cultural value orientations on self-reported emotional expression across cultures. *Journal of Cross-Cultural Psychology* 39, 2 224–229.

Wong, Y. J., Vaughan, E. L., Liu, T. and Chang, K. (2014) Asian Americans' proportion of life in the United States and suicide ideation: the moderating effects of ethnic subgroups. *Asian American Journal of Psychology* 5, 3 237–242.

Wood, J. (2013) On not going home. *New York Review of Books* 36, 4.

Woodgate, R. L. (2006) Siblings' experiences with childhood cancer: a different way of being in the family. *Cancer Nursing* 29, 5 406–414.

Woods, F. (2015, 10 April) Comment: intermarriage is the acid test for migrant integration. *politics.co.uk*. Accessed at: www.politics.co.uk/comment-analysis/2015/04/10/comment-intermarriage-is-the-acid-test-for-migrant-integrati on 26 March 2016.

Woodward, A., Howard, N. and Wolffers, I. (2013) Health and access to care for undocumented migrants living in the European Union: a scoping review. *Health Policy Plan* doi: 10.1093/heapol/czt061.

World Health Organization (WHO) (2006) *The World Health Report*.

World Health Organization (WHO) (2008) Resolution on the health of migrants *Sixty-first World Health Assembly* WHA 61.17 Agenda item 11.9.

World Health Organization (WHO) (2010) *WHO Global Code of Practice on the International Recruitment of Health Personnel*. Accessed at: http://my.ibpinitiative.org/?syla573d on 26 March 2016.

Wu, N. H. and Kim, S. Y. (2009) Chinese American adolescents' perceptions of the language brokering experience as a sense of burden and sense of efficacy. *Journal of Youth and Adolescence* 38, 703–718.

Young, G. (2015, 24 March) As migrants we leave home in search of a future, but we lose the past. *The Guardian:* Immigration Special.

Yngvesson, B. and Mahoney, M. A. (2000) 'As One Should, Ought and Wants to Be' *Theory, Culture and Society* 17, 6 77–110.

Yuval-Davis, N. (1997) *Gender and Nation*. London, Sage.

Zachariah, R., Ford, N., Philips, M. et al. (2009) Task shifting in HIV/AIDS: opportunities, challenges and proposed actions for sub-Saharan Africa. *Transactions of the Royal Society of Tropical Medicine and Hygiene* 103, 6 549–558.

Zimmerman, C., Kiss, L. and Hossain, M. (2011) Migration and health: a framework for 21st century policy-making. *PLoS medicine* 8, 5 e1001034.

Zimmerman, C., Yun, K., Watts, C. et al. (2006) *The Health Risks and Consequences of Trafficking in Women and Adolescents: Findings From a European Study*. London, London School of Hygiene and Medicine.

Zoppi, K. and Epstein, R. (2002) Is communication a skill? Communication behaviours and being in relation. *Communication Techniques and Behaviors* 34, 5 319–24.

INDEX

A

access to health care, 157–158, 162
acculturation
  change from health advantage to
    disadvantage attributed to, 18
  child-rearing in relation to dual
    cultures, 111–114
  in intersection between illness and
    migration, 138
  letting go of the past and, 101
  sibling relationships and, 125
  suicide and, 26
  in understanding responses to
    migration, 103
adolescents
  cancer in, 88
  disciplinary strategies and, 113
  in dual cultures, 111–113
  impact of parental illness on, 56
  language brokering and, 115
  living apart at times of illness,
    139–141, 146–147
  medical migrations, 142–144
  position of, in life cycle, 51
  risky behaviour and, 17
  suicidal ideation and, 25, 27, 113
  trauma as impediment to learning,
    31, 117
adults
  exposure to increased scrutiny,
    148–149
  illness in, 144–149
  older (See elderly)
  parental illness, 56, 145–148
  resilience in the face of trauma,
    44–45
  when adult children leave parents
    behind, 105–107

African-Caribbean
  culture, 51, 79, 86, 178
  doctors, 200
  identity, 77
  migrants, 3, 18, 19, 24–25, 28, 75
African women's clinic, 176
age
  age-appropriate activities and,
    engagement in, 109, 115, 118
  challenges of refugee and asylum
    seeking women and, 34
  children's ability to process what is
    seen and heard, 54
  child's response to illness of parent
    and, 56
  child's response to own illness and,
    53, 54, 138–139
  cultural response to illness and, 76
  dementia and, 28
  divorce and, 120
  effects of trauma influenced by, 43
  ethnicity and, 28
  expectations of caring and, 80–81
  experiences of migration and, 100,
    109–110
  parent's response to illness, 57
  patients' rights and, 209
  positions in life cycle and, 51–52
  racism and, 20
  response to illness and, 53
  suicide and, 26
alcohol abuse, 20, 22, 23, 25, 43, 184
Amsterdam Declaration, 36
antenatal care, 14
anti-gay prejudice, 65–66
anxiety
  in couple relationships, 118
  double culture shock and, 187

2564031